The Doctor *of* Nursing Practice

A Guidebook for Role Development and Professional Issues

Third Edition

Edited by:

Lisa Astalos Chism, DNP, GNP, BC, NCMP, FAANP

Clinical Director, Women's Wellness Clinic
Nurse Practitioner
Certified Menopause Practitioner
Sexual Health Counselor and Educator
Karmanos Cancer Institute
Detroit, Michigan

Adjunct Assistant Professor
Madonna University
Livonia, Michigan

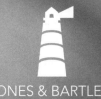

JONES & BARTLETT
LEARNING

World Headquarters
Jones & Bartlett Learning
5 Wall Street
Burlington, MA 01803
978-443-5000
info@jblearning.com
www.jblearning.com

Jones & Bartlett Learning books and products are available through most bookstores and online booksellers. To contact Jones & Bartlett Learning directly, call 800-832-0034, fax 978-443-8000, or visit our website, www.jblearning.com.

Substantial discounts on bulk quantities of Jones & Bartlett Learning publications are available to corporations, professional associations, and other qualified organizations. For details and specific discount information, contact the special sales department at Jones & Bartlett Learning via the above contact information or send an email to specialsales@jblearning.com.

Production Credits

VP, Executive Publisher: David Cella
Executive Editor: Amanda Martin
Associate Acquisitions Editor: Rebecca Myrick
Editorial Assistant: Lauren Vaughn
Production Editor: Sarah Bayle
Senior Marketing Manager: Jennifer Stiles
VP, Manufacturing and Inventory Control:
  Therese Connell
Composition: Cenveo Publisher Services
Cover Design: Kristin E. Parker
Manager of Photo Research, Rights & Permissions:
  Lauren Miller
Cover Image: © Jitka Volfova/Shutterstock
Printing and Binding: Edwards Brothers Malloy
Cover Printing: Edwards Brothers Malloy

Library of Congress Cataloging-in-Publication Data
The doctor of nursing practice: a guidebook for role development and professional issues / edited by Lisa Astalos Chism. — Third edition.
    p. ; cm.
Preceded by The doctor of nursing practice / Lisa Astalos Chism. 2nd ed. c2013.
Includes bibliographical references and index.
ISBN 978-1-284-06625-8
I. Chism, Lisa Astalos, editor.
[DNLM: 1. Education, Nursing, Graduate—United States. 2. Advanced Practice Nursing—United States. 3. Professional Role—United States. WY 18.5]
RT75
610.73071'1—dc23
                          2014034971
6048

Printed in the United States of America
19 18 17 16 15   10 9 8 7 6 5 4 3 2 1

Dedication

This book is dedicated to my father, Paul Astalos, and my mother, Judy Astalos. You were both my inspiration and my cheerleaders. Mom and Dad, you continue to guide me in spirit, and I know you are smiling down on us all.
This book is also dedicated to my husband, Bruce, and my daughter, Isabel. Thank you for your enduring love, support, and friendship. You mean more than you will ever know.

Contents

Preface

I had recently graduated from a doctor of nursing practice (DNP) program in 2007 when I woke up in the middle of the night and thought, now what? I had just spent the past 3 years researching, finding, applying, and finally completing a DNP program. I realized at 2:00 a.m. that day, 2 months after graduation, that I wasn't sure how to integrate my new degree into my professional life. I felt that if I wasn't sure how to integrate my new knowledge and skills into my advanced-practice role or roles, my colleagues probably had the same concerns, questions, and issues.

Since that time I have received wonderful feedback from colleagues and nursing faculty that this was indeed true. The previous editions of this book have served as resources for everyone from prospective and current students to those who have completed their DNP degree. I am very pleased this book has been helpful for so many. Writing and editing the third edition was just as rewarding as the previous editions. From my first query letter to the development of the current edition, this book has been a wonderful adventure.

The American Association of Colleges of Nursing continues to recommend that by 2015 the terminal degree in nursing practice will transition from the traditional master's degrees in nursing to the DNP degree (2004). With the growth of this innovative degree comes the challenge for students and graduates to be able to synthesize the new knowledge and skills they develop in a DNP program and transition into DNP-prepared nurses. What does this mean? That is the question I have attempted to answer. I also strived to share valuable insights pertinent to DNP students, graduates, nurses, and other healthcare professionals who are impacted by the development of this degree.

This book is organized in two parts. Part I reviews the DNP degree and the various roles DNP graduates may assume and integrate. DNP graduates may find themselves developing roles in leadership, clinical practice, research, healthcare policy and advocacy, education, ethics, and information technology. No doubt many nurses who return to school for a DNP degree already possess expertise in these roles. Therefore, the challenge lies in the integration of new knowledge and skills obtained through a DNP program with the intent to improve healthcare delivery in the 21st century.

Part II describes the unique issues DNP graduates may find themselves facing, such as deciding whether to return to graduate school for a DNP degree, the challenges and recommendations related to the BSN-to-DNP degree path, the use of the title *doctor*, educating others about the degree, marketing oneself as a DNP graduate, and, finally, the future of the DNP degree. Case scenarios are used throughout the book to further illustrate the unique situations that DNP graduates may encounter. In addition, I have added personal notes throughout the text about my experiences as a DNP graduate. The interviews have been updated, and new interviews have been added to bring life to the book and describe the wonderful contributions made by many DNP graduates and others, as well as anecdotal accounts of those who helped bring the DNP degree to fruition.

Healthcare delivery and nursing education are evolving, and nursing has responded with the development of the DNP degree. We are practice professionals, and we now have a practice doctorate that is reflective of our heritage. The knowledge and expertise developed through a DNP program have equipped DNP graduates with the skills and perspective necessary to continue to provide high-quality health care and proactively advocate for patients and the nursing profession. DNP graduates will further contribute to health care and nursing in the 21st century through leadership, use of evidence-based practice, expertise in information technologies, involvement in healthcare policy, and mentoring and educating future generations of nurses and healthcare professionals. Whether you are deciding if this degree is right for you, assimilating into your new role as a DNP, or simply seeking information about this innovative degree, it is my hope that this book will prove to be a valuable resource.

REFERENCE

American Association of Colleges of Nursing. (2004). *Position statement on the practice doctorate in nursing*. Retrieved from http://www.aacn.nche.edu/dnp/position-statement

Foreword

The transformational doctorate of nursing practice (DNP) is continuing to cause profound changes throughout much of nursing education, practice, and scholarship. Paralleling the years of the 21st century, we have had 15 years of unprecedented growth in the number of programs and graduates and of professional progress as a recognized and desirable nursing workforce innovation.

Soon after the turn of the century, nursing organizations, such as National Organization of Nurse Practitioner Faculties (NONPF) (O'Sullivan, Carter, Marion, Pohl, & Werner, 2005), American Association of Colleges of Nursing (AACN) (2014), American Academy of Nurse Practitioners (AANP) (2013), and similar groups, drove through agreements and disagreements, collaborations and competitions, actions and counteractions to a fairly common vision in record time. The truest agents of change were the thousands of nurses who enrolled at the first opportunity and have already earned this awesome degree. The positive primary and acute care outcomes of the earliest DNP students' culminating capstone projects foretold the overall impact of nurses with the degree. The rest is history: rapidly evolving organizational positions, roles and scholarship, standards (competencies and essentials), curricula and supports, accreditation, and finally, national policy. Controversies continue to surround the DNP, including the optimal level of scholarship, readiness of the profession for the DNP as an educational requirement for the advanced-practice registered nurse (APRN) designation, and the type of institution qualified to offer the DNP degree.

Lisa Astalos Chism, DNP, GNP, BC, NCMP, FAANP, author of *The Doctor of Nursing Practice: A Guidebook for Role Development and Professional Issues*, completed her DNP in 2007 and enhanced her nurse practitioner (NP) position in several ways as described in her book. Without a background as educator or writer, she miraculously wrote the popular first edition in response to what she felt was a void in understanding the actuality and potential of the DNP: both the degree and the degreed. She covered very important, complex topics such as the NONPF competencies and AACN essentials with amazing accuracy and clarity. She bravely approached controversies, such as the scholarship of the DNP versus the PhD, ethics, the DNP as faculty member, and the BSN-to-DNP path. Already an accomplished NP with a master's degree, she believed the DNP degree prepared and empowered her to practice in new and better ways. She wanted to share her vision and experience as an advanced-practice nurse with a DNP.

Dr. Chism also sought others to help her unfold this DNP movement for new graduates and students. The foreword to the first edition was written by Dr. Carolyn Williams. She was then president (now emerita) of AACN and then dean of University of Kentucky College of Nursing, which offered one of the four practice doctoral programs that existed at the turn of the century. In that foreword, Dr. Williams prepared the reader for the wealth of information to follow. That book included interviews with DNPs who described applications of their new knowledge and skills by a cross section of pioneers with doctoral nursing practice.

The second edition in 2010 captured much of the progress afforded by this practice doctorate. Dr. Chism also chronicled her own growth and forays into new practice arenas, which she attributed to her DNP preparation. The chapters, written by her and others, included the newest information about each topic. Dr. Joan Stanley, senior director of education policy for AACN, wrote the foreword, and she placed that edition in the context of the stakeholder inputs and the Institute of Medicine's (IOM) 2010 *The Future of Nursing* charge to increase education in general and to double the number of nurses with doctorates by 2020. I found the reading fascinating because Dr. Chism reinterviewed most of the first edition DNPs and updated their stories. In a few short years, the interviewees had experienced significant advancements in practice leadership and practice innovation—a study in itself. Between the first and second editions, the number of DNP programs and DNP graduates grew exponentially. For the second edition, Dr. Chism's book was recognized with a 2012 *American Journal of Nursing* Book of the Year award!

It is my honor and pleasure to present to new and returning readers the third edition of *The Doctor of Nursing Practice: A Guidebook for Role Development and Professional Issues*. In 2000 I had a dawning awareness that nursing needed a mainstream practice doctorate. I was on a steep learning curve in two leadership fellowships, two nursing education administrative positions, and responsibilities as NONPF president elect and president. Suddenly, with laser-sharp focus, it became clear that practice doctoral education for advanced nurses would be essential to make full contributions with other doctoral-level members of the healthcare team. The nimble and able NONPF board acted expeditiously, sponsoring the first exploratory webinar and partnering with AACN and nursing specialty groups for summits, committees, and statements. The board members published about the DNP in widely read online journals (Marion et al.,

2003; O'Sullivan et al., 2005), created guiding documents for NP and DNP faculty, and specified DNP advanced-practice nursing competencies for the fully accountable, independent practitioner. In 2004 I joined the faculty of the Georgia Regents University (GRU) College of Nursing, and in 2005 we offered the 10th DNP program in the nation and the 1st in Georgia. Now BS and BA graduates can enter GRU nursing and complete 4 years of accelerated, immersion course work and intensive clinical experiences to earn a DNP degree and national certification as an APRN. Having lived through all these changes, I can attest that Dr. Chism captures the extraordinary essence of 15 years of DNP evolution.

Much has happened since the 2012 award-winning second edition. Although uncertainties still exist, NONPF, AANP, and AACN have affirmed the DNP as the preferred advanced-practice preparation. This affirmation has solidly grounded the future of advanced nursing education. Furthermore, the IOM's *The Future of Nursing* recommendations to double the number of doctorates by 2020, and the Patient Protection and Affordable Care Act demands for more and better health care, have assuredly spurred the new degree's growth and promise. And nurses on their own have increasingly pursued the postmaster's DNP or the post-BSN DNP, which includes advanced-practice preparation. These pioneers have expanded the capabilities and expectations for advanced nursing practice in healthcare delivery and health-related systems. The demand for DNP preparation has resulted in a rush for program implementation. Indeed, as of July 2014 a total of 243 DNP programs were enrolling students nationwide, and more than 70 additional practice doctorates were also under development (AACN, 2014). From 2012 to 2013, the number of students enrolled in DNP programs increased from 11,575 to 14,699. During that same time period, the number of DNP graduates increased from 1,858 to 2,443 (AACN, 2014).

In this context of change, growth, impact, and promise, the third edition presents historical and current facts for each chapter, and two new chapters explore first the DNP graduate as information specialist and then explores the challenges associated with the new BSN-to-DNP pathway. In my view, Dr. Chism's experiences and insights, her interviews with respondents over three editions, and insights from new people make the chapters lively and timely. For example, Dr. Williams's observant and participative perspectives over time are in all three editions. Many of the other stories vividly describe leadership in implementing evidence-based practice, creating safer and more efficient services, mentoring interprofessional teams, and novel healthcare improvements. This third edition has more of Dr. Chism's reflections on her own practice and portrays her extraordinary ability to use her education to reach and push the boundaries of advanced-practice nursing. The person who reads this book will have an excellent understanding of the value of the DNP degree to the patient, to the healthcare system, and to the nurse's own career.

Lucy N. Marion, PhD, RN, FAAN, FAANP
Dean and Professor
Kellett Chair of Nursing
College of Nursing
Georgia Regents University
Augusta, Georgia

REFERENCES

American Association of Colleges of Nursing. (2014). DNP talking points. Retrieved from http://www.aacn.nche.edu/dnp/about/talking-points

American Association of Nurse Practitioners. (2013). Doctor of nursing practice (DNP) discussion paper. Retrieved from http://www.aanp.org/publications/position-statements-papers

Institute of Medicine. (2010). The future of nursing: Leading change, advancing health. Retrieved from http://books.nap.edu/openbook.php?record_id=12956&page=R1

Marion, L., Viens, D., O'Sullivan, A., Crabtree, K., Fontana, S., & Price, M. (2003). The practice doctorate in nursing: Future or fringe? *Topics in Advanced Practice Nursing eJournal.* Retrieved from http://www.medscape.com/viewarticle/453247

O'Sullivan, A., Carter, M., Marion, L., Pohl, J., & Werner, K. (2005). Moving forward together: The practice doctorate in nursing. *Journal for Issues in Nursing.* Retrieved from http://www.nursingworld.org/MainMenuCategories/ANAMarketplace/ANAPeriodicals/OJIN/TableofContents/Volume102005/No3Sept05/tpc28_416028.html

Contributors

Karen McBroom Butler, DNP, RN
Associate Professor
Faculty Associate, Tobacco Policy
    Research Program
University of Kentucky College of
    Nursing
Lexington, Kentucky

Morris A. Magnan, PhD, RN
Clinical Nurse Specialist
Karmanos Cancer Institute
Detroit, Michigan

**Donna Behler McArthur, PhD,
APRN, FNP-BC, FAANP, FNAP**
Professor of Nursing
Vanderbilt University School of
    Nursing
Nashville, Tennessee

Marlene H. Mullin, DNP, APRN, BC
Chair, Legislative Committee
Metro Detroit Chapter, Michigan
    Council of Nurse Practitioners

Catherine Nichols, DNP, APRN, BC
Nurse Practitioner
Women's Wellness Clinic
Karmanos Cancer Institute
Detroit, Michigan

**Mary Ellen Roberts, DNP, APN,C,
FNAP, FAANP, FAAN**
Assistant Professor
Director, Doctor of Nursing
    Practice Program
Seton Hall University
College of Nursing
South Orange, New Jersey

Elizabeth Johnston Taylor, PhD, RN
Professor, School of Nursing
Loma Linda University
Loma Linda, California

Acknowledgments

I wish to first acknowledge God. I am sure that without Your guidance and inspiration, I would not have succeeded in this endeavor. Although I thought this project was bigger than me, You proved to me again that once You planted the seed, You would be with me through it all.

I wish to acknowledge Dr. Elizabeth Johnston Taylor for her immediate encouragement. Dr. Taylor helped me write my first query letter and edited my proposal for the first edition. Her faith and encouragement instilled in me the confidence to push forward with my ideas. She has been a mentor and a friend, and I am thankful for her unending guidance and encouragement. It was so appropriate that Dr. Taylor, a spiritual care expert, wrote a chapter about weighing the decision to go back to school. Her perception regarding decision making is uncanny. She expertly integrated her expertise in spiritual care, which only added to a wonderful, insightful chapter.

I wish to also acknowledge my first mentor, Dr. Morris Magnan. Prior to returning to graduate school for my DNP degree, I am quite sure I had never had a mentor. I initially met Dr. Magnan during my interview for the DNP program. Needless to say, my initial intimidation has grown to true admiration. He is a nursing scholar who impresses me with his level of clinical expertise and overall commitment to the profession of nursing. Through his mentorship I have developed a much broader understanding of nursing as a discipline, science, and profession. Dr. Magnan has not only inspired me to grow as a nurse, but he has also taught me what a true mentor is and should be. I am so thankful to call him a mentor and a friend. It was an honor to have Dr. Magnan write the chapter regarding DNP graduates' expectations for theory, research, and scholarship. He clearly understands the benefit of DNP–PhD partnerships and has supported the need for a practice doctorate in nursing.

I would also like to acknowledge Dr. Karen McBroom Butler. Dr. Butler was an original reviewer of the proposal for this book and not only offered wonderful feedback but also graciously volunteered to assist me with this project. It was an honor that she accepted the task to write the DNP as educator chapter. She is a perfect example of the impact DNP graduates are making in the role of educator. She beautifully articulated the issues and transitions necessary to move nursing education into the 21st century. Her insights into the role of a university faculty member through the eyes of a DNP graduate are invaluable. I am so thankful for her contributions both to the book and to nursing education.

I would also like to acknowledge my good friend and colleague Dr. Marlene Mullin. Dr. Mullin is a champion for the nursing profession. Her commitment to issues such as the homeless crisis and the number of uninsured individuals in this country has motivated her to get involved on a grassroots level by volunteering at a homeless shelter and becoming politically involved. Her dedication to health care and nursing inspires me. I am honored and thankful that she contributed to this project by writing the healthcare policy and advocacy chapter. Dr. Mullin wonderfully describes the rich history of nursing's involvement in policy and political issues. Dr. Mullin exemplifies the importance of addressing healthcare policy issues and continues to be a strong advocate for nursing and for her patients.

I would like to thank my friends and colleagues Dr. Donna McArthur and Dr. Mary Ellen Roberts for contributing a timely chapter about the challenges and recommendations associated with the BSN-to-DNP path. Their insight and candor from the point of view of DNP educators and program directors proved to be very valuable. I truly appreciate their wonderful contribution to this edition of the text as well as their friendship.

I also wish to acknowledge my wonderful friends and colleagues at Karmanos Cancer Institute, especially Ms. Christine Rymal, MSN, APRN, BC, CLT, and Dr. Cathy Nichols, DNP, APRN, BC. You are both incredible examples of exemplary advanced-practice nurses. Your friendship and support are invaluable to me. Dr. Nichols also contributed a valuable chapter in this edition of the text on the DNP graduate as information specialist. She is our resident IT expert, and I am so thankful for her contribution. I also wish to acknowledge my vice president, Ms. Kay Carolin, MSN, RN, for her enduring support and friendship, and for making my clinical and leadership aspirations a reality.

I also want to acknowledge my beautiful "sisters," Ms. Jill Frieders, MS, RN, and Ms. Tonya Schmitt, MS, APRN, BC, DNP student. You inspired me to make sure this book was a practical, useful resource for nurses in every area of practice. I am so thankful for your wisdom, expertise, humor, and, most of all, your friendship.

Thank you to Ms. Suzanne Molter, BSN, RN, for your support and friendship. I truly admire your commitment to pursue your dream to become a nurse.

I also thank Ms. Andrea Rogers, MILS, reference librarian at Beaumont Hospitals and Ms. Margaret Danowski, information specialist, reference librarian, and assistant professor at Madonna University. I would not have been able to revise this book without your expert literature searches and research.

I would also like to thank the editorial and production staff at Jones & Bartlett Learning for their support, expertise, and encouragement, especially Ms. Amanda Martin, Executive Editor, Ms. Rebecca Myrick, Associate Acquisitions Editor, Ms. Jennifer Stiles, Senior Marketing Manager and Ms. Sarah Bayle, Production Editor.

Most important, I would like to acknowledge my family. Thank you to my beautiful daughter, Isabel, who is the greatest joy of my life. Your wisdom and humor are beyond your 14 years. Thank you, Izzy, for your patience and for cheering me on. I am so proud to be your mom. Finally, I would like to thank my husband, Bruce, for being my best friend, my cheerleader, and my champion. I am thankful for your support and guidance and for keeping me on track. Thank you for teaching me to be true to myself and for believing in me.

In closing, I would like to acknowledge all the readers of the previous and current editions of the book. This book is for you. My hope is that the practical, real-life tips, case scenarios, interviews, and information provided in this book will inspire you and guide you on your journey.

PART I

Role Transition

The evolution of a doctor of nursing practice (DNP) degree continues to be a fascinating journey for the profession of nursing. As DNP graduates begin their own journeys, many challenges and issues related to role transition are likely to arise. Today's DNP graduate will engage in a variety of roles that will include leadership, evaluation and translation of research, practice, education, health policy, information technology, and ethics. Often these roles will be integrated and adapted to meet the current needs of healthcare delivery.

As a practice-focused profession, nursing is responding to the healthcare needs of individuals, communities, and systems through the development of a practice-focused doctorate. Most assuredly, as the demands of a complex healthcare environment continue to evolve, nursing will continue to evolve as well. The DNP degree truly exemplifies this evolution and nursing's commitment to the future of health care. Part I of this text specifically discusses the various roles DNP graduates may assume to meet the current and future needs of a complex healthcare environment.

CHAPTER 1

Overview of the Doctor of Nursing Practice Degree

Lisa Astalos Chism

What exactly is a doctor of nursing practice (DNP) degree? As enrollment to this innovative practice doctorate program continues to increase, this question is frequently posed by nurses, patients, and other healthcare professionals both in and out of the healthcare setting. Providing an explanation to this question requires not only defining the DNP degree, but also reflecting on the rich history of doctoral education in nursing. Doctoral education in nursing is connected to our past and influences the directions we may take in the future (Carpenter & Hudacek, 1996). The development of the DNP degree is a tribute to where nursing has been and where we hope to be in the future of doctoral education in nursing.

Understanding the DNP degree requires developing an awareness of the rationale for a practice doctorate. This rationale illustrates the motivation behind the evolution of doctoral education in nursing and provides further explanation of this contemporary degree. The need for parity across the healthcare team, the Institute of Medicine's call for safer healthcare practices, and the need for increased preparation of advanced-practice registered nurses to meet the changing demands of health care are all contributing antecedents of the development of the practice doctorate in nursing (American Association of Colleges of Nursing [AACN], 2006a, 2006b; Apold, 2008; Dracup, Cronenwett, Meleis, & Benner, 2005; Roberts & Glod, 2005). Becoming familiar with the motivating factors behind the DNP degree will aid understanding of the development of this innovative degree.

This chapter provides a definition of the DNP degree and a discussion of the evolution of doctoral education in nursing. The rationale for a practice doctorate is also described. The recipe for the DNP degree, which includes the *Essentials of Doctoral Education for Advanced Nursing Practice* by the AACN (2006b) and the *Practice Doctorate Nurse Practitioner Entry-Level Competencies* by the National Organization of Nurse Practitioner Faculties (NONPF, 2006), is provided in this chapter as well. The pathway to the DNP degree is also discussed. Providing a discussion of these topics will equip one with the information necessary to become familiar with this innovative degree.

Doctor of Nursing Practice Degree Defined

The DNP degree has been adopted as the terminal practice degree in nursing (AACN, 2004, 2006b). The AACN (2004) position statement specifically defines the DNP degree as a "practice focused" doctorate degree, with nursing practice defined as

> any form of nursing intervention that influences health care outcomes for individuals or populations, including the direct care of individual patients, management of care for individuals and populations, administration of nursing and health care organizations, and the development and implementation of health policy. (p. 3)

Preparation at the practice doctorate level is considered the highest level of preparation for nursing practice; hence, it is the terminal degree for nursing practice (AACN, 2004). The DNP degree curriculum is focused on, but not limited to, evidence-based practice, scholarship to advance the profession, organizational and systems leadership, information technology, healthcare policy and advocacy, interprofessional collaboration across disciplines of health care, and advanced nursing practice (AACN, 2006b). It is projected that by 2015 the DNP degree will be the terminal preparation for advanced-practice nursing, and the current master's degree options for advanced nursing practice will be replaced by the DNP degree (AACN, 2006a). A newly developed master's degree, the clinical nurse leader (CNL) degree, will be offered for those who wish to provide healthcare services at the point of care to individuals and cohorts of clients within a healthcare unit or setting (AACN, 2007). This degree prepares the graduate as "a leader in the health care delivery system, not just in the acute care setting but in all settings in which health care is delivered" (AACN, 2007, p. 10). Details regarding the content of the DNP degree curriculum are provided later in this chapter.

Research-Focused Doctorate and Practice-Focused Doctorate Defined

The question, What is a DNP degree? is often followed by the question, What is the difference between a doctor of philosophy (PhD) and a DNP degree? Nurses now can choose between a practice-focused or research-focused doctorate as a terminal degree. Although the academic or research degree, once the only terminal preparation in nursing, has traditionally been the PhD, the AACN now includes the doctor of nursing science (DNS, DNSc, DSN) as a research-focused degree (AACN, 2004).

Further, the AACN Task Force on the Practice Doctorate in Nursing has recommended that the practice doctorate be the DNP degree, which will replace the traditional nursing doctorate (ND) degree (AACN, 2006a). Currently ND programs are taking the necessary steps to adjust their programs to fit the curriculum criteria of DNP degree programs.

The practice- and research-focused doctorates in nursing share a common goal regarding a "scholarly approach to the discipline and a commitment to the advancement of the profession" (AACN, 2006b, p. 3). The differences in these programs include differences in preparation and expertise. The practice doctorate curriculum places more emphasis on practice and less on theory and research methodology (AACN, 2004, 2006b). The final scholarly project differs in that a dissertation required for a PhD degree should document development of new knowledge, and a final scholarly project required for a DNP degree should be grounded in clinical practice and demonstrate ways in which research has an impact on practice.

The focus of the DNP degree is expertise in clinical practice. Additional foci include the *Essentials of Doctoral Education for Advanced Nursing Practice* by the AACN (2006b), which include leadership, health policy and advocacy, and information technology. The focus of a research degree is the generation of new knowledge for the discipline and expertise as a principal investigator. Although the research degree prepares the expert researcher, it should be noted that frequently DNP research projects will also contribute to the discipline by generating new knowledge related to clinical practice and demonstrate the use of evidence-based practice. Please refer to **Table 1-1** for AACN's comparison of a DNP program and PhD, DNS, and DNSc programs.

Evolution of Doctoral Education in Nursing

To appreciate the development of doctoral education in nursing, one must understand where nursing has been with regard to education at the doctoral level. Indeed, nursing has been unique in its approach to doctoral preparation since nurses began to earn doctoral degrees. Even today nurses are prepared at the doctoral level through various degrees, including doctor of education (EdD), PhD, DNS, and now DNP. Prior to the development of the DNP degree, the ND was also offered as a choice for nursing doctoral education.

Examining the chronological development of doctoral education in nursing is somewhat complicated because early doctorates were offered outside nursing. These included the EdD degree and the PhD degree in basic science fields, such as anatomy and physiology (Carpenter & Hudacek, 1996; Marriner-Tomey, 1990). The first nursing-related doctoral program was originated in 1924 at Teachers College, Columbia University, and was an EdD designed to prepare nurses to teach at the college level (Carpenter & Hudacek, 1996). Teachers College was unique in

TABLE 1-1   AACN Contrast Grid of the Key Differences Between DNP and PhD/DNS/DNSc Programs

	DNP	PhD/DNS/DNSc
Program of study	*Objectives:* Prepare nurse specialists at the highest level of advanced practice	*Objectives:* Prepare nurse researchers
	Competencies: Based on *Essentials of Doctoral Education for Advanced Nursing Practice* (AACN, 2006b)*	*Content:* Based on *Indicators of Quality in Research-Focused Doctoral Programs in Nursing* (AACN, 2001)**
Students	Commitment to a practice career	Commitment to a research career
	Oriented toward improving outcomes of care	Oriented toward developing new knowledge
Program faculty	Practice doctorate and/or experience in area in which teaching	Research doctorate in nursing or related field
	Leadership experience in area of specialty practice	Leadership experience in area of sustained research funding
	High level of expertise in specialty practice congruent with focus of academic program	High level of expertise in research congruent with focus of academic program
Resources	Mentors and/or precepts in leadership positions across a variety of practice settings	Mentors/preceptor in research settings
	Access to diverse practice settings with appropriate resources for areas of practice	Access to research settings with appropriate resources
	Access to financial aid	Access to dissertation support dollars
	Access to information and patient-care technology resources congruent with areas of study	Access to information and research technology resources congruent with program of research

TABLE 1-1   AACN Contrast Grid of the Key Differences Between DNP and PhD/DNS/DNSc Programs *(continued)*

	DNP	PhD/DNS/DNSc
Program assessment and evaluation	Program outcome: Healthcare improvements and contributions via practice, policy change, and practice scholarship	Program outcome: Contributes to healthcare improvements via the development of new knowledge and other scholarly projects that provide the foundation for the advancement of nursing science
	Oversight by the institution's authorized bodies (i.e., graduate school) and regional accreditors	Oversight by the institution's authorized bodies (i.e., graduate school) and regional accreditor
	Receives accreditation by specialized nursing accreditor	
	Graduates are eligible for national certification exam	

*American Association of Colleges of Nursing. (2006). *Essentials of doctoral education for advanced nursing practice.* http://www.aacn.nche.edu/publications/position/DNPEssentials.pdf
**American Association of Colleges of Nursing. (2001). *Indicators of Quality in Research-Focused Doctoral Programs in Nursing.* http://www.aacn.nche.edu/publications/position/quality-indicators
Source: Reprinted with permission from AACN DNP Roadmap Task Force Report, October 20, 2006.

that its program was the first to combine both the "nursing and education needs of leaders in the profession" (Carpenter & Hudacek, 1996, p. 5). EdD degrees continued well into the 1960s to be the mainstay of doctoral education for nursing (Marriner-Tomey, 1990).

The first PhD in nursing was offered in 1934 at New York University. Unfortunately, the next PhD in nursing was not offered until the 1950s at the University of Pittsburgh and focused on maternal and child nursing. Incidentally, this degree was the first to recognize the importance of clinical research for the development of the nursing discipline (Carpenter & Hudacek, 1996). The PhD degrees earned elsewhere continued to be in nursing-related fields, such as psychology, sociology, and anthropology. This trend continued until nursing PhD degrees became more popular in the 1970s (Grace, 1978).

Grace (1978) summarized the progression of nursing education over time. Between 1924 and 1959 doctoral education in nursing focused on preparing nurses for "functional specialty" (p. 22). In other words, nurses were prepared to fulfill functional roles as teachers and administrators to lead the field of nursing toward advancement as a profession. The problem with these programs was that they lacked the substantive content necessary to develop nursing as a discipline and a profession. The next shift in doctoral education attempted to fulfill this need and took place between 1960 and 1969. Within this time period, popularity increased for doctoral programs that were nursing related. This included doctorates (PhDs) that were related to disciplines such as sociology, psychology, and anthropology. Grace (1978) noted that the development of these types of programs provided the basic science and research input necessary for the development of future ND programs. Murphy concurred that this stage in the development of doctoral education in nursing led to pertinent questions for the discipline of nursing, such as "(1) What is the essential nature of professional nursing? (2) What is the substantive knowledge base of professional nursing? (3) What kind of research is important for nursing as a knowledge discipline? As a field of practice? (4) How can the scientific base of nursing knowledge be identified and expanded?" (1981, p. 646).

In response to these questions, nursing doctoral education again progressed in the 1970s to include doctorate degrees that are actually in nursing (Grace, 1978). This stage also supported the growth of nursing's substantive structure, hence, the growth of the discipline of nursing. This is where nursing's history of doctoral education becomes more complex. In 1960 the DNS degree originated at Boston University and "focused on the development of nursing theory for a practice discipline" (Marriner-Tomey, 1990, p. 135), hence, the development of the first practice doctorate. The notion of a practice-focused doctorate in nursing is not new. Even as early as the 1970s, it was proposed that the research doctorate (PhD) should focus on preparing nurses to contribute to nursing science, and the practice (or professional) doctorate (DNS) should focus on expertise in clinical practice (Cleland, 1976). Newman also suggested a practice doctorate as the preparation of "professional practitioners" (1975, p. 705) for entry into practice. Grace (1978) noted that it was not sufficient to have a core of nursing researchers building the knowledge base (discipline) without also giving attention to the clinical field. It was also suggested by Grace that nurses prepared through a practice doctorate be titled "social engineers" (1978, p. 26). This seems appropriate given what expert clinicians in nursing are called upon to do.

Although the DNS degree was initially proposed as a practice or professional doctorate, over time the curriculum requirements have become very similar to those for a PhD degree (AACN, 2006a; Apold, 2008; Marriner-Tomey, 1990). Research requirements for this degree have eventually become indistinguishable from that of a PhD in nursing. Because of this, it is not surprising that the

AACN has characterized all DNS degrees as research degrees (2004). With the DNS and PhD degrees so similar in content and focus, the challenge to develop a true practice doctorate remained. An attempt toward this was made in 1979 when the ND originated at Case Western Reserve University, followed by the University of Colorado, Rush University, and South Carolina University. The first ND program was developed by Rozella M. Schlotfeldt, PhD, RN. The ND was different in that the research component was not the general focus of the degree. This degree was designed to be a "pre-service nursing education which would orient nursing's approach to preparing professionals toward competent, independent, accountable nursing practice" (Carpenter & Hudacek, 1996, p. 42). This general theme for a practice doctorate remains consistent even today. Unfortunately, this program did not share the same popularity of DNS or PhD degrees in nursing, and it was less common to find a clinician with this preparation. Further, the curricula in these programs were varied and lacked a uniform approach toward a practice doctorate (Marion et al., 2003).

In 2002 the AACN board of directors formed a task force to examine the current progress of practice doctorates in nursing. Their objective also included comparing proposed curriculum models and discussing recommendations for the future of a practice doctorate (AACN, 2004). To accomplish their mission, the AACN task force (2004) took part in the following activities:

- Reviewed the literature regarding practice doctorates in nursing and other disciplines.
- Established a collaborative relationship with NONPF.
- Interviewed key informants (deans, program directors, graduates, and current students) at the eight current or planned practice-focused doctoral programs in the United States.
- Held open discussions regarding issues surrounding practice-focused doctoral education at AACN's Doctoral Education Conference (January 2003 and February 2004).
- Participated in an open discussion with NONPF along with representatives from key nursing organizations and schools of nursing that were offering or planning a practice doctorate.
- Invited an External Reaction Panel, which involved participation from 10 individuals from various disciplines outside nursing. This panel responded to the draft of the *AACN Position Statement on the Practice Doctorate in Nursing*.

In 2004 the AACN published the *AACN Position Statement on the Practice Doctorate in Nursing* and recommended that the DNP degree would be the terminal degree for nursing practice by 2015. According to NONPF, the purpose of the DNP degree is to prepare nurses to meet the changing demands of health care today by becoming proficient at the following (Marion et al., 2003):

- Evaluating evidence-based practices for care
- Delivering care
- Developing healthcare policy
- Leading and managing clinical care and healthcare systems
- Developing interdisciplinary standards
- Solving healthcare dilemmas
- Reducing disparities in health care

Not only is the development of the DNP degree a culmination of today's emerging healthcare demands; the degree also provides a choice for nurses who wish to focus their doctoral education on nursing practice.

Since its inception the growth of this degree has been astonishing. The University of Kentucky's College of Nursing was the pioneer for this innovative degree and admitted the first DNP class in 2001. In spring 2005, eight DNP programs were offered, and more than 60 were in development. By summer 2005, 80 DNP programs were being considered. In fall 2005, 20 programs offered DNP degrees, and 140 programs were in development. Today there are 243 DNP programs in the United States (AACN, 2014).

It should also be mentioned that in 1999, Columbia University's School of Nursing was formulating plans for a doctor of nursing practice (DrNP) degree that would build on a model of "full-scope, cross-site primary care that Columbia had developed and evaluated over the past ten years" (Goldenberg, 2004, p. 25). This degree was spearheaded by Mary O. Mundinger, DrPH, RN, dean of Columbia University's School of Nursing. The curriculum of a DrNP program is clinically focused with advanced preparation designed to teach "cross-site, full-scope care with content in advanced differential diagnosis skills, advanced pathophysiology and microbiology, selected issues of compliance, management of health care delivery and reimbursement, advanced emergency triage and management, and professional role collaboration and referrals" (Goldenberg, 2004, p. 25). This expanded clinical component is what seems to differentiate a DrNP degree from a DNP degree. The first DrNP class graduated from Columbia University in 2003.

Since the development of the DrNP degree, the Commission on Collegiate Nursing Education (CCNE), the autonomous accrediting body of the AACN, has decided that only practice ND degrees with the doctor of nursing practice title will be eligible for CCNE accreditation (AACN, 2005). This decision was reached unanimously by the CCNE Board of Directors on September 29, 2005 in an effort to develop a process for accrediting only clinically focused NDs (AACN, 2005). The CCNE's decision is consistent with accrediting organizations for other healthcare professions and helps to ensure consistency with degree titling and criteria.

Specific criteria for the DNP degree, including the AACN's *Essentials of Doctoral Education for Advanced Nursing Practice* (2006b) and the *Practice Doctorate Nurse Practitioner Entry-Level Competencies* (NONPF, 2006), are discussed later in this chapter.

Why a Practice Doctorate in Nursing Now?

It has already been mentioned that the notion of a practice doctorate is not new, so why the development of the DNP degree now? It has been noted that the development of the DNP is "more than a mere interruption but rather a response to the need within the healthcare system for expert clinical teachers and clinicians" (Marion, O'Sullivan, Crabtree, Price, & Fontana, 2005, para. 1). Health care needs are not new, yet the growth of this program has been escalating. The question is therefore posed, What are the drivers of this DNP degree, and why is there such urgency?

The Institute of Medicine's Report and Nursing's Response

In 2000 the Institute of Medicine (IOM) published a report titled *To Err Is Human: Building a Safer Health System* (Kohn, Corrigan, & Donaldson, 2000). This report summarized information regarding errors made in health care and offered recommendations to improve the overall quality of care. It was found that "preventable adverse events are a leading cause of death in the United States" (p. 26). In more than 33.6 million admissions to U.S. hospitals in 1997, 44,000 to 98,000 people died as a result of medical-related errors (American Hospital Association, 1999). It was estimated that deaths in hospitals by preventable adverse events exceed the amount attributable to the eighth leading cause of death in America (Centers for Disease Control and Prevention [CDC], 1999b). These numbers also exceed the number of deaths attributable to motor vehicle accidents (43,458), breast cancer (42,297), and AIDS (16,516) (CDC, 1999a). The total cost of health care is greatly affected by these errors as well, with estimated total national costs (lost income, lost household production, disability, healthcare costs) reported as being between $29 billion and $36 billion for adverse events and between $17 billion and $29 billion for preventable adverse events (Thomas et al., 1999).

As a follow-up to the *To Err Is Human* report, in 2001 the IOM published *Crossing the Quality Chasm: A New Health System for the 21st Century*. In an effort to improve health care in the 21st century, the IOM proposed six specific aims for improvement. According to the IOM (2001), these six aims deem that health care should be:

1. Safe in avoiding injuries to patients from the care they receive
2. Effective in providing services based on scientific knowledge to those who could benefit, but services should not be provided to those who may not benefit

3. Patient centered in that provided care is respectful and responsive to individual patient preferences, needs, and values; all patient values should guide all clinical decisions

4. Timely in that wait time and sometimes harmful delays are reduced for those who give and receive care

5. Efficient in that waste is avoided, particularly waste of equipment, supplies, ideas, and energy

6. Equitable in that high-quality care is provided to all regardless of personal characteristics, such as gender, ethnicity, geographic location, and socioeconomic status

The IOM (2001) emphasized that to achieve these aims, additional skills may be required on the healthcare team. This includes all individuals who care for patients. The new skills needed to improve health care and reduce errors are, ironically, many skills that nurses have long been known to exemplify. Some examples of these skills include using electronic communications, synthesizing evidence-based practice information, communicating with patients in an open manner to enable their decision making, understanding the course of illness that specifically relates to the patient's experience outside the hospital, working collaboratively in teams, and understanding the link between health care and healthy populations (IOM, 2001). Developing expertise in these areas required curriculum changes in healthcare education as well as addressing how healthcare education is approached, organized, and funded (IOM, 2001).

In 2003 the Health Professions Education Committee responded to the IOM's *Crossing the Quality Chasm* report (IOM, 2001) by publishing *Health Professions Education: A Bridge to Quality* (Greiner & Knebel, 2003). The committee recommended that "all health professionals should be educated to deliver patient-centered care as members of an interdisciplinary team, emphasizing evidence-based practice, quality improvement approaches, and informatics" (Greiner & Knebel, 2003, p. 45). To meet this goal, the committee proposed a set of competencies to be met by all healthcare clinicians, regardless of discipline. These competencies include the following: provide patient-centered care, function in interdisciplinary teams, employ evidence-based practice, integrate quality improvement standards, and utilize various information systems (Greiner & Knebel, 2003).

As part of the continued effort to advance the education of healthcare professionals, the Robert Wood Johnson Foundation (RWJF) and the IOM specifically addressed advancing nursing education. In 2008 the RWJF and the IOM "launched a two-year initiative to respond to the need to access and transform the nursing profession" (IOM, 2010a, p. 1). The IOM appointed the Committee on the RWJF Initiative on the Future of Nursing. This committee published a report titled *The Future of Nursing: Focus on Education* (IOM, 2010a). In this report, the IOM concluded that "the ways in which nurses were educated during the 20th century are no longer adequate for dealing with the realities of healthcare in the 21st century" (2010a, p. 2). The IOM reiterated the need for the aforementioned competencies, such as leadership, health policy, system improvement, research and evidence-based practice, and teamwork and collaboration. In response to the increasing demands of a complex healthcare environment, the IOM recommended higher levels of education for nurses and new ways to educate nurses to better meet the needs of this population.

The IOM included recommendations in the report that specifically address the number of nurses with doctorate degrees. It was noted that although 13% of nurses hold a graduate degree, fewer than 1% hold doctoral degrees (IOM, 2010a). The IOM concluded that "nurses with doctorates are needed to teach future generations of nurses and to conduct research that becomes the basis for improvements in nursing science and practice" (2010a, p. 4). Therefore, recommendation 5 states that "schools of nursing, with support from private and public funders, academic administrators and university trustees, and accreditation bodies, should double the number of nurses with a doctorate by 2020 to add to the cadre of nurse faculty and researchers, with attention to increasing diversity" (IOM, 2010b, p. 4).

The development of the DNP degree is one of the answers to the call proposed by both the IOM's Health Professions Education Committee and the IOM's and the RWJF's Initiative on the Future of Nursing Committee to redefine how healthcare professionals are educated. Nursing has always had a vested interest in improving quality of care and patient outcomes. Since Florence Nightingale, "nursing education has been directed toward the individualized, personalized care of the patient, not the disease" (Newman, 1975, p. 704). To further illustrate nursing's commitment to improve quality of care and patient outcomes, the competencies described by the Health Professions Education Committee are reflected in the AACN's *Essentials of Doctoral Education for Advanced Nursing Practice* (2006b) and NONPF's *Practice Doctorate Nurse Practitioner Entry-Level Competencies* (2006). Preparing nurses at the practice doctorate level who are experts at using information technology, synthesizing and integrating evidence-based practices, and collaborating across healthcare disciplines will further enable nursing to meet the challenges of health care in the 21st century.

Additional Drivers for a Practice Doctorate in Nursing

In a 2005 report, titled *Advancing the Nation's Health Needs: NIH Research Training Programs*, the National Academy of Sciences (2005) recommended that nursing develop a nonresearch doctorate. The rationale for this initiative included increasing the numbers of expert practitioners who can also fulfill clinical nursing faculty needs (AACN, 2011). The report specifically states that "the need for doctorally prepared practitioners and clinical faculty would be met if nursing could develop a new non-research clinical doctorate, similar to the MD and PharmD in Medicine and Pharmacy, respectively" (National Academy of Sciences, 2005, p. 74). The initiatives of the National Academy of Sciences regarding doctoral education in nursing are reflected in the AACN's development of the DNP degree.

An additional rationale for a practice doctorate is reflected in nursing's educational history when the practice doctorate was first proposed. Newman noted that "nursing lacked the recognition for what it has to offer and authority for putting that knowledge into practice" (1975, p. 704). Starck, Duffy, and Vogler stated that "for nursing to be accountable to the social mandate, the numbers as well as the type of doctorally prepared nurses need attention" (1993, p. 214). NONPF's Practice Doctorate Task Force summarized the most frequently cited additional drivers for a practice doctorate in nursing (Marion et al., 2005):

- Parity with other professionals who are prepared with a practice doctorate. Disciplines such as audiology, dentistry, medicine, pharmacy, psychology, and physical therapy require a practice doctorate for entry into practice.
- A need for longer programs that both reflect the credit hours invested in master's degrees and accommodate additional information needed to prepare nurses for the demands of health care. Most master's degrees require a similar number of credit hours for completion as the number required for practice doctoral degrees.
- Remedy the current nursing faculty shortages. The development of a practice doctorate will help meet the needs for clinical teaching in schools of nursing.
- The increasing complexity of healthcare systems requires additional information to be included in current graduate nursing programs. Rather than further burden the amount of information needed to prepare nurses at the graduate level for a master's degree, a practice doctorate allows for additional information to be provided and affords a practice doctorate to prepare nurses for the changing demands of society and health care.

What Is a DNP Degree Made Of? The Recipe for Curriculum Standards

The standards of a DNP program have been formulated through a collaborative effort among various consensus-based standards. These standards reflect collaborative efforts among the AACN as the *Essentials of Doctoral Education for Advanced Nursing Practice* (2006b), NONPF as the *Practice Doctorate Nurse Practitioner Entry-Level Competencies* (2006), and more recently the National Association of Clinical Nurse Specialists (NACNS) as *Core Practice Doctorate Clinical Nurse Specialist Competencies* (2009). These organizations' strategies for setting the standards of a practice doctorate in nursing demonstrate interrelated criteria that are congruent with all rationales for a practice doctorate in nursing. It should be noted, however, that while maintaining these consensus-based standards, there may be some variability in content within DNP curricula.

AACN *Essentials of Doctoral Education for Advanced Nursing Practice*

In 2006 the AACN published the *Essentials of Doctoral Education for Advanced Nursing Practice*. These essentials are the "foundational outcome competencies deemed essential for all graduates of a DNP program regardless of specialty or functional focus" (AACN, 2006b, p. 8). Nursing faculties have the freedom to creatively design course work to meet these essentials, which are summarized in the following sections.

ESSENTIAL I: SCIENTIFIC UNDERPINNINGS FOR PRACTICE

This essential describes the scientific foundations of nursing practice, which are based on the natural and social sciences. These sciences may include human biology, physiology, and psychology. In addition, nursing science has provided nursing with a body of knowledge to contribute to the discipline of nursing. This body of knowledge or discipline is focused on the following (adapted from AACN, 2006b; Donaldson & Crowley, 1978; Fawcett, 2005; Gortner, 1980):

- The principles and laws that govern the life process, well-being, and optimal functioning of human beings, sick or well
- The patterning of human behavior in interaction with the environment in normal life events and critical life situations
- The processes by which positive changes in health status are affected
- The wholeness of health of human beings, recognizing that they are in continuous interaction with their environments

Nursing science has expanded the discipline of nursing and includes the development of middle-range nursing theories and concepts to guide practice. Understanding the practice of nursing includes developing an understanding of scientific underpinnings for practice (the science and discipline of nursing). Specifically, the DNP degree prepares the graduate to do the following (adapted from AACN, 2006b):

- Integrate nursing science with knowledge from the organizational, biophysical, psychological, and analytical sciences, as well as ethics, as the basis for the highest level of nursing practice.
- Develop and evaluate new practice approaches based on nursing theories and theories from other disciplines.
- Utilize science-based concepts and theories to determine the significance and nature of health and healthcare delivery phenomena, describe strategies used to enhance healthcare delivery, and evaluate outcomes.

ESSENTIAL II: ORGANIZATIONAL AND SYSTEMS LEADERSHIP FOR QUALITY IMPROVEMENT AND SYSTEMS THINKING

Preparation in organizational and systems leadership at every level is imperative for DNP graduates to have an impact on and improve healthcare delivery and patient care outcomes. DNP graduates are distinguished by their ability to focus on new healthcare delivery methods that are based on nursing science. Preparation in this area will provide DNP graduates with expertise in "assessing organizations, identifying systems' issues, and facilitating organization-wide changes in practice delivery" (AACN, 2006b, p. 10). Specifically, the DNP graduate will be prepared to do the following (adapted from AACN, 2006b):

- Utilize scientific findings in nursing and other disciplines to develop and evaluate care delivery approaches that meet the current and future needs of patient populations.
- Guarantee accountability for the safety and quality of care for the patients they care for.
- Manage ethical dilemmas within patient care, healthcare organizations, and research, including developing and evaluating appropriate strategies.

ESSENTIAL III: CLINICAL SCHOLARSHIP AND ANALYTICAL METHODS FOR EVIDENCE-BASED PRACTICE

DNP graduates are unique in that their contributions to nursing science involve the "translation of research into practice and the dissemination and integration of new knowledge" (AACN, 2006b, p. 11). Further, DNP graduates are in a distinctive position to merge nursing science, nursing practice, human needs, and human caring. Specifically, the DNP graduate is expected to be an expert in the evaluation, integration, translation, and application of evidence-based practices. Additionally, DNP graduates are actively involved in nursing practice, which allows for practical, applicable research questions to arise from the practice environment. Working collaboratively with experts in research investigation, DNP graduates can also assist in the generation of new knowledge and affect evidence-based practice from the practice arena. To achieve these goals, the DNP program prepares the graduate to do the following (adapted from AACN, 2006b):

- Analytically and critically evaluate existing literature and other research to determine the best evidence for practice.
- Evaluate practice outcomes within populations in various arenas, such as healthcare organizations, communities, or practice settings.
- Design and evaluate methodologies that improve quality in an effort to promote "safe, effective, efficient, equitable, and patient-centered care" (AACN, 2006b, p. 12).

- Develop practice guidelines that are based on relevant, best-practice findings.
- Utilize informatics and research methodologies to collect and analyze data, design databases, interpret findings to design evidence-based interventions, evaluate outcomes, and identify gaps within evidence-based practice, which will improve the practice environment.
- Work collaboratively with research specialists and act as a "practice consultant" (AACN, 2006b, p. 12).

ESSENTIAL IV: INFORMATION SYSTEMS–TECHNOLOGY AND PATIENT CARE TECHNOLOGY FOR THE IMPROVEMENT AND TRANSFORMATION OF HEALTH CARE

DNP graduates have cutting-edge abilities to use information technology to improve patient care and outcomes. Knowledge regarding the design and implementation of information systems to evaluate programs and outcomes of care is essential for preparation as a DNP graduate. Expertise is garnered in information technology, such as web-based communications, telemedicine, online documentation, and other unique healthcare delivery methods. DNP graduates must also develop expertise in utilizing information technologies to support practice leadership and clinical decision making. Specific to information systems, DNP graduates are prepared to do the following (adapted from AACN, 2006b):

- Evaluate and monitor outcomes of care and quality of care improvement by designing, selecting, using, and evaluating programs related to information technologies.
- Become proficient at the skills necessary to evaluate data extraction from practice information systems and databases.
- Attend to ethical and legal issues related to information technologies within the healthcare setting by providing leadership to evaluate and resolve these issues.
- Communicate and evaluate the accuracy, timeliness, and appropriateness of healthcare consumer information.

ESSENTIAL V: HEALTHCARE POLICY FOR ADVOCACY IN HEALTH CARE

Becoming involved in healthcare policy and advocacy has the potential to affect the delivery of health care across all settings. Thus, knowledge and skills related to healthcare policy are central to nursing practice and are therefore essential to the DNP graduate. Further, "health policy influences multiple care delivery issues, including health disparities, cultural sensitivity, ethics, the internalization of health care concerns, access to care, quality of care, health care financing, and issues of equity and social justice in the delivery of health care" (AACN, 2006b, p. 13). DNP graduates are uniquely positioned to be powerful advocates for healthcare policy through their practice experiences. These practice experiences provide rich influences for the development of policy. Nursing's interest in social justice and equality requires that DNP graduates become involved in and develop expertise in healthcare policy and advocacy.

Additionally, DNP graduates need to be prepared in leadership roles with regard to public policy. As leaders in the practice setting, DNP graduates frequently assimilate research, practice, and policy. Therefore, DNP preparation should include experience in recognizing the factors that influence the development of policy across various settings. The DNP graduate is prepared to do the following (adapted from AACN, 2006b):

- Decisively analyze health policies and proposals from the points of view of consumers, nurses, and other healthcare professionals.
- Provide leadership in the development and implementation of healthcare policy at the institutional, local, state, federal, and international levels.
- Actively participate on committees, boards, or task forces at the institutional, local, state, federal, and international levels.
- Participate in the education of other healthcare professionals, patients, or other stakeholders regarding healthcare policy issues.
- Act as an advocate for the nursing profession through activities related to healthcare policy.
- Influence healthcare financing, regulation, and delivery through the development of leadership in healthcare policy.
- Act as an advocate for ethical, equitable, and social justice policies across all healthcare settings.

ESSENTIAL VI: INTERPROFESSIONAL COLLABORATION FOR IMPROVING PATIENT AND POPULATION HEALTH OUTCOMES

This essential specifically relates to the IOM's mandate to provide safe, timely, equitable, effective, efficient, and patient-centered care. In a multitiered, complex healthcare environment, collaboration among all healthcare disciplines must exist to achieve the IOM's and nursing's goals. Nurses are experts at functioning as collaborators among multiple disciplines. Therefore, as nursing practice experts, DNP graduates must be prepared to facilitate collaboration and team building. This may include both participating in the work of the team and assuming leadership roles when necessary.

With regard to interprofessional collaboration, the DNP graduate must be prepared to do the following (adapted from AACN, 2006b):

- Participate in effective communication and collaboration throughout the development of "practice models, peer review, practice guidelines, health policy, standards of care, and/or other scholarly products" (AACN, 2006b, p. 15).
- Analyze complex practice or organizational issues through leadership of interprofessional teams.
- Act as a consultant to interprofessional teams to implement change in healthcare delivery systems.

ESSENTIAL VII: CLINICAL PREVENTION AND POPULATION HEALTH FOR IMPROVING THE NATION'S HEALTH

Clinical prevention is defined as health promotion and risk reduction–illness prevention for individuals and families, and population health is defined as including all community, environmental, cultural, and socioeconomic aspects of health (Allan et al., 2004; AACN, 2006b). Nursing has foundations in health promotion and risk reduction and is therefore positioned to have an impact on the health status of people in multiple settings. The further preparation included in the DNP curriculum will prepare graduates to "analyze epidemiological, biostatistical, occupational, and environmental data in the development, implementation, and evaluation of clinical prevention and population health" (AACN, 2006b, p. 15). In other words, DNP graduates are in an ideal position to participate in health promotion and risk reduction activities from a nursing perspective with additional preparation in evaluating and interpreting data that are pertinent to improving the health status of individuals (adapted from AACN, 2006b).

ESSENTIAL VIII: ADVANCED NURSING PRACTICE

Because one cannot become proficient in all areas of specialization, DNP degree programs "provide preparation within distinct specialties that require expertise, advanced knowledge, and mastery in one area of nursing practice" (AACN, 2006b, p. 16). This specialization is defined by a specialty practice area within the domain of nursing and is a requisite of the DNP degree. Although the DNP graduate may function in a variety of roles, role preparation within the practice specialty, including legal and regulatory issues, is part of every DNP curriculum. With regard to advanced nursing practice, the DNP graduate is prepared to do the following (adapted from AACN, 2006b):

- Comprehensively assess health and illness parameters while incorporating diverse and culturally sensitive approaches.
- Implement and evaluate therapeutic interventions based on nursing and other sciences.

- Participate in therapeutic relationships with patients and other healthcare professionals to ensure optimal patient care and improve patient outcomes.
- Utilize advanced clinical decision-making skills and critical thinking, and deliver and evaluate evidence-based care to improve patient outcomes.
- Serve as a mentor to others in the nursing profession in an effort to maintain excellence in nursing practice.
- Participate in the education of patients, especially those in complex health situations.

A NOTE ABOUT SPECIALTY-FOCUSED COMPETENCIES ACCORDING TO THE AACN

The purpose of specialty preparation within the DNP curricula is to prepare graduates to fulfill specific roles within health care. Specialty preparation and the eight DNP essentials equip DNP graduates to serve in roles within two different domains. The first domain includes specialization as advanced-practice registered nurses who care for individuals (including, but not limited to, clinical nurse specialist (CNS), nurse practitioner, nurse anesthetist, nurse–midwife). The second domain includes specialization in advanced practice at an organizational or systems level. Because of this variability, specialization content within DNP programs may differ (AACN, 2006b). It should also be noted that postmaster's degree DNP preparation includes doctoral-level content exclusively; however, postbaccalaureate DNP preparation includes both advanced-practice specialty content that was previously covered in master's preparation and doctoral-level content.

NONPF *Practice Doctorate Nurse Practitioner Entry-Level Competencies*

NONPF published *Practice Doctorate Nurse Practitioner Entry-Level Competencies* for nurse practitioner and DNP graduates (2006). These competencies differ somewhat from the AACN's essentials in that they are particular to nurse practitioner roles. However, these competencies are also reflective of the AACN's essentials. The competencies are as follows:

I. Competency Area: Independent Practice

Practices independently by assessing, diagnosing, treating, and managing undifferentiated patients.

Assumes full accountability for actions as a licensed practitioner.

II. Competency Area: Scientific Foundation

Critically analyzes data for practice by integrating knowledge from arts and sciences within the context of nursing's philosophical framework and scientific foundation.

Translates research and data to anticipate, predict, and explain variations in practice.

III. Competency Area: Leadership

Assumes increasingly complex leadership roles.

Provides leadership to foster intercollaboration.

Demonstrates a leadership style that uses critical and reflective thinking.

IV. Competency Area: Quality

Uses best-available evidence to enhance quality in clinical practice.

Evaluates how organizational, structural, financial, marketing, and policy decisions affect cost, quality, and accessibility of health care.

Demonstrates skills in peer review that promote a culture of excellence.

V. Competency Area: Practice Inquiry

Applies clinical investigative skills for evaluation of health outcomes at the patient, family, population, clinical unit, systems, or community levels.

Provides leadership in the translation of new knowledge into practice.

Disseminates evidence from inquiry to diverse audiences using multiple methods.

VI. Competency Area: Technology and Information Literacy

Demonstrates information literacy in complex decision making.

Translates technical and scientific health information appropriate for user need.

VII. Competency Area: Policy

Analyzes ethical, legal, and social factors in policy development.

Influences health policy.

Evaluates the impact of globalization on healthcare policy.

VIII. Competency Area: Health Delivery System

Applies knowledge of organizational behavior and systems.

Demonstrates skills in negotiating, consensus building, and partnering.

Manages risks to individuals, families, populations, and healthcare systems.

Facilitates development of culturally relevant healthcare systems.

IX. Competency Area: Ethics

Applies ethically sound solutions to complex issues.

NACNS *Core Practice Doctorate Clinical Nurse Specialist Competencies*

In 2006 the NACNS consulted with various nursing organizations and nursing accrediting entities regarding the implications of the DNP degree for CNS practice and education (NACNS, 2009). A formal task force, including representatives from

NACNS and 19 other nursing organizations, was charged with developing competencies for the CNS at the doctoral level (NACNS, 2009). Because traditional CNS education has included a master's degree, "the *Core Practice Doctorate Clinical Nurse Specialist Competencies* should be used with the National CNS Competency Task Force's *Organizing Framework and Core Competencies* (2008) and the AACN *Essentials of Doctoral Education for Advanced Nursing Practice* (2006b) to inform educational programs and employer expectations" (NACNS, 2009, p. 10).

The foci of the *Core Practice Doctorate Clinical Nurse Specialist Competencies* are congruent with the AACN's *Essentials of Doctoral Education for Advanced Nursing Practice* and NONPF's *Practice Doctorate Nurse Practitioner Entry-Level Competencies* (**Figure 1-1**). Specifically, graduates of CNS-focused DNP programs should be prepared beyond traditional CNS competencies to "strengthen the already significant contribution that CNSs make in ensuring quality patient outcomes through establishing a practice foundation based on advanced scientific, theoretical, ethical, and economic principles" (NACNS, 2009, p. 11). These competencies ensure that doctoral-prepared CNS graduates are prepared to do the following (adapted from NACNS, 2009):

- Generate and disseminate new knowledge
- Evaluate and translate evidence into practice
- Employ a broad range of theories from nursing and related disciplines

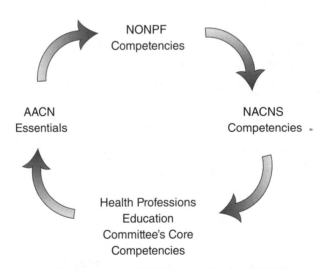

FIGURE 1-1   Relationship among the DNP Essentials, the NONPF Competencies, the NACNS Competencies, and the Core Competencies Needed for Healthcare Professionals per the Committee on Health Professions Education

- Design and evaluate innovative strategies to improve quality of care and safety in all settings
- Improve systems of care
- Provide leadership that promotes interprofessional collaboration
- Influence and shape health policy

CERTIFIED REGISTERED NURSE ANESTHETISTS

As advanced-practice nursing moves toward doctoral preparation for entry into practice, certified registered nurse anesthetists (CRNAs) have debated if this progression is appropriate for this advanced-practice specialty. In 2005 the American Association of Nurse Anesthetists (AANA) Summit on Doctoral Preparation for Nurse Anesthetists convened to discuss and identify potential implications of adopting doctoral preparation (Martin-Sheridan, Ouellette, & Horton, 2006). The summit participants concluded that in the future CRNAs may need additional knowledge and skills that include doctoral preparation. Following the summit, the Task Force on Doctoral Preparation of Nurse Anesthetists was formed to develop recommendations regarding doctoral preparation for CRNAs. In 2007 a decision was made by AANA to transition from master's-level education to doctoral-level education by 2025 (AANA, 2007). To date, the *Standards for Accreditation of Nurse Anesthesia Programs Practice Doctorate* state that "students accepted into accredited entry-level programs on or after January 1, 2022, must graduate with doctoral degrees" (Council on Accreditation of Nurse Anesthesia Programs, 2013, p. 2).

The Path to the DNP Degree: Follow the Academic Road

The path to the DNP degree is currently in transition. Previously DNP preparation included exclusively postmaster's degree preparation. Many postmaster's degree students will have already fulfilled several of the criteria listed in the *Essentials of Doctoral Education for Advanced Nursing Practice* and the *Practice Doctorate Nurse Practitioner Entry-Level Competencies* in their master's degree curricula. Further, as mentioned earlier, the specialization content included in the DNP degree curriculum is currently being fulfilled within the master's degree curriculum. However, a shift is occurring to include postbaccalaureate DNP preparation. This option presents many new challenges for both students and schools of nursing.

Each individual's path to the DNP degree may be unique. Prospective students' program content may be individualized to include the learning experiences necessary to incorporate the described requirements for the DNP degree. Please refer to **Figure 1-2** for an illustration of the pathways to the DNP degree.

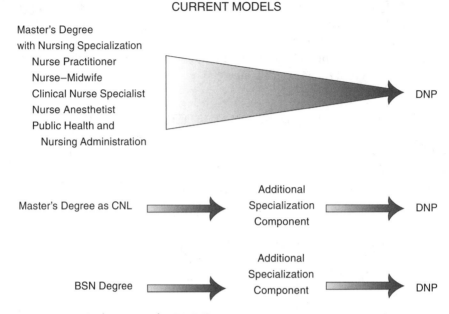

FIGURE 1-2   Pathways to the DNP Degree

Role Transition Introduced

As explained earlier in the chapter, the doctoral-level content of the DNP degree is not intended to provide specialization in nursing practice. The doctoral-level content instead builds on advanced nursing practice specialization and provides additional preparation in the formulation, interpretation, and utilization of evidence-based practices, health policy, information technology, and leadership. Although DNP graduates may function as evaluators and translators of research, health policy advocates, nursing leaders, educators, information specialists, or clinicians, it is entirely likely that these roles will be integrated as well. One DNP graduate may participate in research in addition to practicing as a nurse anesthetist. Another DNP graduate may be a nurse executive in addition to developing health policy. Nursing has always been a profession that involves juggling multiple roles (Dudley-Brown, 2006; Jennings & Rogers, 1988; Sperhac & Strodtbeck, 1997). Within these multiple roles, the fundamental goal of the DNP graduate remains the development of expertise in the delivery of high-quality, patient-centered care, and the graduate utilizes the necessary avenues to provide that care.

Interview with a DNP Cofounder: Then and Now

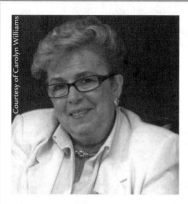

Courtesy of Carolyn Williams

CAROLYN A. WILLIAMS, PHD, RN, FAAN, IS PROFESSOR AND DEAN EMERITUS OF THE UNIVERSITY OF KENTUCKY. She was president of the American Association of Colleges of Nursing from 2000 to 2002 and scholar-in-residence at the Institute of Medicine from 2007 to 2008.

THEN . . . 2008

Dr. Williams, could you please describe your background and current position?

I began my nursing career as a public health nurse at a public health department in a rural area and practiced for 2 years before returning to graduate school. I then received my master's degree in public health nursing. This was a joint master's degree from both the School of Nursing and the School of Public Health from the University of North Carolina at Chapel Hill (UNC, CH). I then went on to earn a PhD in epidemiology from the School of Public Health at UNC, CH. This was met with some controversy in that I did not have a large amount of nursing experience before returning to graduate school. Interestingly, the School of Public Health was supportive of my doctoral studies whereas the School of Nursing seemed to think I needed more nursing experience. This is what I call a "pernicious pattern" in nursing education. I actually had to talk faculty [in nursing] into supporting me to earn a doctorate. However, faculty from other disciplines, e.g., medicine, psychology, and sociology in the School of Public Health, were very supportive. This is where nursing differs from medicine: we don't build in the experience into our educational programs.

Upon finishing my PhD in epidemiology, I took a faculty position at Emory University's School of Nursing. From there, I was asked to return to Chapel Hill to participate in the development and evaluation of a family nurse practitioner program in the School of Nursing and to teach epidemiology in the School of Public Health. The program in the School of Nursing was one of the first six federally funded family nurse practitioner programs in the country. I remained at Chapel Hill for 13 years before accepting an appointment as dean of the College of Nursing at the University of Kentucky. Last year I retired as dean after 22 years in that position and remained as a faculty member.

This year [2007 to 2008] I am a scholar-in-residence at the Institute of Medicine in Washington, DC. My role here includes development of a project, which happens to be interprofessional collaboration. This stems from the view that improvement in quality care depends on people working together in interprofessional teams. Interprofessional collaboration is happening around the margins of education for health care instead of in the mainstream, particularly core clinical components of undergraduate and graduate education for health care. It may be picked up in passing, but frequently it is not a formal part of the curriculum. Part of my project involves identifying the policy changes [that] are needed at the university level to integrate interprofessional collaboration as part [of] an integral component of education in the health professions. Interprofessional collaboration is a necessary part of practice and therefore needs to be integrated into the preparation of healthcare professionals. This leads me to an issue I have always struggled with: too few clinical faculty in nursing actually practice. This is a problem due to the fact that a practice culture is not as visible as I believe it needs to be in most schools of nursing. Some progress in having nursing faculty engaged in practice was achieved with the nurse practitioner movement that started in the 1970s, but it is still a struggle for nursing faculty to engage in practice as part of their faculty role in a manner similar to what happens in medical education. Some faculty attempt to practice on their own, not as a part of their faculty role, and usually faculty practice is not viewed as a priority in schools of nursing. I feel if we want nursing faculty to provide leadership in practice and develop leaders for practice, each school of nursing needs to have a core group of faculty who actually engage in practice as part of their faculty role.

Dr. Williams, could you please describe how your vision for a doctor of nursing practice became a reality?

While on the faculty at the University of North Carolina at Chapel Hill and consulting with a number of individuals in practice settings, I developed some ideas of what nursing education to prepare nurse leaders needs to be. Initially, I viewed the degree as what public health nurses could earn to prepare them to face the challenges of public health nursing. I didn't feel that the master's degrees in nursing offered at that time [1970s through early 1980s] were sufficient for the kind of leadership roles nurses were moving in to. I felt a true practice degree at the doctoral level was needed.

When I went to the University of Kentucky as the dean of nursing, I was charged with developing a PhD in nursing program. While at Chapel Hill I had been very involved in research activity, doctoral education in epidemiology, and was active nationally in research development and advocacy in nursing as chair of the American Nurses Association's Commission on Nursing Research and as the president of the American Academy of Nursing. I proceeded to work with the faculty at the University of Kentucky, and we developed the PhD program in nursing. However, I was still interested in the concept of a practice doctorate and promoting stronger partnerships between nursing practice and nursing education.

As time went on it became clearer and clearer to me that to prepare nurses for leadership in practice, something more in tune with preparing nurses to utilize knowledge, not necessarily generate new knowledge, which was expected in PhD programs, was needed. Thus, I began to talk with and work with my faculty colleagues on the concept of a new practice degree for nurses to prepare for leadership in practice, not in education or research.

I saw practice as the focus with this degree, not research. Working with my University of Kentucky faculty colleagues, particularly Dr. Marcia K. Stanhope and Dr. Julie G. Sebastian, we developed the initial conceptualization of the degree. These foci included four themes that I feel should be central to a practice doctorate in nursing:

1. *Leadership in practice, which included leadership at the point of care. This also includes leadership at the policy level to impact care.*

2. *A population approach and perspective. This involves a broader view of health care, which recognizes the importance of populations when planning and evaluating care processes.*

3. *Integration of evidence-based practice to make informed decisions regarding care.*

4. *The ability to understand change processes and institute positive changes in health care.*

These four themes guided the development of the curriculum of the first DNP program at the University of Kentucky, which when we instituted it was the first in the United States. These themes also influenced and are incorporated in what became the AACN's Essentials of Doctoral Education for Advanced Nursing Practice.

To expand on the development of the DNP program at University of Kentucky, the following is the time line:

1994–1998	*Informal conversations among faculty, people in practice, and others regarding a practice doctorate in nursing*
1998	*Professional Doctorate Task Force Committee formed*
May 1999	*Approval of DNP program by total college faculty*
July 1999	*Medical Center Academic Council approval*
January 2000	*University of Kentucky Board of Trustees approved the program*
May 2000	*Approval by the Kentucky Council of Postsecondary Education*
January 2001	*The first national paper on the DNP degree at the AACN's National Doctoral Education Conference (Williams, Stanhope, & Sebastian, 2001)*
Fall 2001	*Students admitted to the first DNP program in the country.*

In 1998, when the University of Kentucky's DNP task force was created, we decided we didn't want this degree to look like anything else currently in nursing education. We also decided on the name of this degree in this committee. We wanted the degree and the name to focus on nursing practice, and we did not want the degree to be limited to preparing for only one particular type of nursing practice. We decided on the doctor of nursing practice because that describes what the degree is: a practice degree in nursing.

One of the most important things that happened during my presidency of the American Association of Colleges of Nursing was the appointment [of] a task force to look at the issue of a practice doctorate. The task force committee was carefully planned. I wanted to have a positive group of people as well as major stakeholders represented. These stakeholders were credible individuals who had an interest in the development of a practice doctorate. Members of the committee included representatives from Columbia University, the University of Kentucky, a representative from an ND program, as well as a representative from schools that did not have nursing doctoral programs. This committee was chaired by Dr. Elizabeth Lentz, who has written extensively on doctoral education in nursing. As this task force began sorting out the issues, it became the goal that by 2015, the DNP would become the terminal degree for specialization in nursing.

From this point, a group to develop both the essentials of doctoral education in nursing and a roadmap task force were formed. These committees worked together, and we presented together nationally in a series of regional forums. We invited others to engage in discourse regarding the essentials as well as ask questions about the DNP degree. As our presentations across the country came to a conclusion, we noticed an obvious transformation. The DNP degree was beginning to gain more acceptance. By the time we were done, the argument of whether to adopt a practice doctorate in nursing had given rise to how to put this degree in place.

Dr. Williams, are you surprised by the acceptance of the degree and speed with which programs are being developed?

Yes, I am surprised. I thought the DNP degree would be an important development for the field of nursing, and I thought some would adopt a practice doctorate. I certainly did not think things would move so fast. The idea of a DNP really struck a chord with many people.

Dr. Williams, do you think the history of doctoral education in nursing has influenced the development of a practice doctorate in nursing?

Well, we need to have scientists in our field. However, we also need to come to grips with the fact that we are a practice discipline. Over the years, since the late 1970s, many of the leading academic settings in nursing have become increasingly research intensive and [have] not spent as much effort on developing a complementary practice focus. I feel the development of a practice doctorate has more to do with our development as a discipline than the history of doctoral nursing education. Attraction and credibility from the university setting stem from involvement in research. Therefore, it becomes a struggle when handling this practice piece. If nursing wants acceptance as a discipline, we must have research. But we are a practice discipline, and all practice disciplines struggle to some extent in research-intensive university environments.

Dr. Williams, do you agree that nursing should have both a research- and a practice-focused doctorate?

Of course. The ratio between research-focused and practice-focused doctorates may be tipped toward the practice focus due to the practice focus of our discipline.

Dr. Williams, could you describe what you feel is the future of doctoral education in nursing?

Down the pike, some people may move into DNP programs and then discover they want to be researchers and end up also getting a PhD. This would be very healthy for our profession. Essentially, we have lost talented folks due to offering only a research-focused terminal degree. The DNP allows us to accommodate those folks who don't want a research-focused degree. I also feel we need a more intensive clinical component integrated into the degree. This may be in the form of residency programs integrated within nursing degrees or as a postdoctorate option.

Dr. Williams, could you expand on the grandfathering of advanced-practice registered nurses (APRNs) who don't wish to pursue a DNP degree?

The DNP degree will not be required to practice anytime soon. It took a while to require a master's degree to practice as an APRN. There will be a similar transition regarding the DNP degree. If someone is certified and successful as an APRN without a DNP, they should continue to be successful.

Dr. Williams, do you believe the DNP will continue to flourish as a degree option for nursing? If so, what would your advice be regarding nurses earning a DNP degree?

Yes, I do. My advice regarding nurses earning a DNP degree is that it depends on their career choice. Some have been looking for this option for a long time. This may be the right degree for some no matter where they are in practice.

NOW . . . 2014

Dr. Williams, we discussed your nursing background and education the last time we spoke. Could you please describe your current position and what types of projects you are currently involved in?

Since I left the deanship of the College of Nursing at the University of Kentucky in the fall of 2006 I have remained on the faculty as a professor in the college and teach in both our DNP and PhD programs. I spent the 2007–2008 academic year at the Institute of Medicine in DC as the American Academy of Nursing–American Nurses' Foundation's scholar-in-residence. During that year I had the opportunity to be a part of the Health Policy seminars designed for the Robert Wood Johnson Foundation's Health Policy Fellows. It was a unique experience to interact with health policy makers and experts in the national arena.

I continue to teach at the University of Kentucky in the areas of health policy, leadership, and ethics, and I work with students on DNP Clinical Projects and Dissertations. I also continue to serve as a consultant and mentor on issues related to graduate education in nursing and leadership in the field.

Dr. Williams, what is your impression of the current progress of the DNP degree? How does the current progress of the DNP degree compare to your original vision of the DNP degree?

The original vision that my colleagues and I at the University of Kentucky's College of Nursing had for the DNP when we opened the first program of study leading to the DNP in the fall of 2001 was that it would be a postmaster's program for those interested in leadership in nursing practice. Further we saw the DNP as a program of study for clinical nurse specialists, nurse practitioners, and nurse administrators. We conceptualized four key areas which we felt were necessary for leadership in practice and which we felt were not sufficiently dealt with in the master's programs at that time. Those four pillars were: a population approach; the use of the best evidence possible in clinical decision making; understanding how to guide sustainable changes in practice based on the best evidence possible; and leadership at the unit and system level. Our original program was built around those concepts, and I am pleased that those concepts are clearly evident in the DNP essentials developed by the American Association of Colleges of Nursing (AACN, 2006b).

For a program to receive accreditation by the Commission on Collegiate Nursing Education (CCNE) all of the essentials have to be evident in the curriculum. However, one issue that we need to continue to keep in focus and work on, particularly in the emerging BSN to DNP programs preparing nurse practitioners, is how to integrate those concepts into the manner in which the nurse practitioner student conceptualizes their practice. This is tricky since students in such programs focus so much of their efforts on getting comfortable with the assessment and management of individual patients, and time in many programs is limited.

The overall growth of DNP programs has been far more rapid than I expected. The latest data from AACN obtained during the fall of 2013 is that there are now 243 DNP programs in the United States (AACN, 2014). The good news is that access to a DNP program for those interested in such preparation has markedly increased. For those seeking a program, the challenge is to look carefully at what a given program can provide in terms of faculty expertise in key areas—doctoral education, relevant and current practice, and clinical scholarship. Given the national shortage of faculty with the necessary expertise, the very rapid increase in the number of programs makes it imperative that all involved in approving programs and providing them do all that is possible to ensure the quality of DNP programs.

Dr. Williams, why do you think the DNP degree continues to gain acceptance and momentum?

I believe some of the initial momentum for the DNP, particularly among nurse practitioners, was stimulated by AACN's 2015 target. However, I think much of it stems from the recognition that better-prepared nurses can be key players in improving patient outcomes at various levels of care and that the focus of DNP programs is on target with regard to the knowledge base and skills necessary for leadership in improving the quality of patient care and patient outcomes. Finally, the Institute of Medicine's report, The Future of Nursing *(IOM, 2010b), which in recommendation 5 calls for doubling the number of nurses with a doctorate by 2020, has probably added to the momentum.*

Dr. Williams, when we last spoke, you agreed that nursing needed both a research- and practice-focused doctorate. Do you still agree that a research and practice-focused doctorate are beneficial to the profession?

Absolutely. Until the emergence of the DNP the consensus among academic and research leaders in nursing was that the PhD was the route to prepare for leadership in both the academic and practice arena. However, that was an unsustainable course for several reasons. First, too few nurses were seeking PhDs, and too few were being produced. Secondly, most of the PhD programs did not provide content or learning opportunities that directly addressed leadership in the practice arena. Finally, leaders in the field were increasingly recognizing that to be competitive in obtaining grant monies to sustain a viable program of research requires a concentrated focus on research; thus the strongest doctoral programs put their emphasis on how to prepare their graduates to be successful in doing research and obtaining grant support for their work. There was little or no time for preparing for leadership in practice.

In a presentation to the Advisory Council of the National Institute for Nursing Research in 2006 I argued that unless we had practice leaders in nursing who appreciated the need for the best evidence to inform clinical decisions and who knew how to guide evidence-based changes designed to improve nursing practice, the successful efforts of National Institute for Nursing research researchers would not have much impact on the quality of care provided to patients (Williams, 2006). I still hold that view.

Dr. Williams, do you believe that a partnership continues to form between PhD and DNP graduates?

I have been happy to observe some of those partnerships, and I look forward to more. I think all of us concerned about increasing the positive impact that nursing can have on patient outcomes need to encourage and foster such collaboration. I believe those who are faculty in schools and have both a DNP program and a PhD program have a special opportunity and an obligation to work on modeling such behavior by developing collaborative endeavors between DNP and PhD faculty and having students in both programs work with them in their collaborative efforts.

Dr. Williams, are you noticing a transition of roles in nursing as more students graduate from DNP degrees and begin their careers? Are there any specific roles you see evolving as more nurses earn their DNP degree?

I have noticed that a year or two after completing a DNP a number of our graduates have moved into roles that involve assuming more responsibility and demand more organizational leadership. These include moving from providing care as a nurse practitioner to developing a new clinic in a rural area and moving from having responsibility as the nurse leading several clinical programs to becoming the vice president of nursing for a hospital.

In addition to gaining more recognition as expert practitioners and clinical consultants, in the future I think we will see more of our graduates moving into leadership roles traditionally held by individuals with preparation in other fields, such as medicine and management. These include clinic directors, directors of clinical services, directors of quality assurance programs for various types of healthcare organizations and systems, health officers in large health departments, directors of practice initiatives in large healthcare organizations, and chief operating officers in healthcare organizations.

Dr. Williams, what do you think are the most significant contributions the DNP degree has made to nursing education?

I think it has helped to refocus many of our academic leaders in nursing on the essence of our discipline, which is practice, and realistic ways in which we can prepare graduates to provide leadership in improving nursing practice.

Dr. Williams, how would you recommend we continue to move forward with AACN's recommended target date of the DNP for entry into practice by 2015?

The target date was really an aspiration and it has done its work of fostering momentum. Now I think the emphasis should shift to more attention on continuous efforts to ensure program quality and the competence of the graduates in each of the DNP essential areas. Examples of such initiatives include faculty development related to clinical scholarship and partnerships between schools of nursing and practice settings that provide more opportunities for nursing faculty to have meaningful engagement in practice as a part of their faculty role. The DNP will continue to evolve, but for it to continue to be relevant and cutting edge, core DNP faculty who lead in curriculum development and implementation need to be in touch with and understand practice realities and possibilities.

SUMMARY

- The DNP degree is defined as a practice-focused doctorate that prepares graduates as experts in nursing practice.
- Nursing practice is defined by the AACN as "any form of nursing intervention that influences health care outcomes for individuals or populations, including direct care of individual patients, administration of nursing and health care organizations, and the implementation of health policy" (AACN, 2004, p. 3).
- According to the AACN's (2004) position statement, the DNP degree is proposed to be the terminal degree for nursing practice by 2015.
- A nursing PhD degree is a research-focused degree, and a DNP degree is a practice-focused degree.
- The evolution of doctoral education in nursing illustrates where we have been in doctoral education and the direction nursing is taking in the development of doctoral education.
- The concept of a practice doctorate is not new. The idea began in the 1970s with the development of the DNS degree.
- The AACN now designates the DNS and PhD degrees as research-focused degrees, and the DNP and DrNP degrees are designated as practice-focused degrees.
- In 2002 the AACN board of directors formed a task force to examine the current progress of proposed doctorates in nursing.
- In 2000 the IOM published a report titled *To Err Is Human: Building a Safer Health System*, which summarized errors made in the healthcare system and proposed recommendations to improve the overall quality of care.

- In 2003 the Health Professions Education Committee published *Health Professions Education: A Bridge to Quality*, which outlined a specific set of competencies that should be met by all clinicians.
- In 2008 the IOM appointed the Committee on the RWJF Initiative on the Future of Nursing. This committee published a report in 2010 titled *The Future of Nursing: Focus on Education*, which concluded that "the ways in which nurses were educated during the 20th century are no longer adequate for dealing with the realities of healthcare in the 21st century" (IOM, 2010a, p. 2). This committee also recommended doubling the number of nurses with doctorates by 2020.
- In 2004 the AACN published a position statement regarding a practice doctorate in nursing and recommended that by 2015 all nurses pursuing advanced-practice degrees will be prepared as DNP graduates.
- In 2005 the National Academy of Sciences recommended that a nonresearch ND be developed to meet nursing faculty needs.
- In 2006 the AACN described the *Essentials of Doctoral Education for Advanced Nursing Practice*, which represents the standards for DNP curricula.
- NONPF outlined the *Practice Doctorate Nurse Practitioner Entry-Level Competencies* as standards for DNP curricula.
- In 2009 the NACNS developed *Core Practice Doctorate Clinical Nurse Specialist Competencies*.
- In 2007 the AANA stated that nurse anesthetist education would adopt doctoral education as preparation to enter into practice by 2025.
- The DNP degree includes postmaster's degree programs and postbaccalaureate degree programs.
- Graduate students may follow an individualized path to the DNP degree, depending on their current degree preparation.
- DNP graduates may be involved in many different roles that may include, but are not limited to, research evaluator and translator, leader, healthcare policy advocate, educator, information technology specialist, and clinician.

REFLECTION QUESTIONS

1. How do you think nursing's history has contributed to the development of the DNP degree?

2. How do you think the IOM report *To Err Is Human: Building a Safer Health System*, along with the follow-up report *Crossing the Quality Chasm: A New Health System for the 21st Century*, contributed to the development of the DNP degree?

3. Explain why you think the IOM and the RWJF concluded, in their report *The Future of Nursing: Focus on Education*, that nurses need improvement in their educational preparation.

4. Do you think a struggle still exists within nursing today regarding whether doctoral education should be research or practice focused?

5. Do you think nursing doctoral education should be research focused, practice focused, or both?

6. Do you think a DNP degree is the right degree for you?

REFERENCES

Allan, J., Barwick, T., Cashman, S., Cawley, J. F., Day, C., Douglass, C. W., ...Wood, D. (2004). Clinical prevention and population health: Curriculum framework for health professions. *American Journal of Preventive Medicine, 27*(5), 471–476.

American Association of Colleges of Nursing. (2004). *AACN position statement on the practice doctorate in nursing.* Retrieved from http://www.aacn.nche.edu/DNP/pdf/DNP.pdf

American Association of Colleges of Nursing. (2005). Commission on Collegiate Nursing Education moves to consider for accreditation only practice doctorates with the DNP degree title. Retrieved from http://www.aacn.nche.edu/news/articles/2005/commission-on-collegiate-nursing-education-moves-to-consider-for-accreditation-only-practice-doctorates-with-the-dnp-degree-title

American Association of Colleges of Nursing. (2006a). *DNP roadmap task force report.* Retrieved from http://www.aacn.nche.edu/dnp/roadmapreport.pdf

American Association of Colleges of Nursing. (2006b). *Essentials of doctoral education for advanced nursing practice.* Retrieved from http://www.aacn.nche.edu/publications /position/DNPEssentials.pdf

American Association of Colleges of Nursing. (2007). *AACN white paper on the education and role of the clinical nurse leader.* Retrieved from http://www.aacn.nche.edu/publications/ white-papers/cnl

American Association of Colleges of Nursing. (2011). *DNP fact sheet: The doctor of nursing practice (DNP).* Retrieved from http://www.aacn.nche.edu/media-relations/fact-sheets/dnp

American Association of Colleges of Nursing. (2014). *Program directory.* Retrieved from http://www.aacn.nche.edu/dnp/program-directory

American Association of Nurse Anesthetists. (2007). *AANA position on doctoral preparation of nurse anesthetists.* Retrieved from http://www.aana.com/ceandeducation/educationalresources /Documents/AANA_Position_DTF_June_2007.pdf

American Hospital Association. (1999). *Hospital statistics.* Chicago, IL: Author.

Apold, S. (2008). The doctor of nursing practice: Looking back, moving forward. *Journal for Nurse Practitioners, 4*(2), 101–107.

Carpenter, R., & Hudacek, S. (1996). *On doctoral education in nursing: The voice of the student.* New York, NY: National League for Nursing Press.

Centers for Disease Control and Prevention, National Center for Health Statistics. (1999a). Births and deaths: Preliminary data for 1998. *National Vital Statistics Reports, 47*(25), 1–45.

Centers for Disease Control and Prevention, National Center for Health Statistics. (1999b). Deaths: Final data for 1997. *National Vital Statistics Reports, 47*(19), 1–104.

Cleland, V. (1976). Developing a doctoral program. *Nursing Outlook, 24*(10), 631–635.

Council on Accreditation of Nurse Anesthesia Programs. (2013). *Standards for accreditation of nurse anesthesia programs practice doctorate.* Retrieved from http://www.aana.com /newsandjournal/20102019/educnews-0614-p177-183.pdf

Donaldson, S., & Crowley, D. (1978). The discipline of nursing. *Nursing Outlook, 26*(2), 113–120.

Dracup, K., Cronenwett, L., Meleis, A., & Benner, P. (2005). Reflections on the doctorate of nursing practice. *Nursing Outlook, 53*(4), 177–182.

Dudley-Brown, S. (2006). Revisiting the blended role of the advanced practice nurse. *Gastroenterology Nursing, 29*(3), 249–250.

Fawcett, J. (2005). *Contemporary nursing knowledge: Analysis and evaluation of nursing models and theories* (2nd ed.). Philadelphia, PA: F. A. Davis.

Goldenberg, G. (2004). The DrNP degree. *The Academic Nurse: The Journal of the Columbia University School of Nursing, 21*(1), 22–26.

Gortner, S. (1980). Nursing science in transition. *Nursing Research, 29*(3), 180–183.

Grace, H. (1978). The development of doctoral education in nursing: In historical perspective. *Journal of Nursing Education, 17*(4), 17–27.

Greiner, A. C., & Knebel, E. (Eds.). (2003). *Health professions education: A bridge to quality.* Washington, DC: National Academies Press.

Institute of Medicine. (2001). *Crossing the quality chasm: A new health system for the 21st century.* Washington, DC: National Academies Press.

Institute of Medicine. (2010a). *The future of nursing: Focus on education.* Retrieved from http://www.iom.edu/~/media/Files/Report%20Files/2010/The-Future-of-Nursing /Nursing%20Education%202010%20Brief.pdf

Institute of Medicine. (2010b). *The future of nursing: Leading change, advancing health.* Retrieved from http://www.iom.edu/Reports/2010/The-Future-of-Nursing-Leading-Change -Advancing-Health.aspx

Jennings, B., & Rogers, S. (1988). Merging nursing research and practice: A case of multiple identities. *Journal of Advanced Nursing, 13*(6), 752–758.

Kohn, L. T., Corrigan, J. M., & Donaldson, M. S. (Eds.). (2000). *To err is human: Building a safer health system.* Washington, DC: National Academies Press.

Marion, L., O'Sullivan, A., Crabtree, M. K., Price, M., & Fontana, S. (2005). Curriculum models for the practice doctorate in nursing. *Topics in Advanced Practice Nursing eJournal, 5*(1). Retrieved from http://www.medscape.com/viewarticle/500742_print

Marion, L., Viens, D., O'Sullivan, A., Crabtree, M. K., Fontana, S., & Price, M. (2003). The practice doctorate in nursing: Future or fringe. *Topics in Advanced Practice Nursing eJournal, 3*(2). Retrieved from http://www.medscape.com/viewarticle/453247_print

Marriner-Tomey, A. (1990). Historical development of doctoral programs from the middle ages to nursing education today. *Nursing and Health Care, 11*(3), 132–137.

Martin-Sheridan, D., Ouelette, S. M., & Horton, B. J. (2006). Education news: Is doctoral education in our future? *AANA Journal, 74*(2), 101–104.

Murphy, J. (1981). Doctoral education in, of, and for nursing: An historical analysis. *Nursing Outlook, 29*(11), 645–649.

National Academy of Sciences. (2005). *Advancing the nation's health needs: NIH Research Training Programs.* Washington, DC: National Academies Press. Retrieved from http://www.nap.edu/openbook.php?isbn=0309094275

National Association of Clinical Nurse Specialists. (2009). *Core practice doctorate clinical nurse specialist competencies.* Retrieved from http://www.nacns.org/docs/CorePracticeDoctorate.pdf

National CNS Competency Task Force. (2008). *Organizing framework and core competencies.* Retrieved from http://www.nacns.org/docs/CNSCoreCompetenciesBroch.pdf

National Organization of Nurse Practitioner Faculties. (2006). *Practice doctorate nurse practitioner entry-level competencies.* Retrieved from http://c.ymcdn.com/sites/www.nonpf.org/resource/resmgr/competencies/dnp%20np%20competenciesapril2006.pdf

Newman, M. (1975). The professional doctorate in nursing: A position paper. *Nursing Outlook, 23*(11), 704–706.

Roberts, S., & Glod, C. (2005). The practice doctorate in nursing: Is it the answer? *The American Journal for Nurse Practitioners, 9*(11/12), 55–65.

Sperhac, A., & Strodtbeck, F. (1997). Advanced practice nursing: New opportunities for blended roles. *The American Journal of Maternal/Child Nursing, 22*(6), 287–293.

Starck, P., Duffy, M., & Vogler, R. (1993). Developing a nursing doctorate for the 21st century. *Journal of Professional Nursing, 9*(4), 212–219.

Thomas, E., Studdert, D., Newhouse, J., Zbar, B., Howard, K., Williams, E., & Brennan, T. A. (1999). Costs of medical injuries in Utah and Colorado. *Inquiry, 36*(3), 255–264.

Williams, C. A. (2006, January 24). The doctorate of nursing practice: An option for leadership in nursing practice. Presented to the Advisory Council of the National Institute for Nursing Research, National Institutes of Health, Bethesda, MD.

Williams, C. A., Stanhope, M. K., & Sebastian, J. G. (2001). Clinical nursing leadership: One model of professional doctoral education in nursing. In C. M. Golde & G. E. Walker (Eds.). *Envisioning doctoral education for the future* (pp. 85–91). Washington, DC: AACN.

CHAPTER 2

Leadership, Collaboration, and the DNP Graduate

Lisa Astalos Chism

Leadership and collaboration are integral aspects of every potential role a doctor of nursing practice (DNP) graduate may assume. It is well documented in the literature that nurses in all advanced nursing practice roles exhibit leadership and collaboration, whether they are in nurse executive positions, education, or clinical practice (Buonocore, 2004; Carroll, 2005; Joyce, 2001; Mastal, Joshi, & Schulke, 2007). Moreover, leadership is noted to be embedded within less obvious leadership roles, such as advocate, problem solver, idealist, and role model (Garrison & McBryde-Foster, 2004). The changing demands of a complex healthcare environment, the Institute of Medicine's (IOM) call for improved healthcare standards (IOM 2001; Kohn, Corrigan, & Donaldson, 1999), and the Health Professions Education Committee's recommendations (Greiner & Knebel, 2003) collectively support the notion that nurses in all advanced nursing practice roles exemplify leadership across various healthcare settings (American Association of Colleges of Nursing [AACN], 2006; Greiner & Knebel, 2003).

The Health Professions Education Committee has suggested the need for healthcare professionals to exhibit increased collaboration across healthcare disciplines by leading and functioning in interdisciplinary teams (Greiner & Knebel, 2003). Moreover, a systematic review conducted by Wong and Cummings (2007) found that positive leadership behaviors, styles, and practices were significantly associated with increased patient satisfaction and a reduction of adverse events. Therefore, role development as a leader is essential for the DNP graduate. To better prepare nurses as leaders, current DNP curricula include additional preparation in leadership and collaboration. This is evidenced by the standards outlined in the AACN essentials (2006) and the National Organization of Nurse Practitioner Faculties (NONPF) competencies (2006).

This chapter provides a review of the AACN and NONPF curriculum standards for preparation in leadership and collaboration. Leadership attributes and styles that are relevant to the DNP leadership role are also discussed. Collaboration and team styles also have relevance for successful leadership and are reviewed as well. Change as it relates to the DNP graduate is briefly discussed. The reluctant DNP leader—leadership even when one doesn't expect or want it—will also be reviewed. Finally, the responsibility of role-modeling and portraying leadership and collaboration is addressed. Specific case scenarios, including the author's own leadership experience, are included to illustrate how leadership and collaboration may be used to further enhance healthcare delivery at the patient and systems–organizational level.

Curriculum Standards for Leadership and Collaboration

The AACN has outlined curriculum standards in their *Essentials of Doctoral Education for Advanced Nursing Practice* (2006). Essential II: Organizational and Systems Leadership for Quality Improvement and Systems Thinking and Essential VI: Interprofessional Collaboration for Improving Patient and Population Health Outcomes describe specific curriculum requirements that are intended to enhance DNP graduates' leadership and collaboration skills. In summary, the purpose of Essential II is to promote leadership skills to effectively manage patient safety issues, eliminate health disparities, and promote excellence in practice by evaluating evidence-based best practices for healthcare delivery. Further, DNP graduates must become proficient at quality improvement strategies that improve patient outcomes at every level in healthcare delivery (AACN, 2006). Course work that addresses these objectives will enable DNP graduates to gain a broader understanding of leadership attributes and styles. The purpose of Essential VI is to develop expertise in collaborating across the healthcare team to create effective solutions and overcome impediments to healthcare delivery (AACN, 2006). The DNP graduate's proficiency in leadership is also necessary to effectively lead interprofessional teams and promote collaboration within the healthcare team. Therefore, the course work that attends to collaboration will enhance the skills necessary to communicate among various professionals in multiple disciplines. Because leadership depends on effective collaboration, the skills that improve leadership and collaboration are often interrelated.

NONPF has developed specific *Practice Doctorate Nurse Practitioner Entry-Level Competencies* for nurse practitioner–DNP graduates to help guide curriculum standards. The competency area of leadership specifically addresses the need for proficiency in leadership skills for DNP graduates. This competency addresses the need for DNP graduates to garner increased proficiency in assuming additional leadership, to foster interprofessional collaboration, and to demonstrate a reflective, appropriate leadership style (NONPF, 2006).

What's a DNP-Prepared Leader Made Of? The Recipe for Success

Successful leadership encompasses certain individual attributes and qualities, and DNP graduates are encouraged to develop their own unique blends of leadership styles. The following section reviews successful leadership qualities that may enable DNP graduates to thrive in leadership roles.

Leadership Attributes

Although it is agreed that a single definition of leadership may not be sufficient, leadership has been described as "the art and science of influencing a group toward achievement of a goal" (McArthur, 2006, p. 8). It has also been found that a single set of attributes cannot be defined as the exclusive characteristics of an effective leader (Feltner, Mitchell, Norris, & Wolfle, 2008). Although DNP graduates are challenged to lead in a healthcare environment that is rapidly changing due to increased technology, population growth, disparity issues, ethical concerns, and political and economical changes, certain attributes may enhance the DNP graduate's leadership role (Jooste, 2004). Interestingly, research has shown that nurses themselves consider certain attributes to be valuable for effective leadership (Feltner et al., 2008; Joyce, 2001; O'Connor, 2008). It is therefore safe to assume that DNP graduates will have insight regarding the various attributes that are valuable in a leadership role.

Feltner and colleagues (2008) conducted a descriptive study to evaluate what attributes nurses felt were important for effective leadership. Overall, nurses considered communication skills to be the most important attribute of an effective leader. It was found that if communication was effective, the perception of leadership was effective. Additionally, communication should be honest, approachable, open, trustworthy, and reciprocal. Additional attributes noted to be important for leadership were (in rank order) fairness, job knowledge, role model, dependable, participative partnership, confidence, positive attitude, motivating, delegation, flexibility, compassionate, employee loyal, and sets objectives (Feltner et al., 2008). Nurses also mentioned that a leader should be "visionary and give staff members common, challenging, and achievable goals" (Feltner et al., 2008, p. 368). It is interesting that the nurses in this study were able to easily articulate what attributes are valuable in an effective leader. This reinforces the notion that DNP graduates will have insight regarding what attributes are important for leadership.

In a related study, Joyce (2001) evaluated perceptions of leadership among nurse practitioners and described the attributes that were considered relevant for leadership. Joyce stated that the "leadership experiences of nurse practitioners provide a better understanding of the attributes seen as most important for patient care, interacting with colleagues, and influencing health care delivery systems" (2001, p. 24). The four themes that emerged from this study were facilitator, professional, role model, and visionist (Joyce, 2001).

Facilitator was further defined as "the ability to enable individuals or groups to move through tasks" (Joyce, 2001, p. 28). Additional attributes associated with *facilitator* were effective listener, communicator, collaborator, and decision maker. These attributes were demonstrated by the nurse practitioner to achieve mutual goals with clients in the practice setting, in the community, and in the organization (Joyce, 2001).

The attribute *professional* was also found to describe an effective leader. *Professional* was defined as the ability to inspire and enable others to achieve high standards (Joyce, 2001). Additional attributes associated with *professional* were integrity, accountability, competency, capable of managing time, confidence in judgment, ability to set standards, and resourcefulness (Joyce, 2001).

Role model was described as the "ability to demonstrate their profession to others" (Joyce, 2001, p. 28). Interestingly, role model was also noted as a leadership attribute by Feltner and colleagues (2008). Associated attributes were described as abilities to mentor, motivate, and teach. Role-modeling is discussed later in this chapter.

Finally, *visionist* was defined as the "ability to be future oriented" (Joyce, 2001, p. 28). The attributes associated with *visionist* included one who is able to "see the whole picture, take risks, and seek challenges" (Joyce, 2001, p. 28). Visionists also attract others toward their vision and work with others to achieve goals.

Interestingly, the leadership perceptions noted by nurse practitioners also describe how the nurse practitioners defined themselves as leaders. This provides support for the notion that DNP graduates in clinician roles will engage in leadership, sometimes without realizing it. Moreover, Joyce's research demonstrated that nurses have insight regarding the leadership attributes required for healthcare delivery.

O'Connor described a set of attributes developed by the Center for Nursing Leadership and further identified the attributes as "the caring competencies" (2008, p. 21). These attributes are as follows: holding the truth, intellectual and emotional self, discovery of potential, quest for the adventure toward knowing, diversity as a vehicle to wholeness, appreciation of ambiguity, knowing something in life, holding multiple perspectives without judgment, and keeping commitments to oneself (O'Connor, 2008). O'Connor further expanded on these attributes by identifying specific caring behaviors associated with each competency. For example, holding the truth is further described as honest, trustworthy, reliable, and credible. O'Connor also stated that this attribute speaks to the "leader's internal truth" and described the "integrity and authenticity with which he or she does the job" (p. 22). The attribute of intellectual and emotional self is described by O'Connor as the balance between intellect and emotional intelligence. Emotional intelligence is considered more important than intellect, and it is a learned behavior that can be developed and practiced (Goleman, 1995). Emotional intelligence is discussed further in this chapter.

In O'Connor's descriptions of the caring competencies (2008), *discovery of potential* is identified as mentoring. Mentoring encourages others to discover their own path and share their own talents at work. *Quest for the adventure toward knowing* is described as passion, curiosity, and enthusiasm. *Diversity as a vehicle to wholeness* requires the nurse leader to be open minded and committed to improving diversity within an organization. *Appreciation of ambiguity* is described as sharing in decision making with others. This requires the nurse leader to exhibit empowerment, faith, trust, and, importantly, caring. *Knowing something in life* relates to a nurse leader having had many experiences that may be shared with others to encourage and offer support. *Holding multiple perspectives without judgment* speaks to respecting the differences among people with regard to culture, values, beliefs, and ways of life. Further, Joyce (2001) related that the nurse leader must see the differences in people as strengths that can make groups stronger and more diverse. *Keeping commitments to oneself* requires the nurse leader to care for the self. Caring for one's self allows one to be ready and able to care for others.

The caring competencies described by O'Connor (2008) are practical and pertinent to nursing leadership. Further, they speak to the nature of nursing, which is to care (Shelly & Miller, 2006). As nurses, DNP graduates may already possess many of these valuable attributes or competencies, which can further foster their development as nurse leaders.

A discussion of leadership attributes for DNP graduates would not be complete without discussing emotional intelligence. Interestingly, emotional intelligence principles were included in this author's leadership and collaboration DNP course work. Further, it has been noted that nurses are perceived as having high levels of emotional intelligence (Grossman & Valiga, 2005). Emotional intelligence has been suggested to be more important in promoting excellence in leadership than intellect and expertise (Goleman, 1995). Emotional intelligence is defined as "an awareness of and ability to manage emotions and create motivation" (Emotional intelligence, n.d.). Although the definition of emotional intelligence is constantly changing, the basic premise has remained the same. Goleman, Boyatzis, and McKee (2002) expanded on emotional intelligence and described five specific attributes of an emotionally intelligent leader. These attributes are described within four leadership competencies: self-awareness, self-management, social awareness, and relationship management (Goleman et al., 2002) (**Box 2-1**).

BOX 2-1

Emotional Intelligence Leadership Competencies

- Self-awareness
- Self-management
- Social awareness
- Relationship management

Source: Used with permission from *Primal Leadership: Realizing the Power of Emotional Intelligence*, by Daniel Golemen, Richard Boyatzis, & Annie McKee, Harvard Business Review Press, 2002, titles taken from pages 7-10.

Self-awareness describes leaders who have emotional self-awareness the ability to speak openly about emotions regarding their vision. Leaders who possess self-awareness can accurately self-assess areas in which they need to improve, and they pursue self-improvement with grace. The self-aware leader is also self-confident and can stand out in the group (Goleman et al., 2002).

Self-management describes leaders who exhibit emotional self-control by maintaining a calm demeanor even in crisis situations. Self-managed leaders also exhibit transparency, which allows them to openly admit faults or mistakes and remain open to others' feelings and beliefs (Goleman et al., 2002). These leaders can juggle multiple demands without losing focus or energy. They are optimistic and see the glass as half full, not half empty (Goleman et al., 2002). Social awareness describes leaders who express empathy toward others. These leaders can "feel the room" and tune in to what others are thinking or feeling, which allows them to appreciate others' perspectives. Additionally, socially aware leaders have organizational awareness and can understand the unspoken values of others in the organization. This competency also describes leaders who believe in service-oriented behaviors (Goleman et al., 2002).

Finally, relationship management describes leaders who inspire others to be involved in a shared mission. These leaders use influence to engage a group and create enthusiasm. Relationship management includes the ability to promote and facilitate change, especially in an environment with barriers to change. These leaders are skilled at conflict management. Although conflict management may be uncomfortable, these leaders handle it by viewing all sides of an issue then redirecting the energy toward a solution. Finally, these leaders encourage close relationships within the group, which fosters collaboration and the development of strategies and solutions (Goleman et al., 2002).

Following a discussion of pertinent leadership attributes, it becomes clear which attributes DNP graduates should foster (**Table 2-1**). Most, if not all, of these

TABLE 2-1   Leadership Attributes Relevant for DNP Graduates

Leadership Attributes	Examples
Ability to communicate effectively	Communicate effectively across multiple disciplines or teams, such as evaluation of evidence-based practice patterns for development of practice protocols.
Fearlessness	Step into leadership roles when needed, such as instituting and leading a journal club in a practice setting. Also advocate for patients or team members when necessary.
Motivating	Inspire teams/colleagues, such as motivating the team/colleagues to participate in patient satisfaction surveys.
Visionary; looks toward the future	Project future goals and outcomes in a healthcare setting, such as initiating a practice group to include a dietician for onsite consultations for patients.
Role model	Set an example for others, such as mentoring other nurses in the practice setting and encouraging further education.
Knowledge and clinical competence	Maintain and expand current clinical knowledge, such as attending conferences or review journals.
Compassion	Exhibit compassion toward patients and others even when caring for a difficult patient.
Trustworthy	Maintain confidences in a practice setting, such as not sharing information about other team members when issues arise.
Participate in partnerships	Participate in partnerships with patients and others by negotiating with patients when developing a plan of care. Also, partner with other team members to share in the responsibility of problem solving when a difficult patient or team member situation arises.
Honesty about self and others	Openly admit weaknesses and mistakes to others on the team or practice setting, such as admitting to avoiding conflict with others. Also, openly admit areas that need improvement, such as difficulty initiating insulin therapy for patients.
Empathy	Express empathy to patients and team members and share all perspectives. Sense when empathy or understanding is needed in particular situations among team members.

attributes are known by nurses to be valuable attributes for leadership. Further, DNP graduates can develop these leadership attributes by drawing on their previous experiences in leadership and healthcare delivery. This is further elaborated in the case scenarios provided at the end of the chapter.

Although it is important to discuss what leadership attributes are germane and perhaps even instinctive to DNP graduates, it is also necessary to explore leadership styles that may be employed by DNP graduates. Styles of leadership may vary depending on the venue in which they are applied. DNP graduates may also find that their leadership styles fluctuate as they become more experienced leaders. It has been suggested that emotional intelligence is essential for effective leadership; therefore, the leadership styles that are congruent with emotionally intelligent leadership are reviewed next.

Leadership Styles

Goleman et al. (2002) described several styles of leadership and categorized them as resonant or dissonant styles. Resonant styles encourage group members to feel connected to each other and reflect the leader's enthusiasm. These types of leadership styles come naturally to emotionally intelligent leaders; hence, they may be easy for nurses to adopt. The resonant styles are as follows: visionary, coaching, affiliative, and democratic.

When it is engaged, the visionary style motivates the group to a shared dream while allowing others to be free to "innovate, experiment, and take calculated risks" (Goleman et al., 2002, p. 57). This type of style encourages people to stay with the group and the group's mission. The emotional intelligence competency of empathy is most important to a visionary leader. Empathy allows a leader to sense how others feel and understand their perspectives. Interestingly, empathy has long been considered essential to a therapeutic nurse–patient relationship (Bennet, 1995; Kalish, 1973; LaMonica & Karshmer, 1978). One may assume that the visionary style is practiced regularly by nurses. DNP graduates may therefore draw from previous experiences and engage this style of leadership.

The coaching style is another style of leadership that may come naturally to nurses. It involves connecting others to the shared goals of the organization or group. A coaching leader helps others identify what their strengths and weaknesses are and apply them to their own aspirations (Goleman et al., 2002). Coaches also delegate tasks to others that will allow them to be innovative and expand on their potential. This in turn builds confidence in others and helps foster professional development (Goleman et al., 2002). Nurses regularly engage patients in coaching when they provide counseling about health maintenance and prevention (Cook, Ingersoll, & Spitzer, 1999; Lambing, Adams, Fox, & Divine, 2004). Therefore, coaching is another leadership style that may be employed easily by the DNP graduate.

The affiliative style is considered the relationship-builder style. It emphasizes connections among people to bring focus toward a shared goal (Goleman et al., 2002). Nurses are experts at this leadership style. This style is employed whenever nurses share personal stories with each other and when they listen to their patients' and families' concerns. The affiliative leadership style can easily be utilized by DNP graduates when interacting with members of a group or organization.

Occasionally it may not be enough to share with others to create harmony while trying to lead. A democratic leader considers all views when there is conflict or disagreement about what direction to take next (Goleman et al., 2002). This style of leadership is fostered through good communication, which stems from the ability to collaborate, resolve conflict, and influence others (Goleman et al., 2002). Each time a nurse listens to a patient's concerns and considers his or her viewpoint, a democratic style is employed. DNP graduates can draw on their past experiences with this style to employ a democratic style of leadership.

At times leadership may be more challenging for the DNP graduate. This is when the more difficult styles or the dissonant styles may need to be employed. Dissonant styles may make a group feel "off-key" and produce a "lack of harmony" in a group (Goleman et al., 2002, p. 21). These styles include pacesetting and commanding. Further, Goleman and colleagues relate that these styles should be "applied with caution" (2002, p. 53). Although they may be less familiar and less comfortable for nurses, the DNP graduate may need to employ them when necessary.

Pacesetting refers to a style that exhibits extremely high expectations when accomplishing a task is the essential goal. This style can be useful in early phases of organizing a group toward shared goals. However, if it is employed too rigidly and too frequently, this style can backfire and create feelings of mistrust in a group (Goleman et al., 2002). When a plan of care is initially developed for a patient, goals are mutually set for the patient. However, if the patient's healthcare needs change, the plan of care will have to be adjusted in an effort to provide safe, effective care. Similarly, this leadership style may be used by DNP graduates, especially in early planning phases of goal setting or when goals need to be reassessed.

The final leadership style, commanding, is also a dissonant style. The commanding style must also be used with caution, but it may be necessary for specific group goals (Goleman et al., 2002). The commanding style involves the leader taking control of a situation and using a "do it because I said so" attitude (Goleman et al., 2002, p. 76). This style must be used sparingly or goals will not be met. Nurses who have participated in code blue or other emergency situations, whether in or out of the healthcare setting, have experienced or even employed this type of leadership style. In crisis situations, nurses often take charge. DNP graduates will know how to employ this style, but experience will allow them to know when to employ it.

Please refer to **Table 2-2** for a summary of Goleman and colleagues' leadership styles.

TABLE 2-2   Leadership Styles

Resonant Styles	Dissonant Styles
Visionary	Pacesetting
Coaching	Commanding
Affiliative	
Democratic	

Source: Used with permission from *Primal Leadership: Realizing the Power of Emotional Intelligence,* by Daniel Goleman, Richard Boyatzis, & Annie McKee, Harvard Business Review Press, 2002, taken from The Leadership Repertoire, p. 11.

Servant Leadership

This author's own experience as a leader (described later in the chapter) has led to the awareness of additional leadership styles. One of these styles is known as *servant leadership*. In 1970 Greenleaf was the first to describe servant leadership in an essay titled *The Servant as Leader.* This essay was followed by additional essays and publications that related the notion of servant leadership to businesses, education, churches, and society (Greenleaf, 1977). Servant leadership is quite simply leadership in service of others (Autry, 2001). In addition, servant leadership has been described as a calling to be responsible for the psychological, emotional, and financial well-being of others based on the circumstances and environment in which they work (Autry, 2001). Servant leadership could perhaps be considered a holistic approach to leadership. Greenleaf (1977) describes a set of characteristics that are important to the development of service leaders. These characteristics include listening, empathy, healing, awareness, persuasion, conceptualization, foresight, stewardship, commitment to the growth of people, and building community. Listening, empathy, healing, awareness, growth of others, and building community are somewhat self-explanatory. Persuasion speaks to the notion that servant leaders seek to convince rather that coerce others through consensus in a group. Conceptualization speaks to the vision of long-term goals instead of day-to-day issues and problems. Stewardship exemplifies the servant leader's commitment to serving others (Greenleaf, 1977).

Autry (2001) described servant leadership as five specific ways of being: be authentic, be vulnerable, be accepting, be present, and be useful. Being authentic simply means to "be the same person in every circumstance" (Autry, 2001, p. 10). Servant leaders must always be their real self. Being vulnerable speaks to being honest with your feelings, including being honest about your own doubts and fears. Being vulnerable also requires courage and realizing we can't always be in control (Autry, 2001). Being accepting is more than simply approval. Accepting others' ideas and concerns as valid and worthy of discussion exhibits acceptance. Acceptance also means that you accept disagreement as part of the process of work (Autry, 2001). Being present may be very difficult, especially in a busy work environment. However, not being present gives the impression that you are distracted, stressed, and worried, which may cause those around you to feel the same. This requires a servant leader to exercise discipline and stop, focus, and concentrate on the current environment (Autry, 2001). Being useful means being a resource (or providing the resources) for those you are leading. This may be one of the most important attributes of a servant leader (Autry, 2001).

Autry summarized six key points about servant leadership (2001, pp. 20–21):

1. Leadership is not about control; it's about caring for people and being a resource.
2. Leadership is not being the boss; it's about being present.
3. Leadership is about letting go of your territory and being authentic.
4. Leadership should help others find meaning in their work.
5. Leadership requires paying attention.
6. Leadership requires love.

Servant leadership involves many of the attributes previously discussed, such as compassion, trustworthiness, honesty, and empathy. Further, Goleman and colleagues' emotional intelligence leadership competencies will likely foster the philosophy of servant leadership. Self-awareness will enable the servant leader to speak openly and truthfully about their emotions and pursue self-improvement. Self-management skills will enable the servant leader to openly admit their own faults and be open to others' feelings and beliefs. Finally, social awareness, likely the most important emotional intelligence, leadership competency, will encourage the servant leader to express empathy toward others. Social awareness is also associated with the ability to be perceptive of the needs of others. This competency is also related to service-related behaviors (Goleman et al., 2002).

The difference between leadership and management is reviewed later in this chapter, but it is important to mention that servant leadership further illustrates this difference. Authentic servant leadership, unlike management, is not a set of skills or learned behaviors, but rather the modeling of your own way of being through your behavior. That behavior will depend on who you are, your character, and your spirit (Autry, 2001).

DNP graduates may find that the philosophy of servant leadership speaks to their style of leadership. Greenleaf (1977) related that one must work side by side with those they serve to understand the day-to-day issues. Further, working side by side enables direct access to servant leaders and fosters trust through collegiate relationships, mutual respect, and feedback (Howatson-Jones, 2004). Many DNP graduates, much like this author, will find themselves in blended roles working alongside those they lead.

Transformational Leadership

Another type of leadership style that has inspired this author is transformational leadership. Transformational leadership has been described as a "style of leadership in which the leader identifies the needed change, creates vision to guide change through inspiration, and executes the change with the commitment of the members of the group" (Transformational leadership, 2014). Transformational leadership, much like servant leadership, attends to the emotional and spiritual resources of the group. Transformational leaders "inspire others to achieve what might be considered extraordinary results" as "leaders and followers engage with each other, raise each other, and inspire each other" (Marshall, 2011, p. 3). The transformational leader has many of the attributes or characteristics previously discussed, such as emotional intelligence, humility, charisma, visionary, inspiring, and trustworthy (Marshall, 2011).

DNP-prepared nurses may find this style of leadership powerful because they may have opportunities to identify areas that need change by working alongside their colleagues. Further, DNP-prepared nurses may be in a position to affect change or develop innovative practices, and they will need to have vision and the ability to motivate and inspire others.

Collaboration: DNP Graduates Working with Others

Blanchard included a quotation in his book, originally from Blanchard, Carew, and Parisi-Carew: "No one of us is as smart as all of us" (1999). This describes the true purpose of collaboration. The ability to collaborate, defined as working together especially in a joint intellectual effort (Collaborate, 1983), has been identified by the AACN, NONPF, and the Health Professions Education Committee as an essential skill of DNP graduates. Collaboration has been more specifically defined in relation to nursing and health care as "a dynamic, interpersonal process in which two or more individuals make a commitment to each other to interact authentically and constructively to solve problems and to learn from each other to accomplish identifiable goals, purposes, or outcomes" (Hamric, Spross, & Hanson, 2005, p. 344). Given this definition, DNP graduates may build alliances across teams and disciplines in an effort to solve problems, accomplish goals, and improve outcomes. Certain characteristics that promote collaboration will be discussed in the following section. In addition, the Interprofessional Education Collaborative Expert Panel (2011) developed a set of core competencies for interprofessional collaborative practice.

Qualities for Successful Collaboration

Hamric and colleagues (2005) described common purpose as a characteristic that may promote collaboration. Common purpose is similar to the visionary leadership style (Goleman et al., 2002). If the group is striving toward a similar purpose or vision, they will likely be motivated to work together more effectively. Nurses and physicians often work together toward the common purpose of improved patient care. If the DNP graduate can establish a common purpose or vision for the group, the interactions will be more successful and the goals will likely be achieved.

Clinical competence was also identified by Hamric and colleagues as the "most important characteristic underlying a successful collaborative experience among clinicians" (2005, p. 360). These authors related that without this characteristic, trust among collaborative team members is difficult to establish. This can be seen in collaborative relationships between advanced-practice registered nurses and collaborating physicians. A trust in each other's knowledge and abilities must be present for the collaborative relationship to be successful. Therefore, DNP graduates must establish reciprocal trust regarding the clinical competence among team members to ensure effective collaboration.

Interpersonal competence and communication skills were also noted by Hamric and colleagues (2005) to be necessary characteristics for effective collaboration. These characteristics are similar to Goleman and colleagues' (2002) leadership competencies of social awareness and relationship management. As mentioned earlier in the chapter, social awareness includes the ability to exhibit empathy toward others. Relationship management describes leaders who are good at teamwork and collaboration. Therefore, collaboration should include communication among group members that is open, empathic, and cohesive. Nurses are often very effective communicators and exhibit this type of communication. DNP graduates can draw on these communication skills to promote effective collaboration among team members and across disciplines.

Hamric and colleagues (2005) also found trust to be an essential characteristic of effective collaboration. This is evidenced by the collegial relationships across disciplines in the hospital setting. Pharmacy departments trust that nurses are properly dispensing the medications they deliver to the unit. Surgeons trust that nurses are properly assessing patients after a procedure. Nurses trust that physical therapists provide appropriate therapy to a patient after hip replacement surgery. Without trust in each other's knowledge, collaboration and patient care would be compromised. DNP graduates are in a unique position to promote trust within a group. Because nurses are often experts at interacting across disciplines to ensure high-quality care, DNP graduates can lead by example in establishing trust among team members, especially when multiple disciplines are represented.

Valuing and respecting diverse, complimentary knowledge is related to trust because although team members must trust each other's knowledge, this knowledge should also be mutually respected. Hamric and colleagues (2005) related that each discipline complements the other through mutual respect. DNP graduates can promote this characteristic by demonstrating that patient care is centered on the collaborative efforts of multiple disciplines. While working together across disciplines, the common goal of optimal healthcare delivery can be achieved.

Finally, Hamric and colleagues (2005) identified humor as a necessary characteristic for effective collaboration. Interestingly, Goleman and colleagues (2002) also found that humor is an important attribute of an emotionally intelligent leader and is key for effective leadership. Hamric and colleagues stated, "When used with collaboration, humor serves to decrease defensiveness, invite openness, relieve tension, and deflect anger" (2005, p. 362). Further, conflict can be defused and communication can be enhanced when humor is used effectively. DNP graduates are encouraged to recall their own experiences and employ humor to reduce tensions or resolve conflicts.

Styles

Although the preceding characteristics can enhance collaboration, collaboration is also promoted by team interdependence, which is mutually satisfying, positive, and oriented toward problem solving (Smith & Vezina, 2004). Therefore, it is prudent for the DNP graduate to have an awareness about the styles of teams that will promote collaboration and effective results. These types of teams are fostered by leaders who employ the leadership competencies outlined by Goleman and colleagues previously in this chapter. The team styles that enable a team to build and maintain effective relationships with each other and the rest of the organization are identified by Goleman and colleagues (2002) as the self-aware team, the self-managed team, and the empathic team (**Box 2-2**).

Self-aware team members share an awareness of the underlying emotions in the group as a whole. The leader of this group could be a role model for the group

---

BOX 2-2

Team Styles

- Self-aware team
- Self-managed team
- Empathic team

Source: Used with permission from *Primal Leadership: Realizing the Power of Emotional Intelligence*, by Daniel Goleman, Richard Boyatzis, & Annie McKee, Harvard Business Review Press, 2002, taken from Commanding Styles on p. 17.

members by employing empathy toward the emotions of the group, which builds trust and a sense of belonging. This type of scenario sends the message that "we are all in this together" (Goleman et al., 2002, p. 178). This type of team also prioritizes listening to everyone's perspective before decisions are made and stepping in when other members are having difficulty with a task (Goleman et al., 2002). The DNP graduate may foster this type of team by employing the emotional intelligence competencies previously described.

A self-managed team manages itself when it is led by an emotionally intelligent leader. Further, this type of team will hold each member accountable to the positive norms that are already in place (Goleman et al., 2002). The DNP graduate can promote this type of team style by clarifying the team's mission and practicing the team's norms.

The empathic team style is more than just members being nice to each other. The empathic team "figures out what the whole system really needs and goes after it in a way that makes all those involved more successful and satisfied with the outcomes" (Goleman et al., 2002, p. 182). For the DNP graduate, employing empathy across the boundaries between teams, groups, organizations, or disciplines can promote this type of team.

A Discussion About Change

A discussion about DNP graduates and leadership would not be inclusive without a discussion about change. Every DNP graduate, whether he or she is a nurse leader, clinician, researcher, health policy advocate, or educator, will deal with change at some point in his or her career. Obtaining a DNP degree alone presents change for the graduate and his or her colleagues due to the newness of the degree. This author dealt with change simply by being a new DNP graduate in a clinic where she started as a master's degree-prepared nurse practitioner. Her colleagues viewed her a certain way prior to graduating with a DNP degree. Transitioning her colleagues to adjust to the differences, which included adjusting to the title *Dr.*, in addition to educating others about her preparation, was a transition that could have gone poorly if dealt with the wrong way. This situation is perhaps a common one given the number of master's degree-prepared nurses who are returning to school for a DNP degree. Therefore, tips for smooth transitions and promoting change are discussed next.

Effective change has been discussed widely in the literature. One of the most mentioned change theories is Lewin's (1951) process of change, which involves three steps: unfreezing, which occurs as people prepare for change; moving, which occurs when people start to accept and move toward the change; and refreezing, which occurs when people accept the new change and integrate it as the norm. This can best describe the way in which change eventually becomes what is accepted rather than what is rejected.

How do DNP graduates get to the refreezing phase when instituting change? Porter-O'Grady (1998) described certain steps for leaders to apply to the change process that are reflective of the emotional intelligence competencies reviewed previously in the chapter. These steps include the following: (1) be aware of the signs and trends in and out of the organization; (2) construct a vision that will motivate others to become involved in the change process and promote unity; (3) empower others in the group or organization by encouraging all to become involved in the process; (4) provide support that others will need to institute the change and integrate the change as the norm; (5) have a plan of action that will ensure collaboration within and among groups, teams, and organizations; and (6) evaluate the change and be able to adjust the process as necessary (Porter-O'Grady, 1998). These steps are employed every day by nurse leaders, possibly without them realizing it. This author employed these steps in the following way: (1) knew the trends in doctoral education in nursing; (2) shared the benefits of having a DNP-prepared nurse practitioner working in the clinic; (3) educated staff members about the DNP degree; (4) provided education materials explaining the degree; (5) met with the clinic manager regarding the changes associated with her new title and role; and (6) reassessed the clinic staff's understanding of what a DNP degree is and what it means for practice. DNP graduates can employ these steps, along with the leadership attributes and styles discussed, to institute any change, even as simple as returning to the clinic one day after graduating with a DNP degree.

The Reluctant Leader: Unexpected Leadership

Although the DNP degree curriculum has a strong leadership component, it is evident that not every nurse who earns a DNP degree will want to be in a leadership role. Leadership is not always a role that nurses seek or feel comfortable with (Buonocore, 2004; Joyce, 2001; Philpott & Corrigan, 2006). However, as previously noted in the change discussion, leadership will be expected of DNP graduates in all healthcare settings, regardless of the actual role the DNP graduate assumes.

Leadership versus Management

An explanation of the difference between leadership and management may help to alleviate the anxiety that is sometimes felt by DNP graduates when faced with leadership opportunities. Leadership has been defined as "the art and science of influencing a group toward achievement of a goal" (McArthur, 2006, p. 8). Carmen further defined leadership as "to guide and escort" (2002, p. 133). According to Carmen, leadership implies accompaniment and companionship. Management, on the other hand, implies control through supervision and training. Garrison and McBryde-Foster (2004) define management as controlling resources to accomplish organizational goals. In summary, managers wish the people to have faith in the leader, and leaders wish for faith in the people (Carmen, 2002). Additionally, the prior discussion regarding servant leadership may provide more clarification regarding the difference between leadership and management. Given this clarification, DNP graduates can lessen their anxiety about leadership and realize they have the untapped potential within them to lead.

To augment this point, one may reflect on the literature presented earlier in the chapter that illustrates nurses have an instinctive awareness of what attributes are important for effective leadership (Feltner et al., 2008; Joyce, 2001; O'Connor, 2008). DNP graduates have an opportunity to reflect on these attributes, including the emotional intelligence competencies described, and realize that the capacity to lead is within them. Leadership opportunities may be presented in various forms. Self-reflection and honesty will help the DNP graduate to realize his or her true leadership potential when these opportunities are presented.

Role-Modeling: DNP Graduates Setting the Example

Ralph Waldo Emerson is quoted as saying, "What you do speaks so loudly, I can't hear what you are saying." What a perfect way to sum up the act of role-modeling. Although leadership opportunities are presented in various ways, role-modeling may be the most subtle form of leadership. Now more than ever, role-modeling is an extremely important role for DNP graduates. The DNP degree is still a new degree for nursing, and it is definitely new to the healthcare setting. It is therefore imperative that DNP graduates act as role models to their nursing colleagues, other healthcare professionals, and patients to demonstrate the potential of a DNP graduate.

Although it may seem like a daunting task, role-modeling is something nurses do on a regular basis (Coady, 2003; Davies, 1993; Hicks, 2000; Philpott & Corrigan, 2006). Nurses are role models in every aspect of practice, from providing care at the bedside to leading a research study as a principal investigator. Sister Samantha Philpott (Philpott & Corrigan, 2006) wrote about her experiences as a role model senior nurse. Philpott related the general themes she found to be important as a role model: acting fairly, being honest, and communicating effectively. Acting fairly was described as treating patients and others with respect. Philpott stated that "the perception of unfairness is a major cause of poor staff morale" (p. 11). Being honest extended not only to honesty toward patients, but also accepting accountability for one's actions. Communicating effectively included "proactive, honest, and sensitive communication with patients, relatives, and medical staff" (p. 11). Interestingly, Philpott included interpreting body language appropriately as effective communication. Do these themes sound familiar? They are reflective of the leadership attributes that were previously discussed.

Although role-modeling may seem like an immense responsibility, nursing practice embodies immense responsibility. DNP graduates are building on a foundation that is already in place. Therefore, many of the leadership styles and characteristics described in this chapter may be familiar to DNP graduates. Self-reflection and evaluation will enable the DNP graduate to promote effective leadership, collaboration, and role-modeling in every setting.

Case Scenarios Related to the DNP Degree in Leadership and Collaboration

The following case scenarios provide examples of DNP graduates exemplifying roles in leadership.

Case Scenario 1: Leadership in the Clinic Practice Setting

Dr. G. is a women's health nurse practitioner DNP graduate who cares for patients in a suburban outpatient women's health clinic. While seeing a patient who requested an elective pregnancy termination, she overheard the clinic staff speaking loudly about their opinions regarding elective termination. The patient also overheard these comments and became upset. Dr. G. consoled the patient and offered support and a referral for termination. Incidentally, Dr. G. is personally pro-life. After the patient had left the clinic, Dr. G. approached the clinic manager and requested a meeting first alone with the manager and then with the whole clinic staff. In the first meeting with the manager alone, Dr. G. expressed her concerns regarding the incident but requested to handle the situation herself with the staff.

Prior to meeting with the staff, Dr. G. researched sensitivity and diversity training principles and prepared some materials to share with the staff. When she met with the whole staff (providers, staff, and clinic manager), she introduced the notion that more sensitivity should be expressed when dealing with diverse issues that are often presented in the clinic. She related a similar example to the episode that prompted the meeting. Although those who had been involved knew about the episode, they were not aware that they were overheard. They were also not singled out in this meeting. Remorse was later expressed privately by these individuals, who appreciated the opportunity to express more sensitivity to similar issues in the future.

What is the leadership message in this case? Dr. G. could have used a commanding style and verbally expressed her concerns to the staff members involved either privately or in front of others. Instead, she used self-management skills by maintaining a calm demeanor. She also exhibited relationship management skills and involved the whole group in the shared vision of increased sensitivity to diverse issues. Conflict was also diffused because Dr. G. avoided singling out the group members who offended the patient. If they had been confronted differently with the situation, the staff may have acted defensively instead of expressing remorse about the incident.

The leadership attributes exhibited by Dr. G. include empathy, trustworthiness, visionary, effective communication, and compassion. Dr. G. also used significant emotional intelligence. A combination of an affiliative and democratic style was employed regarding this issue. Dr. G. approached the whole group and shared a vision openly (affiliative style), but the differing sides and the consequences were also presented (democratic style) when a specific case involving lack of sensitivity was described. By demonstrating emotional intelligence, the situation was handled effectively and resulted in improved patient care outcomes.

Case Scenario 2: Leadership in the Community

Dr. H. is a clinical nurse specialist (CNS) DNP graduate who works as a CNS at a local hospital and also volunteers at her church as a parish nurse. She began noticing that parish members were not participating in routine health screening events that were sponsored by the parish. Dr. H. approached her parish priest and offered to speak with the congregation after Mass one Sunday. Prior to her presentation, Dr. H. prepared materials for the group that included information regarding the importance of screening and reduced mortality and morbidities resulting from early preventive care. Dr. H. emphasized that health promotion and risk prevention were strongly recommended and that the parish nurses were committed to providing this through health screening to the members of the parish. The parish seemed receptive and appreciative of Dr. H.'s advice and expertise. Further, Dr. H.'s scholarly approach, which included a review of evidence-based practices regarding health promotion and risk reduction, was reflective of her preparation as a DNP graduate.

The leadership attributes that Dr. H. drew from were visionary and motivating in an attempt to inspire the group (the congregation) to buy into a shared vision. Rather than no longer offering the parish health screening, Dr. H. showed compassion and volunteered her time and efforts to educate others and inspire them to take shared responsibility for their healthcare outcomes. Her presentation included evidence from the literature that documented improved outcomes for routine health screening. She also used case studies to further explain the rationale for health screening.

As a result of Dr. H.'s presentation, attendance at the next health screening event nearly tripled, and requests were made for more health education regarding specific topics. Dr. H. started providing educational seminars for her congregation and eventually developed her own consulting health education programs. Her leadership attributes and entrepreneurial skills led her to an additional path in her career that employed the leadership competencies she garnered as a DNP graduate.

Case Scenario 3: Formal Leadership in the Clinical Setting

Dr. C. is a nurse anesthetist DNP graduate who returned to her clinical setting after graduating with a DNP degree. Dr. C. practices at an urban tertiary care hospital. Prior to graduating from a DNP program, Dr. C. had been the lead nurse anesthetist and performed many managerial duties, such as organizing schedules, covering when colleagues were off, and making sure the anesthesia department provided adequate coverage for all operating room cases.

Upon graduation from a DNP degree program, Dr. C. had a clearer understanding of leadership and wanted to become more involved as a leader in the anesthesia department. She wanted to develop more programs of research that investigated the impact nurse anesthetists had on patient care and outcomes. Dr. C. also had a vision that included the nurse anesthetists becoming more involved in nursing education for other nursing departments.

Drawing on her new leadership understanding and past experiences in leadership roles, Dr. C. drafted a proposal for her ideas and scheduled a meeting with the service-line director of surgical services. Although they were appreciated, Dr. C.'s ideas were not initially supported by administration due to financial constraints imposed on the hospital. Instead of giving up, Dr. C. consulted and partnered with her mentor from graduate school (a PhD-prepared nurse), submitted a proposal for a research grant, and obtained funding for a research study in her own department. Upon approval from the hospital internal review board, Dr. C. again approached hospital administration. Now, armed with more resources, Dr. C. eventually was granted approval to conduct the research study. A position was eventually created for Dr. C. within her department (director of research and education for nursing anesthesia), which allowed her to develop more programs of research in the anesthesia department and develop educational programs for nursing.

The leadership attributes exhibited by Dr. C. included courage, the ability to communicate effectively, collaboration, vision, and clinical competence. The leadership style she employed involved an affiliative style. Dr. C. emphasized connections among the anesthesia department, the administration, and a research consultant to bring focus toward a shared goal. Dr. C. also employed a visionary style to motivate those involved to take risks with her and try something new for the anesthesia department. As a result, her leadership skills and abilities allowed Dr. C. to achieve her goals and improve healthcare outcomes.

A Personal Note: A Leadership Case Scenario

I graduated from Oakland University's Doctor of Nursing Practice program in 2007. Upon graduation, I returned to a clinical setting in a small internal medicine practice and wondered how my new degree would impact my practice. I began writing the first edition of this text and realized that I would become an informal leader, sharing my perspectives of the DNP degree and potential roles DNP-prepared nurses could fulfill.

Soon after the first edition was published, my position was eliminated and I was faced with finding a new position as a nurse practitioner. I have always been committed to my role as a clinician and did not have leadership experience, nor did I think I wanted a formal leadership role. I accepted a position in an academic cancer center as a nurse practitioner in a comprehensive breast center. I have always had an interest in women's health, and this seemed like a good fit.

Over the past 5 years in this position, I have grown as a clinician, further developed my scholarship, and transitioned into a formal leadership role. I share my experience because I truly believe my DNP degree has led me to this role.

The clinic in which I practice was called the High-Risk Breast Clinic. The providers consist of three nurse practitioners, including me, and we work closely with radiologists, surgeons, medical oncologists, genetic counselors, other nurse practitioners, physician assistants, and nurses to provide comprehensive breast care. What became apparent is that we truly provide a wellness-focused type of care providing survivorship care, evaluating new breast problems, managing patients with elevated risk for breast cancer, benign breast problems such as pain, and counseling and educating women regarding health promotion and risk reduction. I also developed a specialty menopause clinic to care for patients with menopausal symptoms who are not candidates for hormone therapy, and one of my colleagues has a lymphedema clinic. Eventually the clinic was renamed the Women's Wellness Clinic, which more accurately describes the wellness-focused care we provide.

Throughout this transition I became involved in community events promoting the clinic and educating the community on menopause and breast health. Soon my informal leadership role took on a life of its own. My nursing leadership began consulting me regularly regarding further development and promotion of the clinic. Eventually I approached the vice president with a proposal I wrote for a formal leadership role.

The vice president is truly a servant leader and a transformational leader, and she listened to my ideas. She motivated, inspired, and believed in me. I wrote my own job description and created my title. A few months after I had shared my ideas with her, I was promoted to the position I had created as the clinical director of the Women's Wellness Clinic.

Since that time I have taken on more leadership responsibility working with more nurse practitioners and physician assistants within the center. I never would have thought I would seek out leadership—I was somewhat of a reluctant leader. I credit my DNP degree for the skills and perspective to see the broader view and understand that leadership and clinical practice can be very impactful and rewarding. I am truly committed to servant leadership as my leadership style. I am a work in progress and continually trying to develop as a servant who leads. I maintained my clinical practice and prefer to lead from the trenches. I am able to truly understand, express empathy, and empower others by working with them side by side.

Nursing Leadership's Understanding of the DNP Degree

In 2014 Nichols, O'Connor, and Dunn published the first study that evaluated where, how, and in what capacity DNP-prepared nurses are being employed. Chief nursing officers (CNOs) from academic and public hospitals in Michigan were surveyed regarding their understanding of the role and their expected outcomes of DNP-prepared nurses. These CNOs expressed support toward their employees who are obtaining higher education in general. It was also reported that the respondents would likely hire a DNP-prepared nurse; however, only two reported that DNP-prepared nurses had benefited the system. Interestingly, the CNOs responded that they would not hire a DNP-prepared nurse to do their job. The authors of this study believed this may reflect the CNOs' lack of understanding of the role of the DNP-prepared nurse (Nichols et al., 2014). Therefore, DNP-prepared nurses are called to continue to educate their employers and nursing leadership regarding the value they bring to healthcare outcomes and organizations.

Interviews with Executive Nursing Leaders

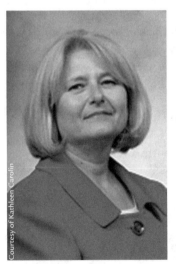
Courtesy of Kathleen Carolin

PERSPECTIVE OF A SENIOR VICE PRESIDENT

Kathleen Carolin, MSA, RN, is senior vice president of Ambulatory Care at Karmanos Cancer Institute. Ms. Carolin has a rich background, including informal and formal leadership, and she also works directly with DNP graduates.

Ms. Carolin, could you describe your current position and your educational background and leadership experiences?

As the senior vice president, Ambulatory and Support Services, I am responsible for the ambulatory clinics and support services. Support services include pharmacy, social work, customer service, concierge, and facility services. The clinics include the multidisciplinary clinics, infusion centers, phase I clinical program, and women's wellness clinic. I began as a diploma graduate RN, then completed my BSN and MSA in hospital administration.

Ms. Carolin, what attracted you to a career in nursing leadership?

For me it was a journey. I definitely did not start out thinking I was going to be a nursing leader. I loved bedside nursing. My clinical experience was as an intensive care nurse and later as a psychiatric nurse. I think the skills I learned as a psychiatric nurse assisted me as a leader. I learned to listen.

When I was approached to take on greater leadership roles I realized how much I cherished the work of nurses. I found I could make a positive impact on people I worked with and through them patient care.

What I have learned through working with other professions is that as a leader I need to respect, support, and facilitate multidisciplinary leaders. We should all strive to work to our full professional potential to meet the needs of our patients in these challenging times.

As a nurse I am ever-inspired by nurses. It is important to me to surround myself with other nursing leaders and visionaries, and together we work to realize excellent professional nursing care.

Ms. Carolin, is there a specific leadership style that you think best describes your leadership style?

I strive to be a transformational leader.

Ms. Carolin, in your opinion, with more than 200 DNP programs and more than 11,000 students enrolled in DNP programs, why do you think the DNP degree has gained sustainability and momentum?

Sustainability has not yet been demonstrated. We need time, perhaps another decade, to see whether it is sustainable in a rapidly changing healthcare environment. As for momentum, it carries great appeal for nurses who want to make a direct impact on changing health care. Nurses tend to see themselves as practitioners more than researchers or academics. The DNP prepares clinicians to translate research and EBP [evidence-based practice] projects into practice that improves patient outcomes and to take on leadership roles in nursing and quality improvement.

Ms. Carolin, do you think the DNP degree adds value to the nursing profession? If so, why?

I think it is adding value to the nursing profession. I see a more scholarly and thoughtful approach to the important questions related to the care of the patient. I have observed this in the collegial discourse with other professions and with the focus on quality improvement related to the delivery of care.

Ms. Carolin, in the future as more nurses earn DNP degrees, what roles do you think DNP-prepared nurses are best prepared to fulfill?

I think their education prepares them as expert clinicians, leaders in clinical services, quality improvement, and administration.

Ms. Carolin, to date, Karmanos Cancer Institute employs four DNP-prepared nurses in the ambulatory care setting. Could you please describe your experiences working with DNP-prepared nurses, especially their leadership ability?

People are different, and even with advanced education some people naturally come with different skill sets.

That being said, I think people who are visionary and strive to be expert clinicians and leaders are inclined to pursue their DNP.

In working with our four DNP-prepared nurses and those pursuing their DNP, I see highly motivated people with a strong drive to pursue nursing excellence for themselves and those they work with. They care deeply for the patients they care for and strive to excel in their clinical practice. They are thoughtful people who reach out to others and want to be included in the vital conversations related to health care. To differing degrees, they all stand out as leaders.

Ms. Carolin, with regard to the DNP degree, what do you think the future holds for nursing leaders?

I think nurses with DNP degrees will continue to thrive as expert clinicians, leaders of clinical practice, and executives in nursing and quality improvement.

I also see a greater presence for the DNP in the interdisciplinary dialogue; more collaboration.

Ms. Carolin, what advice would you give to DNP graduates interested in pursuing nursing leadership?

Be present for the discourse. This sounds simple but it takes courage and a commitment of time. Be willing to ask the hard questions that can change the focus of the dialogue. Bring your scholarly thinking to the discussions, and I think you will naturally move into leadership roles (of course it helps if you are a nice person and can get along with people).

PERSPECTIVE OF A NURSE EXECUTIVE

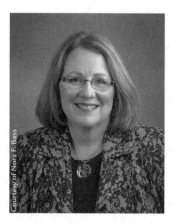

Nora F. Bass, MSN, MBA, APRN, BC, is senior vice president of Surgery Service Line at Parkview Health System in Fort Wayne, Indiana. Ms. Bass is a nurse practitioner and nurse executive with excellent clinical and leadership experience.

Ms. Bass, could you describe your current position and your educational background and leadership experiences?

While working as an NP [nurse practitioner], I was given progressive leadership responsibility and excelled with program development. When a subsequent service line director position opened up, I was given the opportunity and I was promoted. I have continued to grow as a leader and have been given progressive leadership positions ever since that time. As a leader, I am relied upon by nursing staff and physicians to advocate for the right support to get the work done.

Ms. Bass, what attracted you to a career in nursing leadership?

I had always struggled with people making decisions for me as a clinician when they didn't really understand what the barriers were to my practice. I felt that it was critical to have people in place, individuals who could really make a difference in how resources and support were allocated to best support the bedside caregivers. I often saw disconnects between clinicians and administration, issues that arose out of communication deficiencies; deficiencies that arose because of lacking insight.

Ms. Bass, is there a specific leadership style that you think best describes your leadership style?

I would like to believe that I stand for an incredibly high standard as it relates to patient care. I strive for excellence and continuous improvement as it relates to patient care. Anything less than excellence feels intolerable to me.

Ms. Bass, in your opinion, with more than 200 DNP programs and more than 11,000 students enrolled in DNP programs, why do you think the DNP degree has gained sustainability and momentum?

I believe that there has been a great deal of emphasis on the DNP as an alternative provider. I believe advanced-practice nurses have a unique role in patient care, a role that is of its own philosophy and value, one that does not compete with a physician but rather one that complements a physician's practice. As professional organizations strive to bring excellence to the clinical arena, having a voice and a vote are critical to bringing all perspectives into the forefront of patient care. DNPs will bring the nursing perspective and voice to how patients should be cared for in a manner that cannot be minimized.

Ms. Bass, do you think the DNP degree adds value to the nursing profession? If so, why?

The DNP degree allows nurses to practice and care for patients more independently and comprehensively and with greater credibility and with less reliance on the approval of other disciplines.

Ms. Bass, in the future as more nurses earn DNP degrees, what roles do you think DNP-prepared nurses are best prepared to fulfill?

I believe that nurses inherently are best suited for the patient care side of health care. I believe that caring for patients is at the core of who we are and what we do. Nurses, however, regardless of their education, need to step up to leadership roles to ensure that a nursing perspective is honored in the patient care arena. I also believe that DNPs need to be in the forefront relative to advocacy and education, protecting our nursing future both politically and professionally.

Ms. Bass, to date, are there any DNP-prepared nurses employed at your institution? If so, could you please describe your experiences working with DNP-prepared nurses, especially their leadership ability?

I currently work with a DNP who is engaged with quality and clinical effectiveness. She is a champion for better patient care and she has great expertise with regard to problem solving and how to improve clinical outcomes. She is best equipped to tackle both nursing and physician practice to affect how patient care is delivered.

Ms. Bass, with regard to the DNP degree, what do you think the future holds for nursing leaders?

There are challenging times ahead as we head into healthcare reform. There are still too many people without insurance, and health care is too expensive. We need to figure out how to peel out the waste, and waste comes in many forms. I believe that the DNP is a key component to the multidisciplinary team who must contribute to reducing expenses in health care—expenses related to access, diagnostics, supplies, medications, and then hospital admissions. The DNP is key to prevention and wellness tactics; keeping patients healthier will reduce resource consumption.

Ms. Bass, what advice would you give to DNP graduates interested in pursuing nursing leadership?

Having strong leaders in administration is key to preserving the most important care a patient gets, that which is nursing care. Strong advocacy is required so that the voice of nursing is heard and respected. DNPs are poised and educated to lead that charge.

SUMMARY

- Leadership and collaboration are included in the curriculum standards provided by the AACN as evidenced by Essential II: Organizational and Systems Leadership for Quality Improvement and Systems Thinking and Essential VI: Interprofessional Collaboration for Improving Patient and Population Health Outcomes.
- Leadership and collaboration are also included in the NONPF *Practice Doctorate Nurse Practitioner Entry-Level Competencies*.
- Research has shown that nurses are able to identify which attributes are important for leadership. These attributes include communication skills, fairness, job knowledge, ability to role-model, dependability, participative partnership, confidence, positive attitude, motivation, ability to delegate, flexibility, compassion, loyalty toward employees, and ability to set objectives (Feltner et al., 2008).
- Joyce (2001) reported on nurse practitioners' perceptions of leadership attributes and identified four general themes: facilitator, professional, role model, and visionist.
- O'Connor (2008) described several caring competencies that were originally adapted from the Center for Nursing Leadership. These competencies describe pertinent and practical leadership attributes that relate to caring.
- Emotional intelligence has been shown to enhance leadership and includes the leadership competencies of self-awareness, self-management, social awareness, and relationship management.
- Resonant leadership styles encourage the group to work together in harmony and include visionary, coaching, affiliative, and democratic. Dissonant leadership styles—pacesetting and commanding—should be used sparingly (Goleman et al., 2002).
- According to Hamric and colleagues (2005), successful collaboration can be enhanced by the following characteristics: common purpose, clinical competence, interpersonal competence and communication skills, trust, valuing and respecting diversity, complimentary knowledge, and humor.

- The following team styles have been shown to enhance collaboration: the self-aware team, the self-managed team, and the empathic team (Goleman et al., 2002).
- DNP graduates can promote change by applying certain steps that include constructing a vision, empowering others throughout the change, providing support, collaborating with others, and evaluating the change after it is in place (Porter-O'Grady, 1998).
- Leadership and management are defined differently with different goals. Leadership implies accompaniment and companionship, and management implies control through supervision (Carmen, 2002).
- Role-modeling is an important role for DNP graduates and can be accomplished by nurses who draw on many of the leadership attributes and characteristics they already embody.
- Servant leadership is leadership in service of others (Autry, 2001). In addition, servant leadership has been described as a calling to be responsible for the psychological, emotional, and financial well-being of others based on the circumstances and environment in which they work (Autry, 2001).
- Transformational leadership has been described as a "style of leadership in which the leader identifies the needed change, creates vision to guide change through inspiration, and executes the change with the commitment of the members of the group" (Transformational leadership, 2014).

REFLECTION QUESTIONS

1. Do you agree that leadership skills and competencies are necessary for most roles that DNP graduates will assume?
2. What leadership attributes do you think are necessary for a DNP graduate to be an effective leader?
3. What leadership attributes do you possess?
4. What leadership styles do you think you would most likely adopt, as a DNP graduate, when engaged in a leadership role? Why?
5. Do you face conflict or avoid it? Why?
6. Do you think collaboration is an important part of leadership? If so, why?
7. What qualities do you think are important for successful collaborating relationships?
8. As a DNP graduate, what pertinent steps do you think are necessary when instituting change?

9. Do you think you are a role model for nursing practice in your healthcare setting? If so, what qualities enable you to role-model effectively? If not, what qualities would enhance your ability to role-model?

REFERENCES

American Association of Colleges of Nursing. (2006). *Essentials of doctoral education for advanced nursing practice*. Retrieved from http://www.aacn.nche.edu/publications/position/DNPEssentials.pdf

Autry, J. (2001). *The servant leader: How to build a creative team, develop great morale, and improve bottom-performance.* New York, NY: Three Rivers Press.

Bennet, J. (1995). Methodological notes on empathy: Further considerations. *Advances in Nursing Science, 18*(1), 36–50.

Blanchard, K. (1999). *The heart of a leader: Insights on the art of influence.* Colorado Springs, CO: David C. Cook.

Buonocore, D. (2004). Leadership in action: Creating a change in practice. *AACN Clinical Issues, 15*(2), 170–181.

Carmen, T. (2002). *Love em' and lead 'em: Leadership strategies that work for reluctant leaders.* Lanham, MD: Scarecrow Press.

Carroll, T. (2005). Leadership skills and attributes of women and nurse executives: Challenges for the 21st century. *Nursing Administration Quarterly, 29*(2), 146–153.

Coady, E. (2003). Role models. *Nursing Management, 10*(2), 18–21.

Collaborate. (1983). In *Merriam-Webster's collegiate dictionary* (9th ed.). Springfield, MA: Merriam-Webster.

Cook, U., Ingersoll, G. L., & Spitzer, R. (1999). Managed care research, part 1: Defining the domain. *Journal of Nursing Administration, 29*(11), 23–31.

Davies, E. (1993). Clinical role modeling: Uncovering hidden knowledge. *Journal of Advanced Nursing, 18*(4), 627–636.

Emotional intelligence. (n.d.). In Dictionary.com. Retrieved from http://dictionary.reference.com/browse/emotional%20intelligence

Feltner, A., Mitchell, B., Norris, E., & Wolfle, C. (2008). Nurses' views on the characteristics of an effective leader. *AORN Journal, 87*(2), 363–372.

Garrison, D. R., & McBryde-Foster, M. J. (2004). The baccalaureate nurse as a leader in health care delivery. In L. C. Haynes, H. K. Butcher, & T. A. Boese (Eds.), *Nursing in contemporary society: Issues, trends, and transition to practice* (pp. 504–525). Upper Saddle River, NJ: Pearson/Prentice Hall.

Goleman, D. (1995). *Emotional intelligence: Why it can matter more than IQ.* New York, NY: Bantam Dell.

Goleman, D., Boyatzis, R., & McKee, A. (2002). *Primal leadership: Realizing the power of emotional intelligence.* Boston, MA: Harvard Business Review Press.

Greenleaf, R. K. (1970). The servant as leader. Retrieved from https://www.leadershiparlington.org/pdf/TheServantasLeader.pdf

Greanleaf, R. K. (1977). *Servant leadership: A journey into the nature of legitimate power and greatness*. Mahwah, NJ: Paulist Press.

Greiner, A. C., & Knebel, E. (Eds.). (2003). *Health professions education: A bridge to quality*. Washington, DC: National Academies Press.

Grossman, S., & Valiga, T. (2005). *The new leadership challenge: Creating the future of nursing* (2nd ed.). Philadelphia, PA: F. A. Davis.

Hamric, A., Spross, J., & Hanson, C. (2005). *Advanced practice nursing: An integrative approach* (3rd ed.). St. Louis, MO: Elsevier Saunders.

Hicks, D. (2000). Pressure to be a role model. *Nursing Times, 96*(23), 34.

Howatson-Jones, L. (2004). The servant leader. *Nursing Management, 11*(3), 20–24.

Institute of Medicine. (2001). *Crossing the quality chasm: A new health system for the 21st century*. Washington, DC: National Academies Press.

Interprofessional Education Collaborative. (2011). *Core competencies for interprofessional collaborative practice*. Retrieved from http://www.aacn.nche.edu/education-resources /ipecreport.pdf

Jooste, K. (2004). Leadership: A new perspective. *Journal of Nursing Management, 12*(3), 217–223.

Joyce, E. (2001). Leadership perceptions of nurse practitioners. *Lippincott's Case Management, 6*(1), 24–30.

Kalish, B. (1973). What is empathy? *American Journal of Nursing, 73*(9), 1548–1552.

Kohn, L. T., Corrigan, J. M., & Donaldson, M. S. (Eds.). (1999). *To err is human: Building a safer health system*. Washington, DC: National Academies Press.

Lambing, A., Adams, D., Fox, D., & Divine, G. (2004). Nurse practitioners' and physicians' care activities and clinical outcomes with an inpatient geriatric population. *Journal of the American Academy of Nurse Practitioners, 16*(8), 343–352.

LaMonica, E., & Karshmer, J. (1978). Empathy: Educating nurses in professional practice. *Journal of Nursing Education, 17*(2), 3–11.

Lewin, K. (1951). *Field theory in social science: Selected theoretical papers*. New York, NY: Harper & Row.

Marshall, E. J. (2011). *Transformational leadership in nursing*. New York, NY: Springer.

Mastal, M., Joshi, M., & Schulke, K. (2007). Nursing leadership: Championing quality and patient safety in the boardroom. *Nursing Economic$, 25*(6), 323–330.

McArthur, D. (2006). The nurse practitioner as leader. *Journal of the American Academy of Nurse Practitioners, 18*(1), 8–10.

National Organization of Nurse Practitioner Faculties. (2006). *Practice doctorate nurse practitioner entry-level competencies*. Retrieved from http://c.ymcdn.com/sites /www.nonpf.org/resource/resmgr/competencies/dnp%20np%20competenciesapril2006 .pdf

Nichols, C., O'Connor, N., & Dunn, D. (2014). Exploring early and future use of DNP prepared nurses within healthcare organizations. *Journal of Nursing Administration, 44*(2), 74–78.

O'Connor, M. (2008). The dimensions of leadership: A foundation for the caring competency. *Nursing Administration Quarterly, 32*(1), 21–26.

Philpott, S., & Corrigan, P. (2006). Role modeling. *Nursing Management, 13*(1), 10–12.

Porter-O'Grady, T. (1998). The seven basic rules for successful redesign. In E. C. Hein (Ed.), *Contemporary leadership behavior: Selected readings* (5th ed., pp. 226–235). Philadelphia, PA: Lippincott.

Shelly, J., & Miller, A. (2006). *Called to care: A Christian worldview for nursing* (2nd ed.). Downers Grove, IL: InterVarsity Press.

Smith, T., & Vezina, M. (2004). Mediated roles: Working through other people. In L. A. Joel (Ed.), *Advanced practice nursing: Essentials for role development* (pp. 455–472). Philadelphia, PA: F. A. Davis.

Transformational leadership. (2014). In *Business dictionary*. Retrieved from http://www.businessdictionary.com/definition/transformational-leadership.html

Wong, C., & Cummings, G. (2007). The relationship between nursing leadership and patient outcomes: A systematic review. *Journal of Nursing Management, 15*(5), 508–521.

CHAPTER 3

The DNP Graduate as Expert Clinician

Lisa Astalos Chism

M any doctor of nursing practice (DNP) graduates will return to various advanced-practice nursing or clinician roles in clinical settings after they complete their programs. Several years after the development of the DNP degree, one of the most frequently asked questions remains, How will the clinician's role change or benefit from earning a DNP degree? This question is often followed by, If I am in clinical practice, why should I earn a DNP degree? This question may be addressed, in part, by evaluating the many aspects of clinical practice that are enhanced by the expertise garnered through a DNP degree.

The Institute of Medicine (IOM) has recommended that to meet the changing demands of health care, healthcare professionals should gain increased knowledge in evidence-based practice (EBP), information technologies, and interprofessional collaboration (Greiner & Knebel, 2003). To further meet these changing demands of health care, the American Association of Colleges of Nursing (AACN) and the National Organization of Nurse Practitioner Faculties (NONPF) have developed the curriculum standards for the DNP degree, which include guidelines for course work designed to address the evaluation, integration, translation, and implementation of EBP, healthcare information systems, and collaboration across healthcare teams and disciplines (AACN, 2006; NONPF, 2006). In addition, clinical practice may also be improved in more subtle ways through completion of a DNP degree. Mentoring and precepting future nurses and other healthcare professionals are also enhanced through the expertise garnered by earning a DNP degree. Nurses in every setting may frequently be involved in the evaluation and translation of EBP, information systems, interprofessional collaboration, and mentoring or precepting, but the DNP degree serves to augment these experiences and provide additional expertise to further develop skills in these areas. Hence, the expert clinician's knowledge base in these areas is broadened as a culmination of previous experiences and the knowledge and expertise garnered through a DNP degree. Finally, participation in scholarship is expected of all DNP graduates, especially those in clinician roles.

This chapter reviews the AACN essentials, the NONPF competencies, and the National Association of Clinical Nurse Specialists (NACNS) core competencies that pertain to specific areas that are likely to improve the delivery of health care and healthcare outcomes in clinical practice. Advanced nursing practice and advanced-practice nursing may be confusing terms, and therefore clarification is provided. The newly developed APRN Consensus Model will be reviewed because it has implications for advanced-practice registered nurses (APRNs). EBP will be discussed with emphasis on DNP graduates' evaluation and translation of EBP in clinical settings. Information technology is addressed in relation to how newer technologies can enhance clinical practice from a DNP graduate's perspective. Although nurses frequently collaborate with others in various healthcare settings, interprofessional collaboration, as it relates to DNP graduates' and other healthcare professionals' effect on improved healthcare outcomes in clinical practice, is addressed. Additionally, there is a greater responsibility to mentor and precept others when one earns a terminal degree in his or her field. Therefore, DNP graduates' roles as mentors in clinical practice settings are discussed. Finally, personal accounts from DNP graduates who are practicing in clinical settings, and this author's journey to a DNP degree and beyond, are provided.

Curriculum Standards Related to Clinical Practice

The AACN's published *Essentials of Doctoral Education for Advanced Nursing Practice* include specific curriculum requirements that pertain to improving nursing practice. Essential III: Clinical Scholarship and Analytical Methods for Evidence-Based Practice addresses the need for increased expertise in the critical evaluation, integration, translation, and implementation of EBP. This essential also specifies the need for advanced nursing practice professionals to evaluate practice outcomes, design and evaluate methodologies that improve quality of care, develop practice guidelines based on best practice findings, and work collaboratively with research specialists (AACN, 2006). The NONPF competency area that addresses the requirement for this area of practice is scientific foundation (NONPF, 2006). The NACNS also addresses the need for APRNs to evaluate and translate EBP within its published *Core Practice Doctorate Clinical Nurse Specialist Competencies* (NACNS, 2009).

Essential IV: Information Systems–Technology and Patient Care Technology for the Improvement and Transformation of Health Care addresses the need for increased expertise in information technologies that improve overall patient care. Specifically, this essential requires that DNP graduates garner experience in data mining techniques, design and implementation of technologies that improve quality of care, and provision of health consumer information (AACN, 2006). The NONPF competency area that addresses this area of expertise is technology and information literacy (NONPF, 2006). The NACNS also addresses the need for APRNs to "evaluate and improve system-level programs based on the analysis of information from relevant sources such as databases, benchmarks, and epidemiologic data" within the *Core Practice Doctorate Clinical Nurse Specialist Competencies* (NACNS, 2009, p. 13).

Essential VI: Interprofessional Collaboration for Improving Patient and Population Health Outcomes pertains to developing expertise in collaboration across disciplines to improve patient care. Expertise in this area includes analyzing complex practice or organizational issues through participation and leadership of interprofessional teams, acting as a consultant to interprofessional teams, and participating in the development of practice models and policies (AACN, 2006). The NONPF competency area of health delivery system addresses collaboration and related skills to improve healthcare outcomes (NONPF, 2006). The NACNS emphasizes interprofessional collaboration and the role of APRNs in the *Core Practice Doctorate Clinical Nurse Specialist Competencies* (NACNS, 2009).

Finally, Essential VIII: Advanced Nursing Practice addresses the requirements for practicing as an advanced nursing practitioner in various specialty areas. This essential includes development of proficiency in comprehensive health assessment, implementation of therapeutic interventions, development of therapeutic relationships with patients and other healthcare professionals, and development of advanced clinical decision-making skills (AACN, 2006). The NONPF competency area of independent practice requires proficiency in these areas as well (NONPF, 2006). The NACNS includes conducting a "comprehensive assessment of client health care needs, integrating data from multiple sources which include the client and interprofessional team members" within the *Core Practice Doctorate Clinical Nurse Specialist Competencies* (NACNS, 2009, p. 11).

Advanced Nursing Practice and Advanced-Practice Nursing: Let's Clear This Up

The terms *advanced nursing practice* and *advanced-practice nursing* are often used interchangeably (Brown, 1998; Styles & Lewis, 2000); however, these terms actually have different meanings. Providing a definition of nursing will assist in the clarification of these terms. Nursing was defined by Nightingale as having "charge of the personal health of somebody and what nursing has to do is to put the patient in the best condition for nature to act upon him" (1859). In 1980 the American Nurses Association (ANA) defined nursing as "the diagnosis and treatment of human responses to actual or potential health problems" (ANA, 1995, p. 6). The ANA acknowledges that "nursing philosophy and science have been influenced by a greater elaboration of the science of caring and its integration with the traditional knowledge base for diagnosis and treatment of human responses to health and illness" (ANA, 1995, p. 6). Therefore, contemporary nursing practice is defined as these four essential features:

1. Attention to the full range of human experiences and responses to health and illness without restriction to a problem-focused orientation;

2. Integration of objective data with knowledge gained from an understanding of the patient's or group's subjective experience;

3. Application of scientific knowledge to the processes of diagnosis and treatment; and

4. Provision of a caring relationship that facilitates health and healing. (ANA, 1995, p. 6)

Nursing practice describes what nurses do when they provide nursing care (Bryant-Lukosius, DiCenso, Browne, & Pinelli, 2004). To further clarify, advanced nursing practice describes what one does in various specialized roles, such as clinical practice, education, research, and leadership. The domain of advanced nursing practice is defined by the type of specialization area one pursues. Put another way, advancement has been defined in nursing as "the integration of theoretical, research-based, and practical knowledge that occurs as part of graduate nursing education" (ANA, 1995, p. 14). Davies and Hughes expanded on this to further explain that "the term advanced nursing practice extends beyond roles. It is a way of thinking and viewing the world based on clinical knowledge, rather than a composition of roles" (1995, p. 157). Advanced nursing practice is therefore a broad term that describes what nurses do in their various advanced nursing practice roles.

Advanced-practice nursing, on the other hand, describes the "whole field of a specific type of advanced nursing practice" (Bryant-Lukosius et al., 2004, p. 522). Advanced-practice nursing includes several specialty roles in which nurses function at an advanced level of practice (ANA, 1995; Brown, 1998). The APRN "acquires specialized knowledge and skills through study and supervised practice at the master's or doctoral level in nursing" (ANA, 1995, p. 14). APRNs utilize their advanced knowledge and skills within their specialty roles to provide care to individuals, families, and communities.

Hence, the DNP degree is the terminal degree for nursing practice, which includes roles in leadership, clinical practice, education, research, and health policy advocacy. Within the domain of advanced nursing practice are the roles defined as APRNs or clinician roles. These roles include nurse anesthetist, nurse–midwife, clinical nurse specialist, and nurse practitioner. This chapter is primarily focused on the ways in which the DNP degree augments the roles of DNP graduates who are APRNs or are in clinician roles.

APRN Consensus Model

The APRN Consensus Model is a regulatory model for APRNs. The APRN Consensus Model (APRN Joint Dialogue Group, 2008) was developed in 2008 to formally define advanced-practice nursing regulation. This regulatory model defines APRN licensure, accreditation, certification, and education (LACE). The electronic platform created to facilitate the implementation and ongoing communication among the regulatory entities is called the LACE network. This model also formally defines APRN, describes the roles within advanced-practice nursing, and defines APRN educational standards and certification standards. The model was developed by the APRN Consensus Workgroup and National Council of State Boards of Nursing APRN Advisory Committee and has been endorsed by many nursing organizations. It has been proposed that all states adopt this model by 2015.

The APRN Consensus Model defines advanced-practice roles as nurse anesthetists, nurse–midwives, clinical nurse specialists, and nurse practitioners (APRN Joint Dialogue Group, 2008). These roles are related to specific population foci defined as family (across the life span), adult–gerontology, neonatal, pediatrics, women's health, and psychiatric–mental health (APRN Joint Dialogue Group, 2008). Specialty roles are also addressed within the model and are defined as "focus of practice beyond roles and population focus linked to health care needs" (APRN Joint Dialogue Group, 2008, p. 10). Examples of specialty roles include (but are not limited to) oncology, palliative care, orthopedics, and nephrology.

The APRN Consensus Model clearly defines APRN education, certification, and licensure requirements as well. Details can be found within the report (APRN Joint Dialogue Group, 2008). Importantly, the implications for DNP graduates are primarily related to the educational requirement of all APRNs. Broad-based APRN education is defined as formal education with a graduate degree (master's or doctorate) or postgraduate certificate awarded by an academic institution that is accredited by a nursing or nursing-related accrediting organization (APRN Joint Dialogue Group, 2008). The educational requirements for APRNs include preparing the graduate to practice within one of the four delineated APRN roles. Therefore, the APRN Consensus Model will influence the development of DNP degree curricula, particularly the post-BSN DNP curricula for the four APRN roles.

Evidence-Based Practice

Evidence-based practice (EBP) "[denotes] disciplines of health care that proceed empirically with regard to the patient and reject more traditional protocols" (Evidence-based, n.d.). EBP in nursing has been defined as "integration of the evidence available, nursing expertise, and the values and preferences of the individuals, families, and communities who are served" (Sigma Theta Tau International, 2004, p. 69). Congruent with the aims of the DNP degree, Gibbs (2003) related that evidence-based practitioners adopt a process of lifelong learning that involves continually asking clients questions of practical importance, searching for the current best evidence relative to each question, and taking appropriate action that is guided by the evidence. The overall goal of EBP is therefore to promote optimal healthcare outcomes, which are based on critically reviewed clinical evidence, for individual patients, families, and communities.

Even though all DNP graduates are expected to evaluate, integrate, and implement EBP into their settings, DNP graduates in the clinician role have a vantage point of EBP due to their direct impact on care in the clinical setting. Practicing in the clinical setting provides an environment for the DNP graduate clinician to develop and utilize skills pertaining to evaluating, integrating, and implementing EBP. Further, who better to formulate relevant research questions about practice than the clinicians who provide the care? Jennings and Rogers recognized that "while certain aspects of the research process can be shared, it is those nurses in the clinical realm who have the sole opportunity to use research to guide practice" (1988, p. 754).

Barriers to Evidence-Based Practice

It is evident throughout the literature that when EBP is used to deliver care, the best patient outcomes are achieved (Melnyk & Fineout-Overholt, 2005; Melnyk, Fineout-Overholt, Feinstein, Sadler, & Green-Hernandez, 2008). Despite this, EBP is often met with resistance in the clinical setting. Pravikoff, Bartlett, and Herrick (2005) found that when 1,097 nurses were surveyed, approximately half were not familiar with the term *EBP*, and most did not know how to search information databases for literature. This may also be due to the fact that nurses were noted to lack computer and library training that is necessary to adequately search the literature for scientific validation (Fink, Thompson, & Bonnes, 2005; Melnyk, 2005; Pravikoff et al., 2005).

Nurses have also been noted to resist new practice patterns despite evidence that EBP improves patient care outcomes. Nurses regularly practice a certain way because of tradition, past experiences, and intuition rather than utilizing scientific validation (Egerod & Hansen, 2005; Pravikoff et al., 2005). This may be a function of the lack of knowledge about EBP (Melnyk et al., 2004) and lack of belief regarding the influence of EBP on positive outcomes (Melnyk & Fineout-Overholt, 2005). Please refer to **Box 3-1** for a summary of barriers to EBP. DNP graduates have the opportunity to change these barriers and provide education to other healthcare professionals regarding the positive outcomes achieved when EBP patterns are employed. Further, DNP graduates may also improve the perceptions about EBP by role-modeling and adopting EBP patterns themselves. Mentoring others on EBP includes role-modeling and actively engaging healthcare professionals in activities that promote the use of EBP.

> ### BOX 3-1
>
> #### Summary of Barriers to Evidence-Based Practice
>
> - Lack of computer training
> - Lack of library resources and library training
> - Resistance to change due to reliance on tradition, past experience, and intuition
> - Lack of knowledge about the positive influence of EBP on outcomes
> - Lack of belief that EBP will positively influence outcomes
> - Poor motivation to investigate EBP

Reducing Barriers to Evidence-Based Practice

Although employing EBP methods in their own clinical practice is paramount, DNP graduates in clinician roles also have a responsibility to reduce the EBP barriers within their practice settings. Further, DNP graduates' expertise in information systems technology, leadership, clinical decision making, and EBP evaluation, integration, and implementation places them in the perfect position to reduce EBP barriers in the clinical setting. Therefore, the challenge for DNP graduates in the clinician role lies not only in overcoming their own barriers regarding the adoption of EBP patterns, but also in providing the leadership and role-modeling necessary to promote EBP in the clinical setting.

What interventions will enable DNP graduates to foster the use of EBP in their own practice settings and overcome the barriers to EBP? Research has shown that defining EBP for all who provide care is essential (Hudson, Duke, Haas, & Varnell, 2008). In addition to providing a clear definition of EBP, DNP graduates must provide the knowledge and skills necessary to critically evaluate EBP. Hudson and colleagues state, "Nurses must have the knowledge and skills to critically question and assist with correcting misguided, inaccurate, or insufficient guidelines in practice" (2008, p. 414). Others have also agreed that barriers to EBP can be overcome with additional education that strengthens knowledge regarding methods to critically evaluate and integrate EBP (Melnyk & Fineout-Overholt, 2005; Melnyk et al., 2004; Sheriff, Wallis, & Chaboyer, 2007). Specifically, learning how to navigate information systems databases is a valuable tool to locate and evaluate pertinent EBP information (Melnyk et al., 2004). In their programs, DNP graduates gain proficiency in information technologies and are therefore ideal consultants in this area. Research also suggests that interactive workshops were shown to be effective pedagogical techniques to increase knowledge and understanding of EBP (Sheriff et al., 2007). DNP graduates' leadership and collaboration skills facilitate the development and provision of in-service programs and workshops regarding EBP in the clinical setting.

The literature also suggests that it is not enough to have knowledge about EBP; one must believe that EBP actually has a positive effect on outcomes (Melnyk, 2002; Melnyk & Fineout-Overholt, 2005). Hence, DNP graduates in the clinician role may convince others through specific exemplars that adopting EBP patterns is worth the effort. Increasing belief in EBP may also be achieved through mentoring and role-modeling the use of EBP. In a study by Melnyk and colleagues, nurses reported increased use of EBP was directly influenced by "support from faculty, clinical nurse specialists, nurse practitioners, library resources and personnel, administrators, research departments, peer researchers, and specific mentors or clinical experts, as well as time for discussion and use of current research" (2004, p. 191). DNP graduates are often viewed as mentors and role models and are therefore in an ideal position to influence others regarding the use of EBP. **Box 3-2** provides tips for DNP graduates to reduce barriers to EBP.

DNP Graduates Evaluating and Translating Evidence-Based Practice

DNP graduates in clinician roles are perfectly positioned to ask questions directly from the clinical setting. Asking questions is the first and most important step toward integrating EBP into clinical practice. Further, asking clinically relevant questions is essential to the development of new knowledge in a field. After the question has been asked, answers may be evaluated in the clinical setting, which allows for direct implementation of EBP. It has been suggested in various dialogues about EBP that it may take up to 18 years to adopt practices based on clinical evidence. Reducing this amount of time to evaluate and translate EBP is essential and well within the domain of DNP graduates. Further, activities such as evaluating research articles in journal clubs, developing in-service programs and workshops that teach evaluation and implementation of research findings,

---

BOX 3-2

Tips for DNP Graduates to Reduce Barriers to Evidence-Based Practice

- Define EBP to others in the healthcare setting.
- Provide education regarding EBP that emphasizes positive outcomes through in-service training and workshops.
- Provide consultation regarding information systems, including searching databases for pertinent answers to clinically formulated questions.
- Increase belief in the benefits of EBP by mentoring others in the healthcare setting and providing exemplars through case studies.
- Mentor others in EBP methods, such as searching databases and critically reviewing and evaluating research findings.

and conducting and reviewing literature searches of the most current evidence will further encourage the adoption of EBP in the clinical setting and foster the improvement of healthcare outcomes.

It was previously mentioned that DNP graduates are positioned to ask questions directly from the clinical setting. Asking questions may also lead to the identification of gaps in service. These gaps may take on the form of an unmet need in health care and society. DNP graduates are well equipped to create evidence-based solutions, such as the development of new practice programs that fulfill unmet healthcare and societal needs. **Box 3-3** provides tips for DNP graduates to evaluate and translate EBP within their own practices.

Case Scenario of a DNP Graduate Clinician's Experience with Evidence-Based Practice

Dr. C. is a DNP graduate clinician (certified nurse practitioner) working in a hospital-based internal medicine ambulatory care setting. Dr. C. was a graduate student in a DNP program when she accepted this position. While in school, Dr. C. inquired about resources within the institution that might help her apply the latest research findings to patient care. Dr. C. received assistance from the reference librarian at this institution and began obtaining literature regarding pertinent patient issues.

BOX 3-3

Tips for DNP Graduate Clinicians to Employ Evidence-Based Practice Within Their Own Practices

- Formulate questions when providing care, especially when you don't know if the treatments or recommendations are based on clinical evidence.
- Conduct literature reviews regarding treatments or topics you are interested in or if you question the best practices.
- Start a journal club in your area of clinical practice and meet regularly to discuss pertinent literature.
- If you are in an organization with a library or related resources, ask the reference librarian to conduct searches or automatically alert you regarding pertinent topics you encounter in practice.
- Communicate with other healthcare professionals and ask questions about whether certain practices are based on evidence or if they are simply what has always been done.
- Organize in-service programs for staff and others about how to search for evidence and find the best answers to questions.
- Identify unmet healthcare and societal needs and develop evidence-based solutions to fulfill these unmet needs.

Initially, sifting through the information was difficult. The myriad results, discussions, and literature reviews made it difficult to decipher what information was accurate and pertinent to best practice recommendations. Through her graduate program, Dr. C. attended a methodology workshop (part of the DNP curriculum) that clarified how to critically review a research article and determine whether the information was indeed valuable. Upon finishing her DNP program, Dr. C. became more proficient at locating and evaluating EBP information. Now, when Dr. C. reviews EBP articles, she critically evaluates the information for sample sizes, accuracy of statistical analyses, and ability to generalize the results to the given population. As a clinician, Dr. C. is able to apply the EBP patterns she researches and validate effectiveness in her setting.

Taking this knowledge and added expertise a step further, Dr. C. suggested to the physician she practices with that they start a journal club in their setting. Dr. M. was enthusiastic about this and offered to assist with presentation of pertinent topics, even contributing his "Journal Watch" articles for review. Dr. C. also regularly precepts students from various advanced-practice nursing programs and now integrates the review of EBP techniques as part of her students' clinical experiences. Dr. C. has found that as she becomes more proficient at reviewing the information, it actually takes her less time to incorporate EBP activities into her day.

A PERSONAL NOTE: DISCOVERING AN UNMET NEED AND DEVELOPING A SPECIALTY CLINIC

I had been practicing in a comprehensive breast center for approximately 2 years when I identified an unmet healthcare and societal need in the population I was caring for. Many breast cancer patients and survivors experience menopausal symptoms either as a result of breast cancer treatments or age. Women as young as 30 years may experience induced menopause through certain treatments or therapies. These women may not safely use traditional hormone therapies to treat their menopausal symptoms, and their menopausal symptoms were frequently not assessed or treated.

I became certified as a menopause practitioner through the North American Menopause Society and began developing my knowledge regarding menopause. I also immersed myself in the literature regarding nonhormonal and nonpharmacologic therapies to reduce the symptoms of menopause, including vulvavaginal atrophy (VVA). I participated in community outreach programs through my institution to spread awareness of menopause symptom management in this population. I also spoke at peer-reviewed conferences and published in peer-reviewed journals on the topic of menopause, VVA, and breast cancer.

In addition, I approached my nursing leadership regarding the development of a dedicated menopause specialty clinic within the Women's Wellness Clinic (WWC). I developed a business plan and a set of clinic goals. This program was approved and has been successfully growing for more than 2 years. The clinic goals also received multiprofessional approval from the breast multidisciplinary team. Currently, patients are referred to this specialty clinic by oncology, surgery, and the community.

Caring for patients in this specialty clinic has identified another unmet health-care and societal need in this population: sexual health. Many patients suffering from menopausal symptoms also have sexual health concerns that have not been addressed. I have completed a sexual health certificate as a sexual health counselor and educator at the University of Michigan. This program prepared me with evidence-based information to assess, educate, and counsel patients regarding sexual health. I am currently developing a specialty practice clinic to meet the sexual health needs of the population for which I care.

The development of this specialty clinic is the result of the identification of an unmet healthcare and societal need. I believe that my preparation to evaluate, translate, and implement EBP equipped me to identify the unmet need and develop a specialty practice as a solution.

Information Technology

Following a discussion about EBP, the literature is clear that proficiency in information technology is essential to foster the use of EBP (Carroll, Bradford, Foster, Cato, & Jones, 2007; Peck, 2005; Zytkowski, 2003). Others refer to the "knowledge explosion" taking place in health care and state that "there has been increasing pressure for health care systems to improve efficiency while standardizing and streamlining organizational processes and maintaining care quality" (Carroll et al., 2007, p. 39). The amount of information now being accessed to improve quality and health care outcomes requires that nurses embrace nursing informatics in every healthcare setting. Curran relates that "health and knowledge are increasing at a rapid rate. Both the ability to manage information and skilled use of technology are basic tools for practice" (2003, p. 320).

Information technology is also referred to in the nursing literature as nursing informatics. Nursing informatics is defined as "a combination of computer science, information science, and nursing science designed to assist in the management and processing of nursing data, information, and knowledge to support the practice of nursing and the delivery of nursing care" (Graves & Corcoran, 1989, p. 227). The International Medical Informatics Association's Nursing Informatics Special Interest Group offers a similar definition that includes the "integration of nursing, its information, and information management with information processing and communication technology, to support the health of people worldwide" (1998). From these definitions it may be extrapolated that the purpose of nursing informatics is to develop systems that manage, organize, and process health information (Zytkowski, 2003) in an effort to improve quality of care and healthcare outcomes.

Nursing informatics has become so essential to improving quality and healthcare outcomes that in 1992 the ANA designated nursing informatics as an approved nursing specialty (Zytkowski, 2003). The ANA refers to nursing informatics as "a specialty that integrates nursing science, computer science, and information science to manage community data, information, and knowledge in nursing practice" (2001, p. vii). For the purpose of this discussion, the broader term *information technology*, which includes nursing informatics, is used.

Is Nursing Overcoming Technophobia? Embracing Information Technology

Traditionally nursing has been somewhat reluctant to embrace information technology (Gaumer, Koeniger-Donohue, Friel, & Sudbay, 2007; Peck, 2005; Simpson, 2004). However, due to the need for improvement in quality and healthcare outcomes, nursing has begun the challenge of integrating information technologies into patient care. Further, the IOM's call for improvement in quality and healthcare outcomes specifically designates proficiency in information systems as a requirement for healthcare professionals (IOM, 2001). The IOM's report *To Err Is Human: Building a Safer Health System* (Kohn, Corrigan, & Donaldson, 1999) was the initial call for a decrease in medical errors. *Crossing the Quality Chasm: A New Health System for the 21st Century* (IOM, 2001) followed this report and specifically called for an emphasis on information technology to improve healthcare outcomes and reduce errors. In 2003 the IOM published a report outlining the requirements for healthcare professionals' education and recommended that information technologies be included as a core competency for all healthcare professionals (Greiner & Knebel, 2003). These reports, and nursing's desire to improve patient care outcomes, have contributed to nursing's increasing acceptance of information technology.

Consequently recent research has shown that nursing noted improved care through the adoption of information technology. A study by Gaumer and colleagues (2007) described the use of information technologies by APRNs. Seventy percent of the APRNs surveyed reported that they were able to perform their jobs better due to information technologies. Eighty-seven percent of the APRNs stated that their time was more efficiently spent because of information technology. Further, 81% perceived that patient safety was improved through information technologies. Overall, 75% responded that their caregiving was improved by the use of information technologies.

Simpson also stated that information technology improves nursing practice by "counteracting human error, by improving human behavior, and by putting nurses where they need to be more effective" (2004, p. 303). Further, information technology has the potential to improve more specific aspects of nursing. Recruitment and retention are improved due to increased job satisfaction through information technologies, such as electronic charting, electronic mobile devices, and innovative devices such as smart intravenous pumps (Simpson, 2005). Patient care is improved by information technologies that facilitate the "data-to-information-to-knowledge continuum" (Simpson, 2005, p. 346). EBP is more accessible via information technologies and is therefore more quickly adopted by nursing. Overall, the use of information technology to evaluate and implement EBP improves quality and patient care outcomes.

Specific to advanced nursing practice, Zytkowski relates that information technology has an impact on nurse practitioners' practices by influencing "access to individual health information, reimbursement, and practice based on evidence from research" (2003, p. 278). Further, nurse practitioners are responsible for improving patient care while adhering to organizational standards for scope of practice. These demands are dependent on access to real-time resources and information (Zytkowski, 2003). Information technology provides this information in the most up-to-date fashion through Internet resources.

More Than Just Nuts and Bolts: Technology Used to Improve Clinical Practice

Information technology is used by nurses in many specialty areas related to nursing practice, such as leadership roles (computer software for management of health information), education roles (distance education technologies), and clinician roles (personal digital assistants or PDAs). The employment of information technology in nursing practice is becoming commonplace. Further, many nurses, especially in the clinical environment, are using various information technologies and do not realize they are doing so.

Nursing leaders may be found using information technology to perform data mining. This technique enables the sorting of data from large populations to reveal healthcare-related patterns that may improve the quality of care and healthcare outcomes. Nursing leaders may also use software that organizes large amounts of systems information to streamline the management of systems issues. Information technology through the Internet may also be used by nurse leaders to communicate information to large groups of people who are not in the same location.

Nursing educators may also be found using information technologies to share information with students. Online course work, email, and interactive live meetings are now essential aspects of distance education. These technologies allow the sharing of information to those previously not able to attend courses on campus.

Nurses in the clinical setting are inundated with data related to patient care and frequently use very innovative types of information technologies. PDAs are often found in the pocket of many nurses in the clinical setting. They may be loaded with software such as Epocrates, 5-Minute Clinical Consult, and various other programs that are available on the Internet and are designed to provide information in the palm of one's hand. Some of these programs are free and may be downloaded immediately. Clinical pharmacists endorse the use of PDAs by nurses in the clinical setting and find that they provide general management and data collection, drug referencing for side effects, adverse reactions, compatibility, dose-specific reactions, and clinical references relating to diagnoses, disease management, and laboratory referencing (Shneyder, 2002). Software programs such as Epocrates offer pharmacology, diagnostic, and symptom information. Epocrates also offers a medical dictionary and International Classification of Diseases (ICD) and Current Procedural Terminology (CPT) codes for accurate terminology and billing codes for diagnoses and procedures.

Another example of clinical nurses employing informatics is the use of telehealth technologies. Telehealth is defined as "the use of electronic information and telecommunication technologies to support long-distance clinical health care, patient and professional health-related education, public health, and health administration" (Sharp, 1998, pp. 68–69). Nursing tends to prefer telehealth because of the emphasis on patients' long-term wellness, self-management, and health (Peck, 2005). Telehealth can be used as an interactive technique or as a method to track patient data. As access to patient care data improves, patient care improves as well (Peck, 2005). Telehealth also includes care that is provided despite distance. Collaboration between physicians and APRNs frequently takes place between locations. Home care companies are also employing telehealth by providing nurses in the field with PDAs so they can take photos of wounds and upload them to a website so an APRN can view the photos through an online portal. The patient's status is evaluated and care is provided without the APRN leaving his or her clinical setting.

APRNs may also integrate information technology into patient education. Internet resources can provide patient information quickly and easily. However, patients are often intimidated by the Internet and are not sure how to accurately search for information. APRNs can access this information for patients quickly and print patient education resources that are frequently available on various health-related websites. Further, APRNs can decipher information for patients while advising them what information is accurate and appropriate for patient education. Knowing what information is appropriate and deciphering it for patients is a form of information technology (Curran, 2003).

DNP Graduates Navigating the Information Highway

As information technology specialists, how do DNP graduates in clinician roles utilize nursing informatics to improve quality and health care outcomes? Many of the answers are reviewed in this chapter. It should also be mentioned that nurses in all clinical settings frequently use information technology. However, of the information technologies reviewed, some are essential proficiencies for DNP graduates who are most directly involved in patient care.

The use of PDAs is vital for the provision of up-to-date, efficient, and accurate information to DNP graduates in the clinician role. The use of this technology improves access to information regarding medications, treatment regimens, and billing and coding information. This information improves quality of care, safety, and cost.

Techniques to provide patient information that can be accessed on the Internet are also essential for DNP graduates in the clinician role. Advising patients about accurate health-related websites is appreciated by patients who do not feel comfortable looking for this information themselves. Simply utilizing a search engine to print information for patients, in their language, is a nursing informatics skill that is often overlooked as information technology. However, this skill improves patient education, and therefore quality and patient care outcomes are improved.

The use of telehealth is also a valuable tool to improve nursing practice by allowing care to be more accessible. APRNs can utilize Internet portals to view patient data and modify care as the data change to allow for seamless, efficient, and improved care. Telehealth as a means to share information is also essential for DNP graduates in clinician roles. Physician–DNP graduate collaboration may be improved through telehealth technologies by providing consultation in rural areas.

Partnering with nursing administration to perform data mining techniques also allows DNP graduates in clinician roles to observe patterns in large amounts of patient data. This information provides insights about patient patterns regarding their health status and facilitates solutions to improve patient care. Data mining also facilitates the development of EBP patterns.

Finally, exhibiting an overall comfort with the utilization of information technology will enable DNP graduates in clinician roles to influence others' comfort with technology. Teaching others how to access information on the Internet, sharing information obtained on personal data devices (laptops, tablets), and participating in the development of in-service training regarding nursing informatics will encourage others to become involved in learning about and using these technologies. It is widely known that participation in the design, development, and use of information technology will increase the likelihood that it is accepted (Carroll et al., 2007; Courtney, Demiris, & Alexander, 2005).

Please refer to **Box 3-4** and **Box 3-5** for lists of ways that DNP graduates can use information technology and websites regarding information technology.

Case Scenario: A DNP Graduate Clinician's Experiences with Information Technology

As one can see, information technology can be integrated into the clinical setting in various ways to improve quality and patient outcomes. Dr. A. is a DNP

BOX 3-4

Utilization of Information Technology for DNP Graduates in Clinician Roles

- Use laptops or tablets to access up-to-date information regarding medications, diagnostics, and symptoms.
- Use Internet search engines to access patient information materials.
- Review websites for patients to determine if the most accurate and appropriate information is being relayed.
- Utilize reference librarians at your institution or locally to obtain information technology resources and assist with literature searches.
- Partner with administration to become involved in data mining to evaluate patterns in patient data.
- Provide in-service training to other healthcare professionals regarding information technology.
- Role-model and utilize information technologies in your clinical setting, and share what technologies improve your clinical practice.

BOX 3-5

Websites for Information Technology in Nursing

- Healthcare Information and Management Systems Society (HIMSS) (www.himss.org/ASP/topics_nursinginformatics.asp): This website provides information from the Healthcare Information and Management Systems Society Nursing Informatics Task Force.
- Computers Informatics Nursing (CIN) (www.cinjournal.com): This is the website for the *Computers, Informatics, Nursing* journal.
- Online Journal of Nursing Informatics (www.ojni.org): This is the website for the *Online Journal of Nursing Informatics*.
- Nursing Informatics Online (www.informaticsnurse.com): This website lists informatics nursing jobs and miscellaneous nursing informatics information.
- Nursing Informatics (www.nursinginformatics.com): This website provides information regarding education and continuing education courses about nursing informatics.
- American Nursing Informatics Association (www.ania.org): This is the website for the American Nursing Informatics Association.

graduate nurse practitioner who works in an off-site hospital outpatient setting. Dr. A. utilizes various information technologies throughout his day while seeing patients.

Dr. A. frequently utilizes his hospital reference librarian to obtain new information technologies that are available within his system and in any healthcare setting.

Additionally, when caring for patients, Dr. A. frequently uses a search engine to obtain patient information while patients are in the clinic. Dr. A. believes this empowers patients and provides much-needed information at a time when patients are vulnerable.

Dr. A. also uses a laptop loaded with Epocrates software. He uses Epocrates regularly to check for medication interactions and obtain information about specific diagnoses. In addition, Dr. A. recently upgraded his Epocrates software and can obtain ICD and CPT codes to ensure accurate billing.

Recently Dr. A. became aware of a local home care company that equips its nurses with laptops to document patient care while at the bedside. These home care nurses also have the capability to photograph wounds, upload the photos to the home care secure site, and provide a portal for healthcare professionals to view the photos from the clinical setting. Interestingly, Dr. K., the physician who works with Dr. A., was not interested in sampling this website with the home care agency until Dr. A. convinced him to view the wound photos on the site. Both Dr. A. and Dr. K. now regularly consult this home care company and are able to update the plan of care while they are still in their clinical setting.

Because of the expertise in information technology Dr. A. garnered while in a DNP program, he is comfortable discovering and utilizing new information technologies within his clinical setting. Prior to his DNP program, Dr. A. shared some of the same reluctance many others express with regard to information technologies. However, Dr. A.'s awareness of the IOM's call for improved health care through the utilization of information technologies and the importance of obtaining up-to-date information that is available through information technologies confirmed for him that it is necessary to become comfortable with these technologies.

Interprofessional Collaboration in the Clinical Setting: More Than Just Getting Along

Interprofessional collaboration was discussed previously as it relates to DNP graduates in leadership or potential leadership roles. The current discussion regarding interprofessional collaboration relates specifically to DNP graduates in clinician roles. The recognition that one caregiver alone is unable to support the complexity of current healthcare delivery led to the IOM's recommendation that interprofessional collaboration be included in the educational standards of healthcare professionals in the future (Greiner & Knebel, 2003). Given the additional preparation in this area garnered through a DNP program, the DNP graduate in a clinician role is in a perfect position to influence and exemplify interprofessional collaboration.

Interprofessional collaboration from the clinician's perspective involves more than just getting along with your collaborating physician. The word *collaborate* is derived from the Latin word *collaborare*, which means "to work with one another" (Collaborate, 2004). The ANA has defined collaboration as a partnership with shared power, recognition and acceptance of separate and combined practice spheres of activity and responsibility, mutual safeguarding of the legitimate interests of each party, and a commonality of goals (1995).

The Interprofessional Education Collaborative Expert Panel published a report titled *Core Competencies for Interprofessional Collaborative Practice* (2011). This set of core competencies was supported by various organizations, such as the AACN, American Association of Osteopathic Medicine, American Association of Colleges of Pharmacy, American Dental Education Association, Association of Medical Colleges, and Association of Schools of Public Health. These organizations used the IOM's five core competencies for all healthcare professionals when they developed these core competencies (2011).

The *Core Competencies for Interprofessional Collaborative Practice* are organized into four domains (Interprofessional Education Collaborative Expert Panel, 2011):

- Values–ethics for interprofessional practice
- Roles–responsibilities
- Interprofessional communication
- Teams and teamwork

Within these domains, general and specific competency statements are included to guide proficiency. DNP graduates are encouraged to review the *Core Competencies for Interprofessional Collaborative Practice* because they are pertinent to clinical practice and systems leadership.

Interprofessional collaboration has repeatedly been shown to decrease healthcare costs and improve both quality of care and healthcare outcomes. Cowan and colleagues (2006) found that collaborative relationships between physicians and nurse practitioners reduced hospital length of stay without altering readmissions or mortality. McKay and Crippen (2008) also found that instituting a collaborative practice model decreased length of hospital stay and overall healthcare costs. Schmalenberg and colleagues (2005) also noted that interdisciplinary collaborative relationships between nurses and physicians were linked to improved quality of care. Finally, Knaus, Draper, Wagner, and Zimmerman (1986) reported that when collaborative relationships were present in hospitals, 41% lower mortality occurred than the predicted number of deaths.

Although evidence clearly supports interprofessional collaboration, others have reported barriers. Stein-Parbury and Liaschenko (2007) reported that interprofessional collaboration was hindered when physicians dismissed nurses' knowledge, clinical assessment skills, and concerns about patients. Another frequently noted barrier was lack of recognition regarding other healthcare professionals' roles or knowledge base (Yeager, 2005). The overwhelming solution presented in the literature regarding these barriers was improved communication among healthcare professionals (Gerardi & Fontaine, 2007; McKay & Crippen, 2008; Rossen, Bartlett, & Herrick, 2008; Stein-Parbury & Liaschenko, 2007). Other antecedents to interprofessional collaboration included shared vision among healthcare professionals (Hallas, Butz, & Gitterman, 2004; Yeager, 2005) and trust and respect regarding fellow healthcare professionals' knowledge and expertise (Stein-Parbury & Liaschenko, 2007).

Creating the Bridge: The Challenge for DNP Graduate Clinicians

What does this all mean to the DNP graduate clinician? Although fostering collaboration is related to leadership, one may begin to see how the roles of DNP graduates are truly integrated. The DNP graduate in a clinician role may not be in a formal leadership position; however, the same set of skills is required to promote interdisciplinary collaboration in the clinical setting. These skills will enable DNP graduates in a clinician role to create a bridge between all members of the healthcare team.

Gerardi and Fontaine (2007) described collaboration in relation to the American Association of Critical-Care Nurses publication titled *Standards for Establishing and Sustaining Healthy Work Environments* (2005). Six key components were found to be essential for a healthy work environment, including true collaboration. Gerardi and Fontaine state that "true collaboration is a way of being and a way of working" (2007, p. 10). These are words for DNP graduates to live by. Gerardi and Fontaine also related that true collaboration is a "continuum of engagement" that involves "self-reflection, information sharing, negotiation, feedback, conflict, engagement, conflict resolution, and finally forgiveness and reconciliation" (2007, p. 10).

DNP graduates in clinician roles engage in balancing acts daily when collaborating with other healthcare professionals. Communication techniques that include open listening, understanding multiple perspectives, and developing patient-oriented solutions negotiated together within a team have been repeatedly noted to foster interdisciplinary collaboration (Goleman, Boyatzis, & McKee, 2002; Hamric, Spross, & Hanson, 2005).

Apker, Propp, Zabava Ford, and Hofmeister (2006) explored how nurses communicate professionalism while collaborating with other healthcare team members. These authors noted that displaying professionalism can lead to beneficial outcomes for patients, nurses, and organizations. Moreover, these authors found that four specific types of communication fostered collaboration and enabled nurses to display professionalism. They were named the "Four C's of Professional Nurse

Communication in Health Care Team Interactions" and included collaboration, credibility, compassion, and coordination (2006, p. 183).

Collaboration was further elaborated on as updating team members regularly and preparing appropriately before presenting the information. Nurses who had their ducks in a row when collaborating were viewed as being professional as well. Further, nurses who engaged in dialogue with physicians to identify solutions for problems and shared in decision making also displayed professionalism and effective collaboration.

Credibility was further described as how nurses display their proficiency while collaborating with other healthcare team members. Establishing credibility when collaborating may also reduce barriers to collaboration associated with lack of recognition of team members' knowledge and expertise. Interestingly, nurses who effectively displayed credibility while adjusting their communication style depending on the varied roles, personalities, and situations were viewed as effectively collaborating with other healthcare team members. Terms such as "sensing the environment" and "adapting to the situation" were used to describe nurses who displayed credibility while collaborating (Apker et al., 2006, p. 184). These terms are similar to emotional intelligence competencies that improve communication and leadership.

Compassion was described as showing consideration for all team members, especially those who were considered novices (Apker et al., 2006). Mentoring and demonstrating social support to newer team members were key to displaying professionalism and compassion. Advocacy was another behavior noted to be associated with compassion. Respondents stated that when other team members were advocated for, compassion was displayed. Finally, communication that included an optimistic, supportive, and positive attitude was noted to display compassion (Apker et al., 2006).

The final communication skill set included coordination. The manner in which nurses coordinate healthcare delivery speaks to nurses being the center "hub" of the healthcare team (Apker et al., 2006, p. 185). This communication skill demonstrates the leadership nurses must assume every day when providing care. The ability to coordinate care while collaborating with the healthcare team also demonstrates nursing professionalism.

With regard to DNP graduates, Apker and colleagues' work (2006) describes valuable insights for collaboration and professionalism in nursing. DNP graduates have earned the terminal degree in their field. Therefore, demonstrating professionalism through effective collaboration is vital to their success in every role they assume.

Realizing that "true collaboration is a way of being" (Gerardi & Fontaine, 2007, p. 10) will enable DNP graduates to successfully build bridges among all healthcare disciplines. Knowing how to effectively communicate while collaborating will enable

BOX 3-6

Tips for Building Bridges among Healthcare Disciplines

- Respect the knowledge and expertise of other members of the healthcare team in the clinical setting.

- Frequently seek out input and feedback from other members of the healthcare team, especially members in other disciplines.

- Provide accurate and complete information when discussing patients or patient care issues with members of the healthcare team.

- Organize team meetings with members of the healthcare team to focus on new treatment guidelines and EBP.

- Communicate effectively by utilizing active listening, compassion, and empathy.

- Use emotional intelligence competencies to accurately assess the needs of the healthcare team and feel the room's emotional environment.

- Mentor new team members and provide social support through compassion and empathy.

DNP graduates to effectively collaborate and build bridges among healthcare disciplines. Building these bridges will facilitate interprofessional collaboration and enable DNP graduates to continually improve quality and healthcare outcomes in an ever-changing, complex healthcare environment. Please refer to **Box 3-6** for bridge-building tips.

Case Scenarios of Interprofessional Collaboration

The following case scenarios describe two types of interprofessional collaboration: one in which the DNP graduate is unsuccessful in building a collaborative relationship and one in which the DNP graduate experiences interprofessional collaboration.

CASE SCENARIO 1: AN ATTEMPT TO BUILD A BRIDGE

Dr. L. is a new graduate from a BSN-to-DNP program. His experience with collaboration involves working with physicians in a small rural emergency room (ER) setting. His specialization in his DNP program prepared him to become certified as an acute care clinical nurse specialist. Upon graduating, Dr. L. took a position as an ER nurse practitioner and began working with the same healthcare team he previously worked with.

Early on, Dr. L. attempted to develop a grand rounds program in the ER that would include case presentations with input from all disciplines in the ER setting, including pharmacy, nursing, and medicine. Unfortunately, this idea was met with much resistance from the ER staff physicians. Additionally, when attempting to collaborate with the physicians regarding patient care, Dr. L. was treated poorly and was frequently questioned in an accusatory fashion when he suggested different evidence-based treatments. Dr. L. overheard staff physicians making statements such as, "Who does he think he is recommending this treatment?" The medical staff treated him disrespectfully in front of other staff members and patients. As a result, the nursing staff did not exhibit trust in his abilities.

Dr. L. approached the nurse manager of the ER and was again met with resistance regarding additional educational programs for the staff. Instead of the physicians and nurse manager providing mentoring, Dr. L. was left to fend for himself. Hospital administration offered no assistance and did not have previous experience dealing with the issues related to advanced nursing practice. Eventually Dr. L. left the hospital and relocated to work in a large university setting with other APRNs. Dr. L. felt he would get the support and mentoring he needed to grow as an APRN and a valued member of the healthcare team. Sadly, the small rural hospital lost a DNP graduate who attempted to improve quality of care and patient outcomes through collaboration.

CASE SCENARIO 2: A BRIDGE BUILT

Dr. N. is a DNP graduate working as a nurse–midwife in a university-affiliated outpatient clinic. Dr. N. began to notice that she had been caring for an increasing number of patients who had previously undergone bariatric surgery and are now pregnant. Upon doing a literature search to obtain information regarding caring for this unique population, Dr. N. noted that there was a paucity of EBP guidelines available pertaining to pregnant postbariatric surgery patients.

Dr. N. took the first step to integrating EBP and asked a question: What are the increased risks to both mother and baby when the mother has had bariatric surgery? Dr. N. requested a grand rounds meeting with the departments of obstetrics, surgery, and dietary. She contacted her reference librarian, who provided her with literature regarding bariatric surgery and postsurgical complications, including risks that persist well after surgery. Dr. N. also contacted the information technology department, and with their assistance she was able to arrange a satellite meeting with another teaching institution that had recently begun a clinical trial involving pregnant patients who had previously undergone bariatric surgery.

The grand rounds meeting was well attended by nursing, medicine, obstetrics, surgery, and dietary. Many questions were raised regarding how to care for this population, including how to address their unique nutritional needs. The team initiated steps to develop a research program in their institution, and Dr. N. was able to actively participate in this endeavor. Dr. N. used the knowledge she had garnered in her DNP program to integrate EBP, utilize information technologies, and build a bridge between disciplines. This process had started with her simply asking a question while caring for a patient.

A Personal Note: Interprofessional Collaboration Improving Practice

As stated earlier in this chapter, I practice in a comprehensive breast center within an National Cancer Institute–certified cancer center in a clinic called the Women's Wellness Clinic (WWC). My practice includes assessing and diagnosing patients who have a new breast concern. I also care for breast cancer survivors, patients with elevated risk for developing breast cancer, and patients with benign breast problems. My practice depends on breast imaging and related modalities, such as breast biopsy. Therefore, the breast imaging specialists (radiologists) are located within the comprehensive breast center in an embedded reading room. The diagnostic imaging equipment and technicians are also located within the comprehensive breast center. This allows for seamless care and a wonderful opportunity for interprofessional collaboration.

The radiologists and I are colleagues and discuss patient care multiple times per day. My practice depends on these relationships and this type of care. As a result, I can assess a new patient in the comprehensive breast center and order the appropriate breast imaging; then the patient has the testing done within the center. The radiologists and I review the imagery, and I discuss the findings with the patient. If needed, the patient will then proceed to biopsy within the center and return 1 week later so we can discuss the findings from pathology. This type of model results in seamless care and improved patient satisfaction (Gagliardi, Grunfeld, & Evans, 2004; Gui et al., 1995; Searles & Mecklenburg, 2013).

Through close collaboration between the WWC and the radiologists, another program has been developed by the Department of Radiology. If a patient undergoes a breast biopsy within the center, that patient is scheduled to see a nurse practitioner in the WWC 1 week later to discuss the results and receive a referral for further treatment if necessary. This eliminates the risk that the pathology results are not communicated to the patient from the referring provider, and it expedites care. This program is a quality initiative that depends on interprofessional collaboration between the WWC and radiology.

Finally, Dr. Sharon Helmer (director of breast imaging), Dr. Morris Magnan (PhD-prepared clinical nurse specialist from this center), and I have collaborated on a publication describing the model we use to provide seamless, interprofessional care within this center. This article describes the process the WWC uses to provide care with the radiologists acting as expert consultants. At the time of this writing, the article is in press for the *Journal of Interprofessional Care*.

Mentoring: DNP Graduates Shaping the Future of Clinician Roles

Mentor has been defined as a trusted counselor or guide (McKinley, 2004; Mentor, 2004). The term originated in Greek mythology and refers to Odysseus's trusted counselor, who became his son Telemachus's teacher (Mentor, 2004). Odysseus entrusted the care of his son to Mentor while he went to fight in the Trojan War. Mentor's job was not just to teach Telemachus, but also to help him develop as a man and prepare him for the responsibilities he would assume (McKinley, 2004). In the professional realm, mentoring involves helping others achieve goals and offering support in a nonthreatening way. Hence, the clinical setting is an ideal place for DNP graduates to mentor and shape the future of nursing.

DNP Graduates: From Experts to Novices and Back to Experts

Mentoring involves the mentor having a certain level of expertise. A discussion about expertise and mentoring would not be complete without mentioning Patricia Benner's book *From Novice to Expert* (1984). Dr. Benner's work is derived from the Dreyfus Model of Skill Acquisition. This model posits that while developing a set of skills, one progresses through five levels of proficiency: novice, advanced beginner, competent, proficient, and expert (Benner, 1982; Dreyfus & Dreyfus, 1980). Dr. Benner has purported that these levels of skill development may be used to describe how nurses develop proficiency as experts. Dr. Benner's premise was that experience results in expertise. Nurses begin their careers as novices and move through the levels by gaining experience in the clinical setting. Expertise has been characterized as knowing the vision of what is possible (Benner, 1982). In other words, knowing the goals and possible outcomes from an expert's interventions is what allows a nurse to move from proficiency to expertise.

By definition, DNP graduates are in a position of expertise. DNP graduates are acutely aware of the goals of healthcare delivery and various interventions to improve these goals. However, many of the new skills that are introduced (or reinforced) to DNP graduates place them in the position of novice after spending perhaps years in the position of expert. Concepts such as EBP, information technologies, leadership skills, interprofessional collaboration, and research methodology may be less familiar to many DNP graduates who may be functioning at high levels of expertise in the clinical setting. Therefore, garnering newer, sophisticated skills in a DNP program may make many DNP graduates feel less like experts and more like novices.

Despite this, many DNP graduates will find themselves in the role of mentor. However, the wealth of clinical expertise many DNP graduates possess may allow them to move from novice to expert quite easily. The new skills DNP graduates garner in their programs are integrated into their nursing practice. Further, the skills acquired in a DNP program enable graduates to develop an enlarged view of healthcare delivery and design ways to improve healthcare outcomes, which will foster expertise in nursing practice. Dracup and Bryan-Brown relate that "the expert has gone beyond the tasks and responds to the whole picture" (2004, p. 449). DNP graduates are well beyond the tasks of nursing and are able to envision the whole picture.

The Robert Wood Johnson Foundation Executive Nurse Fellows program has identified five competencies that are essential for mentoring (Thomas & Herrin, 2008). These competencies may be related to ways in which DNP graduates increase their level of expertise and eventually provide mentoring. The first competency is the ability to translate a strategic vision into a motivating message. Each time a DNP graduate expresses why he or she returned to school for a DNP degree, a strategic vision is shared, which serves to motivate others. This author is often told that she has inspired others to return to school either for nursing or for a graduate degree in nursing.

The second competency is risk taking and creativity. Again, earning a new, innovative degree demonstrates risk taking and creativity. Further, the ability to complete a research project that is grounded in clinical practice displays creativity.

The third competency is the ability to understand and develop oneself with regard to self-knowledge and individual motivation. DNP graduates are challenged through their DNP programs to know themselves and their individual motivation, as well as their own personal leadership styles. The choice to earn a DNP degree illustrates awareness of the need for additional knowledge to meet the changing demands of health care. Further, the additional leadership skills they garner enable DNP graduates to develop awareness regarding their own strengths and weaknesses. DNP graduates are experts at knowing what they do not know and discovering ways to enrich their knowledge base.

The fourth competency is inspiring and leading change. DNP graduates will be leaders regardless of their area of expertise. They will be called on to inspire and guide others in times of change.

The final competency is effective communication and interpersonal effectiveness. DNP graduates will mentor through their ability to engage in mutual and equal relationships. Many DNP graduates have had previous experiences that involved hierarchical relationships with other healthcare professionals. These experiences will serve to remind DNP graduates that successful mentoring relationships are built on empathy, compassion, respect, and nurturing behaviors. Therefore, DNP graduates will have sensitivity regarding what type of mentoring relationship is mutual and equal.

Precepting: The Ideal Opportunity to Mentor

For the DNP graduate in a clinical setting, precepting is often integrated into the clinical role. Precepting is a time-limited commitment that evolves into a teaching-learning relationship between student and preceptor. However, "mentoring is more than just training or precepting" (McKinley, 2004, p. 207). Mentoring has been described as a way to assist in human development, where one invests time, energy, and personal knowledge to enable another to grow and develop (McKinley, 2004). Although precepting differs from mentoring, precepting offers a perfect opportunity for DNP graduates in clinical settings to become mentors.

Hayes (1998) studied the stories of students who felt they had experienced a mentoring relationship with their clinical preceptor. Specific descriptors were cited by the students related to their experiences. These descriptors included the following: a vested interest in the student; a love for teaching; openness; friendship; trust; acting as a life jacket; patience; sharing job advice; and role-modeling kind, empathetic, competent patient care (Hayes, 1998). These characteristics mirror many leadership attributes. Further, when they think of a teacher, preceptor, or clinical instructor who inspired, led, and truly made a difference in their lives, many DNP graduates recall similar experiences. Hence, self-reflection, previous experiences, and the skills garnered in a DNP program will enable DNP graduates to seize the opportunity to build mentoring relationships in the clinical setting.

McKinley (2004) wrote about mentoring in nursing and related three steps to the mentoring process that may foster successful mentoring relationships both in and out of the clinical setting: reflecting, reframing, and resolving. Reflecting involves the creation of the relationship (McKinley, 2004). This includes sharing personal information to build common ground and discussing the goals of the relationship. DNP graduates in a preceptor role may share their personal journeys in nursing as a way to inspire and guide. Also, DNP graduates may ask students what their expectations are for the semester and share what they hope to accomplish while teaching. This author often advises students she precepts to ask all the silly questions, not just questions about clinical scenarios. Frequently questions about certification, relationships with staff, and how to interview for a job are cited among the most valuable pointers students received during a clinical rotation.

Reframing encourages connecting and allows the mentor to challenge the student (McKinley, 2004). DNP graduates may use their broadened knowledge base about information technologies to encourage students to look outside the box for information. This may also be done by challenging students to integrate EBP when developing a plan of care. At this time the DNP graduate may demonstrate these skills to the student and reinforce learning in an ongoing process. Melnyk and colleagues (2004) found that EBP increased with mentorship from others who utilize EBP. These behaviors strengthen the relationship between mentor and student and allow the student to grow (McKinley, 2004). Resolving involves the mentor empowering the student to develop solutions (McKinley, 2004). This is when the foundation built by reflection and reframing is put into action. The DNP graduate allows the student to examine the options and consequences of the options. Previously it was mentioned that expertise means knowing the vision of what is possible

(Benner, 1982). DNP graduates may have experienced this type of learning from mentors while acquiring new skills in their DNP programs. These experiences will allow DNP graduates to let the students own their solutions. This process is similar to DNP graduates developing and owning their solutions through their own evidence-based research projects—a process that came to fruition through the mentoring they once received.

A Word about Scholarship

The DNP-prepared clinician most assuredly has a very complex role. DNP-prepared clinicians may also blend additional roles, much like this author. The challenge lies in integrating scholarship into these roles. The DNP degree may open the clinician's eyes and be their springboard to scholarship. DNP graduates' perspectives will change and their views will be broadened. Therefore, scholarship may be the avenue to share this enhanced perspective and broadened view with the discipline of nursing and the world. DNP-prepared clinicians have a responsibility to maintain scholarship as it applies to their clinical practice or other areas of interest.

Conclusion

The ways in which DNP graduates may shape the future of nursing through mentoring are numerous (please refer to **Box 3-7**). In the clinical setting DNP graduates are in the forefront of health care and therefore in a position to improve quality and healthcare outcomes. Mentoring new nurses, APRNs, and other healthcare professionals will ensure that the DNP graduates' focus on improved healthcare delivery will be a priority of the future of nursing practice.

BOX 3-7

Tips for DNP Graduates Mentoring in the Clinical Setting

- Express an interest in students personally.
- Share personal experiences, especially personal setbacks or failures.
- Express a love for teaching.
- Stay open to ideas, input, and suggestions.
- Be willing to give advice about jobs, interviewing, and creating good staff relations.
- Role-model empathetic and compassionate patient care.
- Motivate students to have a vision, especially a vision of themselves when they complete their degree.

(continues)

BOX 3-7 (continued)

- Challenge students to come up with their own solutions and empower them to own their solutions.
- Allow students to be wrong, and give constructive, noncritical feedback when they are wrong.
- Create opportunities to be creative and utilize EBP or information technology to develop solutions.
- Role-model effective interdisciplinary collaboration by demonstrating or role-playing the discussion of care with other disciplines.

Interviews with DNP Clinicians

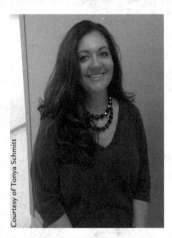

Courtesy of Tonya Schmitt

The following interviews with DNP students and graduates provide invaluable insight from practicing clinicians.

PERSPECTIVE OF A PEDIATRIC NURSE PRACTITIONER IN A CARDIAC TRANSPLANT DEPARTMENT

Tonya Schmitt, MS, APRN, BC, is a pediatric nurse practitioner and DNP student at the University of Michigan.

Ms. Schmitt, could you please describe your current position?

I am a pediatric nurse practitioner working in a cardiac transplant department, the Division of Cardiovascular Surgery. I have recently transitioned into this role after 12 years of working in a primary care setting. My role involves direct patient care in an ambulatory setting and the coordination of services for pediatric transplant patients, both inpatient and outpatient. This role requires a mesh of clinical and administrative functions, perfect for a DNP-prepared nurse practitioner! The curriculum from my DNP program has provided me with a strong foundation to transition into this new clinical area.

With my new role have come new challenges. I find myself learning to navigate the healthcare system with a completely different focus. I am now involved in hospital policy and process development as well as quality and patient safety initiatives. It is exciting to be part of program development; it gives me a chance to apply evidence-based nursing to my everyday work. It is also a chance for me to express to hospital administration that nursing professionals do contribute scholarly work.

Ms. Schmitt, what made you decide to return to school to earn your DNP degree?

The decision to embark on this DNP journey came after a great deal of reflection and prayer. The future of my career as a pediatric nurse practitioner was dependent upon the decision I would make. As I was entering what I consider to be the second half of my career, I realized the importance of advancing my education now. I needed to reflect on my previous accomplishments and set new career goals. I felt that if I stayed in my current role I would feel stifled and have little opportunity for growth and career advancement.

The DNP seemed to align with my desire to remain committed to clinical practice and the advancement of nursing. I wanted to enrich my critical thinking skills and learn what it means to be a nursing leader. I am hopeful that advanced leadership skills will help me to be a voice for nursing and advocate for the profession.

Further motivation for the DNP degree comes from my interest in the advancement of evidence-based practice. I believe that the nursing research is crucial to the development of best-practice guidelines and safe patient care outcomes. I believe that attaining a terminal degree in the field of nursing will help me with the professional development needed to become more involved in nursing research.

Ms. Schmitt, as a DNP student, how do you think your degree will impact your practice as a pediatric nurse practitioner?

The DNP program has already enhanced my professional growth as a pediatric nurse practitioner. I have had the opportunity to apply newly gained knowledge to my clinical practice. For instance, I have worked with the director of quality and safety to use information technology to improve staff communication and increase patient safety outcomes. I have also been involved in the development of hospital system clinical practice guidelines and policy development.

As a DNP-prepared pediatric nurse practitioner, I will work very hard to be an expert in my field of practice. I feel that I have an obligation to nursing to lead by example. The DNP degree will prepare me do this by giving me the skills necessary to evaluate, interpret, and implement evidence-based nursing research into clinical practice.

Ms. Schmitt, how do you feel your perspective is changing as a DNP student?

Since starting the DNP program my perspective of nursing and the future of the profession has evolved. I am beginning to see much clearer now the value of advanced education and the advantage of the DNP role in clinical practice. Initially I was focused on the way in which the advanced degree would benefit me personally; now I see things on a much larger scale.

I recognize the way nursing can impact health care at systems level. For example, with the enactment of the healthcare reform act, doctoral-prepared advanced-practice nurses have an opportunity to make significant contributions to the progression of health care. As many Americans find themselves navigating the healthcare arena, nurse practitioners will be at the forefront providing safe quality care.

I feel it is important to mention that after working with a DNP student, many of my physician colleagues and hospital administrators have changed their perspective of the doctoral-prepared nurses. They recognize the value of having a DNP on their team and encourage me as I continue with my program. As an advanced-practice nurse at the Detroit Medical Center, I feel my contributions to health care are validated. I am greatly supported by both management and the chief of our department, Dr. Henry Walters III. I foresee a future of interdisciplinary collaboration regarding research and patient care guidelines.

Ms. Schmitt, what are your goals for the next 5 years after obtaining your DNP degree?

Upon completion of the DNP program I hope to utilize my degree in my current role as a transplant coordinator. I am dedicated to the ongoing advancement of this hospital becoming a cardiac transplant center of excellence. I am also interested in future research surrounding adolescent heart transplant and the transition to adult care. In the future I would like to develop a research based, theory-driven protocol surrounding this topic. I am hopeful that this research will benefit other hospitals nationally and provide solid guidelines for practitioners.

In addition to my work in the heart transplant center, I would like to explore an opportunity within nursing administration. I am particularly interested in developing a role for a director of advanced-practice nurses. I feel it would be beneficial to have a clinical director to advocate for advanced-practice nurses at our medical center.

Ms. Schmitt, do you have any advice for other clinicians regarding returning to school to earn a DNP degree?

I would encourage future students to take their time when choosing a program. It is beneficial to investigate all your academic options. Make sure that your personal goals relate to the vision and mission of the program you chose. I would also suggest that students make sure that the timing is right to return to school! The DNP program is rigorous and will demand a great deal of time. It is important to have the support of your family and friends; you will rely on them for encouragement and strength when you are experiencing a low moment.

I think students need to understand that doctoral education is not an extension of your master's program. The program is meant to enhance your overall clinical practice and prepare you to be an expert in your clinical field. As a new student it is also important to communicate closely with your academic advisor and faculty; do not be afraid to ask for clarity and direction. Do not be discouraged when you fall short of the goal. Learn from your errors and push forward.

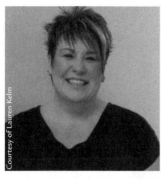

Courtesy of Lauren Kelm

PERSPECTIVE OF A PEDIATRIC NURSE PRACTITIONER IN ACUTE CARE

Lauren Kelm, MSN, APRN, CCRN, BC, is a pediatric nurse practitioner and DNP student at Madonna University.

Ms. Kelm, could you please describe your current position?

I am a pediatric nurse practitioner with an extensive background in pediatric acute care and intensive care. Recently I decided to make a transition to the Division of Cardiovascular Surgery as a pediatric cardiac transplant coordinator. The role is quite different than the role of an acute care NP [nurse practitioner] in a critical care setting. In addition to caring for acute care transplant patients, I now must utilize my knowledge of caring for children with chronic conditions, provide anticipatory guidance, and coordinate an extensive group of pediatric specialists involved in the care of transplant patients. I manage all immunosuppression related to our patients. I am actively involved in program and policy review, quality and safety initiatives, and research within the department.

Because of my love for teaching, I am also employed as part-time clinical faculty for the acute care PNP [pediatric nurse practitioner] program at a major urban university. I am responsible for placement of students in their clinical assignments and provide feedback to students using a clinical database when evaluating their clinical coursework.

Ms. Kelm, what made you decide to return to school to earn your DNP degree?

I am the girl who received the calling to be a nurse. I had never been sick, had never been in the hospital, or had a sick family member. However, it was something I just needed to do. After working many years as a nurse at the bedside in critical care, I was determined to return to school to advance my practice. After completing my master's degree as a pediatric nurse practitioner, I was hired directly back into my PICU [pediatric intensive care unit] as one of the first nurse practitioners to work for the critical care medicine team at my institution. I was thrilled to achieve this role, and it was a natural transition for me. I was a leader on the unit, and I was received with open arms by my critical care colleagues as an advanced-practice nurse. In addition to clinical care, I was involved in many quality and safety initiatives in the PICU. I developed many educational programs and was actively involved in critical care research. My work was being recognized by hospital administrators, yet I felt I was not yet advancing the discipline of nursing with my small contribution. My desire to return for my DNP was formulated before I even finished my master's program. There was no question that I would return for my DNP. I am eager to continue my contribution to nursing . . . as a leader . . . a researcher . . . an educator . . . and as a role model for new nurses entering this amazing profession.

Ms. Kelm, as a DNP student, how do you think your degree will impact your practice as a pediatric nurse practitioner?

The courses that I have completed thus far in my DNP program have made a significant impact in my practice as a pediatric cardiac transplant coordinator. After just several weeks in this new position, I was able to recognize many quality and safety concerns, workflow disruption, and major communication and infrastructure concerns. I have been working diligently with my partner (who is also working to obtain her DNP) on process improvement projects, policy creation, and changes in our department healthcare information technology.

Ms. Kelm, how do you feel your perspective is changing as a DNP student?

As a DNP student, I am now able to see nursing as a much larger discipline, one involving hospital systems, quality improvement, healthcare informatics, policy, and academia. I feel I am developing the skills necessary to incorporate all of these areas into my daily practice and make significant contributions to my workplace. I feel much more comfortable using evidence-based literature to guide my practice and work closely with my physician colleagues and nursing leaders to implement change.

Ms. Kelm, what are your goals for the next 5 years after obtaining your DNP degree?

In addition to my role as a pediatric cardiac transplant coordinator, I hope to continue my work in research, the education of students, and projects involving process improvement. I hope to become more proficient in healthcare informatics, meaningful use, and data mining. This is an educational area I feel is not fully studied until the DNP level. I also feel it is necessary to become actively involved in my national organizations and speak publically at national conferences about the work we are doing in my institution.

Ms. Kelm, do you have any advice for other clinicians regarding returning to school to earn a DNP degree?

Research multiple DNP programs and speak with their faculty. It is important to find the program that fits well with your personal philosophy and educational objectives. Though the content of these programs must incorporate the DNP essentials, each program is a bit unique in its educational content. Interview current students regarding their likes and dislikes of each program. While in school, try not to get overwhelmed by coursework assignments. Set small goals to achieve as you progress through larger projects. Budget your time as you balance your work and your courses. Take time for yourself and your family.

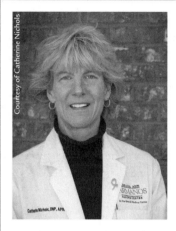

Courtesy of Catherine Nichols

PERSPECTIVE OF A DNP-PREPARED NURSE PRACTITIONER

Catherine Nichols, DNP, APRN, BC, is a nurse practitioner.

Dr. Nichols, could you please describe your educational background and current position?

Nursing is actually a second career for me. I received a bachelor's degree in communications, and journalism was my initial bachelor's degree, and I worked in radio for several years. I had a major life change of mind and heart, and I wanted to contribute to society in a different manner. It was then I decided to become a nurse. I went back to school in an accelerated BSN [bachelor of science in nursing] program at Wayne State University, and I went on to receive an MSN [master of science in nursing] in the Adult Nurse Practitioner program. I continued my nursing education with my pursuit of a doctorate in nursing practice form Madonna University, and I currently practice as a nurse practitioner at the Women's Wellness Clinic in the Walt Breast Clinic at Karmanos Cancer Institute in Detroit. I am privileged to practice at Karmanos as it is one of only 41 designated National Cancer Institutes in the United States. My practice consists of diagnosing breast cancer, treating benign and malignant breast disease, and treating cancer survivors throughout their lifetime recovery. I also treat women with menopausal and women's specific health needs.

Dr. Nichols, what motivated you to return to school to earn a DNP degree?

When I was an undergrad in the BSN program, as a second career student, I was dumb-founded to learn of the fragmentation of the nursing profession. The lack of educational and practice standards for nursing across the board was incredible to me.

It was at this early stage in my nursing career that I knew I needed to further my education to not only develop excellence in my personal practice, but to become an advocate and voice for the unity and pursuit of excellence and standardization of the nursing profession. The pursuit of excellence is embodied in the doctor of nursing practice. The DNP is just one way nursing can unify and use its collective voice to act as a key agent in guiding, developing, and leading our profession as well as our nation's healthcare delivery methods.

Dr. Nichols, could you describe your experience in a DNP program?

Obtaining a DNP was one of the most challenging and rewarding experiences of my life.

I obtained my DNP at Madonna University. I selected that university, first, because of its Christian foundations, second, because of the unique curriculum, and third, because of its adaptability with my full-time position as an NP. Madonna's DNP program is one-half on-campus didactic program, and one-half online, offering flexibility for the practicing APRN. Because of its unique nature, Madonna attracts students from all over the country. My cohort included a student from Canada. I was fortunate to have the opportunity to develop a network of colleagues from a vast array of practices and practice sites, and I was able to broaden my vision of nursing and our healthcare delivery system because of the exposure to that wonderful cohort. The DNP program challenged me to expand my view of nursing and was a catalyst for ongoing research and education.

Dr. Nichols, how do you think the DNP has impacted your role as a clinician?

The DNP vision broadens my clinical vision and empowers me to practice on a level on par with my fellow colleagues. I believe the DNP has changed my colleagues' perceptions of my current clinical role and has ushered in a more collaborating and reciprocal relationship.

I believe the DNP has facilitated a view as a colleague and collaborating consultant to many of my collegial physicians and other advanced-practice clinicians. Interprofessional collaboration is key to the success of all health care, and it is essential in my particular arena of oncology. The DNP has also revolutionized my systems thinking and has improved the quality and productivity of my personal practice as I am able to navigate patient and healthcare systems with newfound expertise.

Dr. Nichols, how has your view of nursing as a discipline and a practice changed since earning a DNP degree?

The process of acquiring a DNP resulted in a clearer vision of the discipline of nursing. It brought me back to the roots of nursing as an independent discipline. This vision has had a huge impact on my understanding of the power and value nursing can offer, from the bedside to the boardroom. We, as nurses, are the largest workforce division in health care, and we have the potential to change our current healthcare system and the provision of quality healthcare delivery in this country.

Before earning a DNP, I never fully owned the nursing profession or grasped the totality of the knowledge, depth, and breadth that nursing can bring to health care as an independent discipline. After experiencing a DNP education, I not only proudly own nursing as the invaluable discipline it is, but I see health care through new eyes. This new vision has impacted my practice with the knowledge and skills only an APRN can provide in guiding, directing, and treating both acute and chronic diseases amid the complexity of our healthcare system. Navigating the intricate and often confusing healthcare system is a barrier to patient care, and the DNP has given me the tools and systems understanding to help break those barriers for my patients. Practicing as an APRN, fully embracing nursing, facilitates a much broader and holistic and effective approach to the care of all my patients.

The DNP provides me with a vehicle through which I can actively and effectively be involved in health care and patient advocacy groups to affect change both within the nursing profession and in my own environment. The DNP has changed my perspective of nursing and health care from one within the context of a current setting to seeing my piece of care delivery as part of an overall whole of interprofessional collaboration of care and systems.

Dr. Nichols, would you encourage other advanced-practice registered nurses to return to school for a DNP degree? If so, why?

The answer is resoundingly yes!

As I went through the DNP program I became acutely aware that we are far more than just nurses. Gone are the days of nursing as a servant to other disciplines. The DNP has given me a clear vision of the discipline of nursing. We can no longer remain silent, waiting for direction from other disciplines, but we must speak collectively as nurses to become powerful change agents in health care.

Moreover, as APRNs we need not only a unifying degree for our profession, but parity with our clinical colleagues in physical therapy, occupational therapy, audiology, and pharmacy, who have adopted a doctoral degree as educational options or requirements for practice. The DNP is the unifying answer to our fragmented history of multiple degrees and preparation for practice. It is an answer to the nation's critical lack of primary care providers and delivery of quality health care. The DNP is the answer to the age-old question, What is an advanced-practice nurse, and how is that different from a PA [physician assistant] or MD? It answers the accusation, Why don't you just become a doctor? I am a doctor . . . of nursing practice, and I am first and foremost a nurse.

Dr. Nichols, what are your goals for the next 5 years related to nursing and nursing practice?

A main goal is to be an advocate for the nursing profession on several fronts.

My first goal is to champion new APRNs in their pursuit of excellence in obtaining the DNP for the unification of our profession and to deliver the highest quality of nursing care possible, and to be a change agent in our nation's healthcare system. I am engaging in this goal now as a clinical preceptor of NP students at various universities. This affords me the opportunity to guide, teach, and empower new APRNs in the DNP direction.

My second goal is to continue my doctoral research and dissemination concerning the utilization of DNPs in clinical settings and their effect on the quality of healthcare outcomes and healthcare system impacts. I began this research as my capstone project, surveying

CNOs [chief nursing officers] from Michigan's public and teaching hospitals. The study has been published in the Journal of Nursing Administration *(February 2014) as an early exploration in this area. I plan to continue this research with the CNOs already surveyed because of an initial low response rate, and because of the general lack of knowledge about DNPs and our degree and talents. I also plan to access DNPs through APRN and DNP organizations to determine how and in what manner they are utilized in their healthcare environments. The dissemination of this research will be invaluable to educational and practice standards of the DNP.*

My third goal is to be a coach, teacher, and guide to aspiring nurses on every level, and to encourage ownership and pursuit of nursing as the professional discipline it is. I am pursuing this as a mentor to nurses and APRNs in my institution and plan to continue mentoring and teaching at a university level. Encouraging love, pride, and commitment to our discipline is the foundation of nursing practice on every level, and I plan to foster that love in as many aspiring nurses as I can.

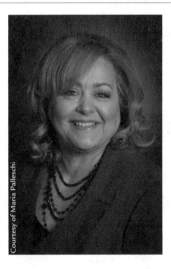

Courtesy of Maria Palleschi

PERSPECTIVE OF AN ADVANCED PRACTICE NURSE PRACTITIONER IN A LEADERSHIP ROLE

Maria Palleschi, DNP, APRN-BC, CCRN, is a nurse practitioner.

Dr. Palleschi, could you please describe your educational background and current position?

I graduated with a diploma from Harper Hospital School of Nursing in 1977, went on to receive my BSN in 1992 and MSN in 1996 from Wayne State University, and my DNP in 2012 from Madonna University. I worked at Harper University Hospital in critical care as a staff RN, charge nurse, and preceptor from 1977–1996, at which time I became the critical care clinical nurse specialist (CNS). For the first 18 months as an APRN, I was placed on a project that standardized critical care across the four adult Detroit Medical Center hospitals. This project, led by a consultant firm, shaped my vision for critical care. During the project I learned to value the financial aspect of health care and the rigor necessary to facilitate evidence-based change across a service line. I helped facilitate 13 work groups that developed standards for mechanical ventilation, nutrition, infection control, pressure ulcer prevention and management, as well as vascular and neurosurgical pathways.

Early in my APRN career I was responsible for the medical intensive care unit and the surgical intensive care unit. For the past 5 years I have been covering all four of the intensive care units, including neuroscience and cardiovascular. The CNS position is challenging, and every day brings something new. I am the APRN advisor for the hospital and unit-based critical care shared governance councils as well as unit-based performance improvement. I have many roles from the unit, hospital, system, and enterprise position. From a system perspective, Dr. Safwan Badr and I cochair the DMC Critical Care Committee. This interprofessional committee implements strategies and policy from the Tenet Critical Care Committee, of which I am a member. From an enterprise perspective, I serve as the chair of a number of work groups, including seda-tion, mobility, and pressure ulcer. I am the site chair for sepsis and serve as a member for the Tenet Sepsis Committee. I am also site lead for the Surviving Sepsis Campaign acute care collaborative. Sinai-Grace and Harper University Hospital are the only two hospitals in Michigan on the national collaborative. My role is very complex and would take a few pages (or days) to describe. My responsibilities span across all APRN role components, from clinical rounding daily with the intensivist team to a leadership role for the entire nursing staff.

Dr. Palleschi, what motivated you to return to school to earn a DNP degree?

In retrospect, I didn't even consider the 14-year gap since graduating from Wayne State before starting my DNP. Most APRNs do not wait very long to further their education. I think my family, working in an academic center, maintaining my certification in critical care, and all the committee projects kept me busy enough that I didn't consider returning to school. My motivation to return to school was totally internal. I felt the need, the itch, to go back to school and obtain my doctorate. My children were out of the house and I had some time to invest in myself again. I wanted to do more research and further expand my portfolio. I thought that earning my DNP would prepare me for the future and provide me an opportunity to teach. Also, having a peer in the program helped push me to make the decision. Dr. Sue Sirianni started in the program the year before I did and encouraged me to return to earn a DNP degree. We ended up doing our capstone research together on sepsis across four hospitals in the Detroit Medical Center.

Dr. Palleschi, could you describe your experience in a DNP program?

My experience was very positive. I was one of 15 students in my DNP cohort. The full-time program afforded students the opportunity to graduate in 2 years. Not many of my peers reached that goal, but I really pushed to finish in 2 years. Madonna University faculty mem-bers are all very caring, compassionate, and intelligent people. I think the Madonna program is exceptional and should be a model for all DNP programs. Unlike some DNP programs,

Madonna's is strictly based on the DNP essentials and incorporates them into each class and assignment. The classroom and online structure supported me to learn in an environment that suited my lifestyle and work schedule. The course work was intense and invigorating.

Dr. Palleschi, how do you think the DNP has impacted your role as a clinician?

I think I am more of a global and enterprise thinker. I am able to articulate the impact of healthcare policy on the local hospital system. I am able to apply the evidence and technology to design systems that will improve patient outcomes for conditions such as sepsis. I also think that the system and hospital leadership value my doctoral preparation and often acknowledge the accomplishment. I think having a DNP made me more credible as a clinician and leader to the staff and physicians.

Dr. Palleschi, how has your view of nursing as a discipline and a practice changed since earning a DNP degree?

I think my view has remained that nursing is integral to superior patient outcomes. Without substantial nursing care, health promotion, restoration, and patient comfort are impacted. What has changed is my view is the role the nurse plays in interprofessional relationships. Coordination of care is essential to providing high quality care. I think nurses must learn to be active participants and lead interprofessional teams to initiate, incorporate, and monitor change. Team members who work together efficiently and collaboratively facilitate the best patient outcomes. My vision is to empower and nurture nurses to lead teams and engage physicians and providers in an effort to improve communication. I think communication and processes that support communication among team members foster an environment of high reliability.

Dr. Palleschi, would you encourage other advanced-practice registered nurses to return to school for a DNP degree? Why or why not?

I encourage staff every day to continue their education and advance to a DNP degree. I think it is imperative for nursing that we continue to further our advancement through research and embrace a more collaborative approach to patient care.

Dr. Palleschi, what are your goals for the next 5 years related to nursing and nursing practice?

I hope to continue to mentor and motivate nurses to transform their practice into a more collaborative one where they can work together and strive for excellence with other healthcare professionals. I want to have a larger practice role in the corporate environment, whether with Tenet or another healthcare system. I plan on doing more research on sepsis, mobility, and sleep in the ICU.

Why a DNP for Clinicians?

In the beginning of the chapter, the question was posed, How will the clinician's role change or benefit from earning a DNP degree? After a discussion regarding the many aspects of the DNP graduates' role as clinician, it is this author's anticipation that a broader understanding has developed. Many readers will turn to this section to discover why clinicians should seek a DNP degree. As a DNP graduate who finished her degree 7 years ago, this author has realized the answer to this question is somewhat complex. Healthcare delivery is improved through expertise in evaluating, translating, and implementing EBP, information technology, interprofessional collaboration, and mentoring. However, one may not fully appreciate the benefits of the DNP degree until some time after graduation. The experience of doctoral study also shapes and defines how clinicians' roles are actualized after graduation. Clinicians should understand that realizing the benefits of a DNP degree is a process that will continue to unfold years after graduation. Be assured, however, that this process is worthwhile, rewarding, and exciting. Nursing is uniquely positioned to improve health care through increased knowledge and education. As a colleague, Dr. Kathleen Payson, so accurately stated, "Education is power and the highway to make a difference." (K. Payson, personal communication, May, 2008).

A Personal Note: Why a DNP?

I always knew I would go back to school after earning a master's degree in nursing. I was impatiently waiting for a true practice doctorate to become a reality. I intended to stay involved in nursing practice as an APRN. Therefore, when the opportunity to earn a DNP degree in the first program in Michigan presented itself, I was the first student to apply. In graduate school I wasn't quite sure what the result would be upon completing my degree; I just knew I needed to learn more. Now, as a DNP graduate clinician, I am beginning to understand how a DNP degree enhances my ability to deliver and improve health care. I am more aware of the needs of my patients as individuals and members of communities, and I have developed more complex skills to meet their needs. Moreover, I have a more acute awareness of the needs of my profession and the increasing complexities in health care today.

The skills I developed through the DNP program are reflected in how I care for my patients. I regularly evaluate and translate EBP for my patients and seek new ways to integrate this information into the plan of care, as evidenced by the development of a specialty practice. When patient care is not optimal due to systems or organizational issues, I use my leadership and collaboration skills to develop solutions to improve care. It is even clearer to me now that earning a DNP degree prepared me for a formal leadership role and enabled me to develop my new position. I continue to mentor others in nursing who wish to pursue a DNP degree and have developed a specialty preceptor program within my clinical setting. Finally, I am committed to promoting nursing, the nurse practitioner role, servant leadership, and the DNP degree through pedagogical methods that will increase others' understanding.

I believe I knew a great deal about nursing when I was prepared at the master's degree level. Earning a DNP degree not only broadened this knowledge base, but also made me more aware of my role in nursing practice and healthcare delivery. I am also more aware of where nursing—as a practice profession—has been, where we are going, and where we need to be. Now, 7 years after graduating with a DNP degree, I realize the impact this degree will have on health care. As leaders and practice experts, DNP graduates are shaping the future of health care by influencing healthcare policy, providing leadership, and evaluating, translating, and implementing EBP. I am very proud to be a DNP graduate and am more fully committed to promoting the DNP degree.

SUMMARY

- Advanced-practice nursing and advanced nursing practice are often used interchangeably but actually have different meanings. Advanced nursing practice describes what nurses do when they provide nursing care. Advanced-practice nursing describes the whole field of specific types of nursing practice (Bryant-Lukosius et al., 2004).
- The APRN Consensus Model defines advanced-practice nursing and the regulations for LACE of APRNs.
- EBP serves to promote optimal healthcare outcomes, which are based on critically reviewed clinical evidence for individual patients, families, and communities.
- Although all DNP graduates are expected to evaluate, translate, and implement EBP into their particular settings, DNP graduates in clinician roles have a vantage point of EBP due to their direct impact on care in the clinical setting.
- Barriers to EBP exist and include resistance to change, lack of preparation regarding EBP, lack of resources for EBP, lack of belief in EBP, and poor motivation to investigate EBP.
- DNP graduates in the clinical setting and other settings can reduce barriers to EBP by defining EBP to others, providing education regarding EBP, providing consultation in researching EBP, and mentoring others regarding EBP outcomes.
- DNP graduates can evaluate and translate EBP by asking relevant questions in the clinical setting, reading literature reviews regarding pertinent topics,

starting a journal club in their practice setting, communicating to others regarding EBP, and organizing educational programs to increase the knowledge of other healthcare professionals in their setting.

- Information technologies serve to manage, organize, and process health information (Zytkowski, 2003) in an effort to improve the quality of care and healthcare outcomes.

- IOM reports in 2000, 2001, and 2003 expressed an increased need for healthcare professionals to increase their proficiency in information technologies to meet the complex demands of health care.

- Nursing uses information technologies to improve care, improve care delivery, and provide accurate, up-to-date information to patients. This is done through the use of PDAs, telehealth technologies, and reference librarians for consultation regarding information technology resources.

- Interprofessional collaboration is more than just getting along. DNP graduates are perfectly positioned to influence and exemplify interprofessional collaboration.

- The Interprofessional Education Collaborative Expert Panel (2011) published its *Core Competencies for Interprofessional Collaborative Practice*.

- Improved communication has been shown to be the most effective avenue to decrease barriers to interprofessional collaboration.

- DNP graduates will be looked to as mentors in health care. This involves DNP graduates in clinician roles displaying expertise, even when they may feel like novices regarding the new skills they have garnered in their DNP programs.

- Precepting students presents the ideal opportunity for DNP graduates in the clinical setting to act as mentors.

- DNP graduates may shape the future of nursing and influence the improvement of healthcare outcomes by mentoring others in the healthcare arena.

- The DNP degree may open the clinician's eyes and be their springboard to scholarship. DNP-prepared clinicians have a responsibility to maintain scholarship as it applies to their clinical practice or other areas of interest.

REFLECTION QUESTIONS

1. Do you think you understand the importance of EBP in nursing and in health care?

2. Do you think you evaluate and translate EBP into your nursing practice?

3. What ways can you think of to further evaluate and translate EBP into your nursing practice?

4. Do you think nursing has embraced information technologies?

5. In what ways do you think you could utilize information technologies in your nursing practice?

6. Do you think interprofessional collaboration is important to meet the demands of a complex healthcare system?

7. In what ways can you improve interprofessional collaboration in your setting?

8. Do you think you have, or have had, a mentor? If so, how can your experience with a mentor improve your ability to mentor others?

9. In what ways do you think DNP graduates in clinician roles, and other roles, have the opportunity to shape the future of nursing?

10. Do you think scholarship can be developed while in a clinical practice? If so, how? What are your scholarship interests?

REFERENCES

American Association of Colleges of Nursing. (2006). *Essentials of doctoral education for advanced nursing practice.* Retrieved from http://www.aacn.nche.edu/publications/position/DNPEssentials.pdf

American Association of Critical-Care Nurses. (2005). *AACN standards for establishing and sustaining healthy work environments: A journey to excellence.* Retrieved from http://www.aacn.org:88/WD/HWE/Docs/HWEStandards.pdf

American Nurses Association. (1995). *Nursing's social policy statement.* Washington, DC: Author.

American Nurses Association. (2001). *Scope and standards of nursing informatics practice.* Washington, DC: Author.

Apker, J., Propp, K., Zabava Ford, W., & Hofmeister, N. (2006). Collaboration, credibility, compassion, and coordination: Professional nurse communication skill sets in health care team interactions. *Journal of Professional Nursing, 22*(3), 180–189.

APRN Joint Dialogue Group. (2008). *Consensus model for APRN regulation: Licensure, accreditation, certification & education.* Retrieved from http://www.aacn.nche.edu/education-resources/APRNReport.pdf

Benner, P. (1982). From novice to expert. *American Journal of Nursing, 82*(3), 402–407.

Benner, P. (1984). *From novice to expert: Excellence and power in clinical nursing practice.* Menlo Park, CA: Addison-Wesley.

Brown, S. J. (1998). A framework for advanced practice nursing. *Journal of Professional Nursing, 14*(3), 157–164.

Bryant-Lukosius, D., DiCenso, A., Browne, G., & Pinelli, J. (2004). Advanced practice nursing roles: Development, implementation, and evaluation. *Journal of Advanced Nursing, 48*(5), 519–529.

Carroll, K., Bradford, A., Foster, M., Cato, J., & Jones, J. (2007). An emerging giant: Nursing informatics. *Journal of Nursing Management, 38*(3), 38–42.

Collaborate. (2004). *Webster's concise English dictionary*. New Lenark, Scotland: David Dale House.

Courtney, K., Demiris, G., & Alexander, G. (2005). Information technology: Changing nursing processes at the point-of-care. *Nursing Administration Quarterly, 29*(4), 315–322.

Cowan, M., Shapiro, M., Hays, R., Abdelmonem, A., Vazitani, S., Ward, C., & Ettner, S. (2006). The effect of a multidisciplinary hospitalist/physician and advanced practice nurse collaboration on hospital costs. *Journal of Nursing Administration, 36*(2), 79–85.

Curran, C. (2003). Informatics competencies for nurse practitioners. *AACN Clinical Issues, 14*(3), 320–330.

Davies, B., & Hughes, A. M. (1995). Clarification of advanced nursing practice: Characteristics and competencies. *Clinical Nurse Specialist, 9*(3), 156–160.

Dracup, K., & Bryan-Brown, C. (2004). From novice to expert to mentor: Shaping the future. *American Journal of Critical Care, 13*(6), 448–450.

Dreyfus, S., & Dreyfus, H. (1980). *A five stage model of the mental activities involved in directed skill acquisition* (Unpublished doctoral study supported by the Air Force Office of Scientific Research, USAF, contract F49620-79-C0063). University of California, Berkeley.

Egerod, I., & Hansen, G. M. (2005). Evidence-based practice among Danish cardiac nurses: A national survey. *Journal of Advanced Nursing, 51*(5), 465–473.

Evidence-based. (n.d.). In E. McKean (Ed.), *New Oxford American Dictionary* (2nd ed.) [Computer software]. New York, NY: Oxford University Press.

Fink, R., Thompson, C. J., & Bonnes, D. (2005). Overcoming barriers and promoting the use of research in practice. *Journal of Nursing Administration, 35*(3), 121–129.

Gagliardi, A., Grunfeld, E., & Evans, W. K. (2004). Evaluation of diagnostic assessment units in oncology: A systematic review. *Journal of Clinical Oncology, 22*(6), 1126–1135.

Gaumer, G., Koeniger-Donohue, R., Friel, C., & Sudbay, M. (2007). Use of information technology by advanced practice nurses. *Computers, Informatics, Nursing, 25*(6), 344–352.

Gerardi, D., & Fontaine, D. (2007). True collaboration: Envisioning new ways of working together. *AACN Advanced Critical Care, 18*(1), 10–14.

Gibbs, L. (2003). *Evidence-based practice for the helping professions: A practical guide with integrated multimedia*. Pacific Grove, CA: Brooks/Cole Thomson Learning.

Goleman, D., Boyatzis, R., & McKee, A. (2002). *Primal leadership: Realizing the power of emotional intelligence*. Boston, MA: Harvard Business Review Press.

Graves, J., & Corcoran, S. (1989). The study of nursing informatics. *Image: Journal of Nursing Scholarship, 21*(4), 227–231.

Greiner, A. C., & Knebel, E. (Eds.). (2003). *Health professions education: A bridge to quality*. Washington, DC: National Academies Press.

Gui, P. P., Allum, W. H., Perry, N. M., Welles, C. A., Curling, O. M., McLean, A., ... Carpenter R. (1995). One-stop diagnosis for symptomatic breast disease. *Annals of the Royal College of Surgeons of England, 77*, 24–27.

Hallas, D., Butz, A., & Gitterman, B. (2004). Attitudes and beliefs for effective pediatric nurse practitioner and physician collaboration. *Journal of Pediatric Health Care, 18*(2), 77–86.

Hamric, A., Spross, J., & Hanson, C. (2005). *Advanced practice nursing: An integrative approach* (3rd ed.). St. Louis, MO: Elsevier Saunders.

Hayes, E. (1998). Mentoring and self-efficacy for advanced practice nursing practice: A philosophical approach for nurse practitioner preceptors. *Journal of the American Academy of Nurse Practitioners, 10*(2), 53–57.

Hudson, K., Duke, G., Haas, B., & Varnell, G. (2008). Navigating the evidence-based practice maze. *Journal of Nursing Management, 16*(4), 409–416.

Institute of Medicine. (2001). *Crossing the quality chasm: A new health system for the 21st century.* Washington, DC: National Academies Press.

International Medical Informatics Association Nursing Informatics Special Interest Group. (1998). *Nursing informatics definition.* Retrieved from http://www.imiani.org

Interprofessional Education Collaborative Expert Panel. (2011). *Core competencies for interprofessional collaborative practice: Report of an expert panel.* Washington, DC: Author. Retrieved from http://www.aacn.nche.edu/education-resources/ipecreport.pdf

Jennings, B. M., & Rogers, S. (1988). Merging nursing research and practice: A case of multiple identities. *Journal of Advanced Nursing, 13*(6), 752–758.

Knaus, W., Draper, E., Wagner, D., & Zimmerman, J. (1986). An evaluation of outcome from intensive care in major medical centers. *Annals of Internal Medicine, 104*(3), 410–418.

Kohn, L. T., Corrigan, J. M., & Donaldson, M. S. (Eds.). (1999). *To err is human: Building a safer health system.* Washington, DC: National Academies Press.

McKay, C., & Crippen, L. (2008). Collaboration through clinical integration. *Nursing Administration Quarterly, 32*(2), 109–116.

McKinley, M. (2004). Mentoring matters: Creating, connecting, empowering. *AACN Clinical Issues, 15*(2), 205–214.

Melnyk, B. (2002). Strategies for overcoming barriers in implementing evidence-based practice. *Pediatric Nursing, 28*(2), 159–161.

Melnyk, B. (2005). Advanced evidence-based practice in clinical and academic settings. *Worldviews on Evidence-Based Nursing, 2*(3), 161–165.

Melnyk, B., & Fineout-Overholt, E. (2005). *Evidence-based practice in nursing and healthcare: A guide to best practice.* Philadelphia, PA: Lippincott Williams & Wilkins.

Melnyk, B., Fineout-Overholt, E., Feinstein, N., Li, H., Small, L., Wilcox, L., & Kraus, R. (2004). Nurses' perceived knowledge, beliefs, skills, and needs regarding evidence-based practice: Implications for accelerating the paradigm shift. *Worldviews on Evidence-Based Nursing, 1*(3), 185–193.

Melnyk, B., Fineout-Overholt, E., Feinstein, N., Sadler, L., & Green-Hernandez, C. (2008). Nurse practitioner educators' perceived knowledge, beliefs, and teaching strategies regarding evidence-based practice: Implications for accelerating the integration of evidence-based practice into graduate programs. *Journal of Professional Nursing, 24*(1), 7–13.

Mentor. (2004). *Webster's concise English dictionary.* New Lenark, Scotland: David Dale House.

National Association of Clinical Nurse Specialists. (2009). *Core practice doctorate clinical nurse specialist competencies.* Retrieved from http://www.nacns.org/docs/CorePracticeDoctorate.pdf

National Organization of Nurse Practitioner Faculties. (2006). *Practice doctorate nurse practitioner entry-level competencies.* Retrieved from http://c.ymcdn.com/sites/www.nonpf.org/resource/resmgr/competencies/dnp%20np%20competenciesapril2006.pdf

Nichols, C., O'Connor, N., & Dunn, D. (2014). Exploring early and future use of DNP pre-pared nurses within healthcare organizations. *Journal of Nursing Administration, 44*(2), 74–78.

Nightingale, F. (1859). *Notes on nursing: What it is and what it is not.* London, England: Harrison and Sons.

Peck, A. (2005). Changing the face of standard nursing practice through telehealth and telenursing. *Nursing Administration Quarterly, 29*(4), 339–343.

Pravikoff, D., Pierce, S., & Tanner, A. (2005). Evidence-based practice readiness study sup-ported by academy nursing informatics expert panel. *Nursing Outlook, 53*(1), 49–50.

Rossen, K., Bartlett, R., & Herrick, C. (2008). Interdisciplinary collaboration: The need to revisit. *Issues in Mental Health Nursing, 29*(4), 387–396.

Schmalenberg, C., Kramer, M., King, C., Krugman, M., Lund, C., Poduska, D., & Rapp, D. (2005). Excellence through evidence: Securing collegial/collaboration nurse–physician relationships, part 1. *Journal of Nursing Administration, 35*(10), 450–458.

Searles, C., & Mecklenburg, R. (2013). Nurse practitioner-staffed clinic offers same day, comprehensive appointment for breast symptoms, leading to faster diagnosis and lower costs. Retrieved from http://www.innovations.ahrq.gov/content.aspx?id+3895

Sharp, N. (1998). From "incident to" to telehealth: New federal rules and regulations affect NPs. *Nurse Practitioner, 23*(8), 68–69.

Sheriff, K., Wallis, M., & Chaboyer, W. (2007). Nurses' attitudes to and perceptions of knowl-edge and skills regarding evidence-based practice. *International Journal of Nursing Practice, 13*(6), 363–369.

Shneyder, Y. (2002). Personal digital assistants (PDAs) for the nurse practitioner. *Journal of Pediatric Health Care, 16*(6), 317–320.

Sigma Theta Tau International Evidence-Based Practice Task Force. (2004). Evidence-based nursing: Rationale and resources. *Worldviews on Evidence-Based Nursing, 1*(1), 69–75.

Simpson, R. (2004). The softer side of technology: How IT helps nursing care. *Nursing Administration Quarterly, 28*(4), 302–305.

Simpson, R. (2005). From tele-ed to telehealth: The need for IT ubiquity in nursing. *Nursing Administration Quarterly, 29*(4), 344–348.

Stein-Parbury, J., & Liaschenko, J. (2007). Understanding collaboration between nurses and physicians as knowledge at work. *American Journal of Critical Care, 16*(5), 470–477.

Styles, M., & Lewis, C. (2000). Conceptualizations of advanced nursing practice. In A. Hamric, J. Spross, & C. Hanson (Eds.), *Advanced nursing practice: An integrative approach* (pp. 33–51). Philadelphia, PA: Saunders.

Thomas, J., & Herrin, D. (2008). The Robert Wood Johnson Executive Nurse Fellows Program: A model for learning in an executive master of science in nursing program. *Journal of Nursing Administration, 38*(3), 112–115.

Yeager, S. (2005). Interdisciplinary collaboration: The heart and soul of health care. *Critical Care Nursing Clinics of North America, 17*(2), 143–148.

Zytkowski, M. (2003). Nursing informatics: The key to unlocking contemporary nursing practice. *AACN Clinical Issues, 14*(3), 271–281.

CHAPTER 4

The DNP: Expectations for Theory, Research, and Scholarship

Morris A. Magnan

The words *theory*, *research*, and *scholarship* are inextricably linked to the notion of doctoral study. Of these three, *theory* and *research* seem to be the most troublesome for doctor of nursing practice (DNP) hopefuls. For some reason these two words tend to stimulate affective responses ranging from ennui to mild anxiety to panic, but rarely exhilaration. Undoubtedly, some DNP hopefuls have skipped over this chapter or decided to read it last simply because the words *research* and *theory* appear in the title. It is for this group, especially, that the chapter is written. It is hoped that the information provided will serve as a resource that increases the reader's capacity to succeed in being and becoming a DNP.

The chapter is divided into two major sections to provide information that might be helpful to DNP hopefuls: (1) during doctoral study and (2) beyond graduation. The first major section of the chapter begins with a brief discussion of theory and highlights the importance of learning how to work with middle-range theory to guide observation and plan interventions. Then research expectations are discussed, with particular attention given to what is needed to support evidence-based practice. A section on scholarship follows, which provides detailed information about skills of scholarship that must be developed to succeed in doctoral study. In addition, the scholarship section includes information about the DNP final project—what it is, how to choose a topic, and how to choose a committee. This first major section of the chapter ends by providing tips on getting the DNP final project published.

The second major section of the chapter focuses on scholarship and research beyond graduation. This section opens with a discussion of scholarship expectations and barriers to scholarship that DNPs who work in academic or clinical service settings may encounter. The discussion then turns to mentorship and the role it might play in achieving scholarship and research goals. The chapter ends by providing some pointers on building a network of support for research and scholarship.

The DNP and Theory

Human beings invest a great deal of time and effort in trying to understand how the world works. When this effort is characterized by systematic, rigorous, and reproducible modes of inquiry, it is referred to as science. Scientists in a field strive to provide systematic and responsibly supported descriptions and explanations about phenomena (objects and events) in the world of human experience. The overall goal is to advance these descriptions and explanations to the level of theoretical formulations. Thus, theory is a valued product of scientific inquiry. Some authors have even taken the position that the aim of science is theory (Kerlinger, 1973) and that the aim of nursing science is to produce practice-relevant nursing theory (Jacobs & Huether, 1978). Doctoral programs in nursing prepare doctor of philosophy (PhD) students to develop theory for nursing practice, whereas DNP students are prepared to use theory in practice.

The complexities of doctoral-level practice require that DNP students have a broad base of knowledge gleaned from a number of sciences, not just nursing. To be adequately prepared to address current and emerging practice issues, the DNP essentials (American Association of Colleges of Nursing [AACN], 2006) recommends a foundation in biology, genomics, the science of therapeutics, the psychosocial sciences, and the science of complex organizational structures. In addition, there is a clear expectation that DNP graduates will have some facility in using theory from nursing and other sciences to, for example, determine the nature and significance of health-related phenomena; describe strategies to ameliorate health-related phenomena; address problems related to the delivery of health care; and develop and evaluate new approaches to practice (AACN, 2006). The implications of these expectations seem clear: DNP graduates need to be proficient in applying theory to diverse practice situations. The application of theory to practice may extend along a number of lines, such as using relevant theories to address patient-centered clinical problems, conceptualize quality improvement initiatives, or address organizational problems related to the uptake and diffusion of well-tested, innovative approaches to clinical practice.

There are many definitions of theory. One useful definition comes from Kerlinger, who defined theory as "a set of interrelated constructs (concepts), definitions, and propositions that present a systematic view of phenomena by specifying relations among variables, with the purpose of explaining and predicting the phenomena" (1973, p. 9). The utility of a theory comes from the organization it provides for thinking, observing, and interpreting what is observed (Fawcett, 2005).

Historically nursing theory has provided both a guide for practice and a basis for research. Nursing theory consists of concepts connected by relational statements that describe, predict, or explain phenomena that are consistent with nursing's perspective (Donaldson & Crowley, 1978). Attempts have been made to classify nursing's theoretical formulations into a hierarchy consisting of conceptual models, grand theories, and middle-range theories (Fawcett, 2005). The purpose of conceptual models is often to communicate knowledge that is useful to the whole discipline of nursing. Grand theories are more delimited in scope than conceptual models and tend to focus on developing one aspect of a conceptual model, such as health or self-care. In contrast, middle-range theories describe, explain, or predict concrete and specific phenomena (Fawcett, 2005). Thus, middle-range theories, unlike grand theories, are narrower in scope, more amenable to validation through empirical testing (Lenz, Suppe, Gift, Pugh, & Milligan, 1995), and more immediately applicable to clinical practice (Fawcett, 2005; Lenz, 1998a, 1998b).

Over the past 2 decades a burgeoning interest in middle-range theory has led to the publication of several books on the topic. Some of these books provide a compendium of middle-range nursing theories, and others present middle-range theories from nursing and middle-range theories from other disciplines that have had some utility in addressing problems encountered in clinical practice. DNP students might want to consider adding to their library one or both of the following resources: *Middle Range Theories: Application to Nursing Research* (Peterson & Bredow, 2004) and *Handbook of Stress, Coping, and Health: Implications for Nursing Research, Theory, and Practice* (Rice, 2000). These and other compendia should be viewed as introductory, secondary sources of information about the theories discussed. If a decision is made to use a particular middle-range theory as the conceptual framework for a scholarly project (e.g., the DNP capstone project), it is always best to access and have a thorough understanding of the theorist's original work rather than relying on interpretations offered by other authors.

In a book chapter titled "Nursing Science for Nursing Practice," Donaldson (1995) discusses the importance of taking a pragmatic approach to using theory in practice. From Donaldson's perspective, the pragmatist nurse will use knowledge from nursing, nursing science, and other disciplines only if it has utility for achieving the desired clinical outcomes. Extending Donaldson's views to the application of middle-range theory in practice, it could be argued that middle-range theories that facilitate a straightforward approach to the conceptualization of clinical problems and patient outcomes, delineate effective interventions, and point to appropriate modes of measuring patient outcomes are likely to be more useful in addressing clinical problems encountered in doctoral-level practice than conceptual models and grand theories (Donaldson, 1995).

Nursing science can generate some, but not all, of the theory needed to inform nursing practice (Donaldson & Crowley, 1978). Therefore, introducing DNP students to middle-range theories from nursing and other health-related disciplines will help them build an armamentarium of theory from which they can draw upon. Some theories (not all are middle range) that DNP students have found to be immediately applicable to problems encountered in the clinical setting can be found in **Box 4-1**.

BOX 4-1

Theories DNP Students Have Found to Be Applicable to the Clinical Setting

Health Belief Model (Rosenstock, 1990)

Theory of Planned Behavior (Ajzen & Madden, 1986)

Self-Efficacy (Bandura, 1977, 1997)

Transtheoretical Model of Behavioral Change (Prochaska & DiClemente, 1983)

Interaction Model of Client Health Behavior (Cox, 1982)

Theory of Unpleasant Symptoms (Lenz, Pugh, Milligan, Gift, & Suppe, 1997)

Uncertainty in Illness (Mishel, 1990)

Middle-Range Theory of Empathy (Olson & Hanchett, 1997)

In a very practical sense, exposing DNP students to a large number of middle-range theories may be of lesser importance than helping them acquire skills needed to apply middle-range theory to practice. The ability to apply middle-range theory to practice should be viewed as an important, learned, transferable skill. In other words, acquiring skill at applying one middle-range theory to a practice situation should transfer to the application of other middle-range theories to practice situations. To acquire this skill, DNP graduates will need to have a foundation in the language of theory (e.g., concepts, relational statements); learn how to distinguish modifiable from nonmodifiable predictors and understand the meaning this has for planning theory-based interventions; and understand how to interpret the research literature to determine the level of empirical support for relationships among theoretical concepts. In addition, DNP graduates need to understand thoroughly how to frame a health-related phenomenon (e.g., a clinical problem) within a theoretical perspective and then use the selected theory as a guide for theory-driven assessment, to select theory-based interventions, and to develop theoretically congruent measures for predicted outcomes.

According to the DNP essentials, the DNP program should prepare the graduate to "develop and evaluate new practice approaches based on nursing theories and theories from other disciplines" (AACN, 2006, p. 9). The importance of having DNPs prepared to develop and evaluate theory-driven interventions cannot be overstated. In *Nursing's Social Policy Statement* (American Nurses Association, 2003), society is promised nursing interventions that are based on theoretical and evidence-based knowledge. Thus, society's confidence in the profession depends, in part, on nursing's ability to deliver on this promise. DNP graduates are functioning at the highest level of professional practice. Moreover, their education prepares them to bridge the gap between theory and practice. Therefore, DNP graduates are well positioned to help nursing fulfill its promise.

The DNP and Research

The DNP is not a research degree. The DNP essentials clearly state that practice-focused doctoral programs leading to the DNP place "less emphasis … on research methodology and statistics than is apparent in research-focused programs" (AACN, 2006, p. 3). However, it is important that DNP hopefuls understand that less emphasis on research methodology and statistics does not mean no emphasis. In fact, it is expected that DNP graduates will play a pivotal role in nursing's research enterprise, particularly at the juncture of providing leadership for evidence-based practice (AACN, 2006; Lenz, 2005). In addition, it is expected that DNP graduates will have a foundation in research sufficient to support participation in translational research, initiate practice inquiry, and collaborate effectively in knowledge-generating research (AACN, 2006).

Curriculum standards for research and statistics are not stated explicitly in the DNP essentials document (AACN, 2006). However, the DNP essentials does make it clear that "DNP curricula are designed so that all students attain DNP end-of-program competencies" (AACN, 2006, p. 7). The term *curriculum* can be understood broadly as all the learning that is planned and guided by a school. Designing DNP curricula and making decisions about what courses and learning activities should be included in a DNP program are the responsibility of the academic unit that offers the DNP program. Therefore, each school develops its own DNP curriculum and includes courses in research and statistics based on the faculty's understanding of what is needed to achieve competencies outlined in the DNP essentials. A careful review of the entire DNP essentials document suggests that a foundation in research ethics, the fundamentals of research methodology, core statistical principles, and critical appraisal of research literature is needed to achieve some of the DNP competencies listed under Essentials I, II, IV, V, VII, and VIII and all of the DNP competencies listed under Essential III. The extent to which DNP curricula—planned learning activities—facilitate the creation of a solid foundation in research ethics, research methods, core statistical procedures, and the critical appraisal of literature will vary from school to school. Given the newness of DNP programs, there are, understandably, no data available to compare the research capabilities of DNP graduates across programs. This absence of comparative information places a greater responsibility on DNP hopefuls to shop carefully for a DNP program that will help them meet competencies that require a foundation in research. A thorough understanding of the research foundations specified or implied in the DNP essentials document can facilitate making a wise choice. In addition, DNP hopefuls may find Magyar, Whitney, and Brown's (2006) article on the research foundations of the practice doctorate particularly helpful as they strive to more fully understand the research expectations of DNPs.

Research Capabilities for Evidence-Based Practice

In nursing there is a general consensus that practitioners can no longer rely solely on experience, pathophysiologic rationale, or opinion-based processes to achieve high-quality, contextually relevant patient outcomes. Dramatic changes in healthcare delivery, with an increased focus on containing costs while promoting patient safety and achieving high-quality outcomes, have intensified the demand for evidence-based health care. Evidence-based medicine (EBM) is widely understood as "the conscientious, explicit, and judicious use of current best evidence in making decisions about the care of patients," whereas the practice of EBM "integrating individual clinical expertise with the best available external clinical evidence from systematic research" (Sackett, Rosenberg, Gray, Haynes, & Richardson, 1996, p. 71). Evidence-based nursing practice (EBNP) differs from EBM. In the medical model, evidence from randomized clinical trials (RCTs) is weighted more heavily than all other forms of evidence (Sackett et al., 1996). In nursing, practitioners take into account evidence from RCTs but cast a much wider net to inform their clinical decision making by taking into account evidence from both qualitative and quantitative research, clinician expertise, the patient's clinical state, the clinical setting and circumstances, and patient values, preferences, and beliefs (DiCenso, Guyatt, & Ciliska, 2005; Melnyk & Fineout-Overholt, 2005). One useful definition describes EBNP as "the conscientious integration of best research evidence with clinical expertise and patient values and needs in the delivery of quality, cost-effective health care" (Burns & Grove, 2005, p. 736).

Essential III of the DNP essentials explicitly states that curricula should prepare DNP graduates to "use analytic methods to critically appraise existing literature and other evidence to determine and implement the best evidence for practice" (AACN, 2006, p. 12). In the current healthcare climate, adequate preparation in the area of evidence-based practice is likely to carry more weight with DNP prospective employers than capabilities related to participating in translational research, initiating practice inquiry, or collaborating effectively in knowledge-generating research. Moreover, research has shown that employers expect advanced-practice registered nurses (APRNs) to be aware of the most current practice information so they can serve as a resource for others (McDiarmid, 1998; Stetler & DiMaggio, 1991). Thus, DNP hopefuls may want to pay particular attention to developing knowledge, skills, and habits of inquiry needed to build competencies for evidence-based practice.

The critical appraisal of research literature is particularly relevant to evidence-based practice. In nursing, the research literature is broadly divided into two dominant paradigms: quantitative research and qualitative research (Weaver & Olson, 2006). Quantitative research is characterized by objectivity and the use of numerical data to obtain information about the world (Burns & Grove, 2005). Qualitative research is characterized by the use of subjective, interactive approaches to describe life experiences and give meaning to them (Burns & Grove, 2005). Both approaches employ systematic modes of inquiry, and both require rigor in implementation. Criteria have been established for evaluating the rigor of quantitative and qualitative research (Burns & Grove, 2005). To critically appraise the research literature emanating from these two paradigms, DNP graduates need to know about and understand the paradigm-specific criteria used to evaluate quantitative and qualitative studies. Then analytical methods, such as comparison, can be used to critically evaluate whether and to what extent attributes of rigor are evident within a particular study. Greater confidence can be placed in decisions to change practice patterns when evidence to support the decision comes from more rigorous studies.

Decisions about how best to prepare DNP students for evidence-based practice are the curricular concerns of schools that offer DNP programs. However, the level of competency attained at the end of the program and beyond will largely depend on the DNP student. The student's commitment to developing learning skills for the immediate future, the ability to adapt these skills to meet the requirements of changing circumstances, and, above all, the ability and willingness to apply learning to action will likely play a critical role (Titmus, 1999). With respect to evidence-based practice, one learning skill that must be mastered by all DNP students is the ability to access relevant information using computer information technology (CIT). Getting connected to the right web-based resources is critical. Popular search engines, such as Google and Yahoo!, are a starting point, but learning how to navigate these search engines is no substitute for developing the skills needed to use library CIT efficiently to glean information from electronic sources and bibliographic databases, such as CINAHL, ProQuest Nursing Journals, MEDLINE, PsycINFO, and others.

University students now learn how to search computerized bibliographic databases as part of their undergraduate education. Thus, library literacy is an a priori expectation for all graduate-level students. DNP hopefuls who have not yet learned how to search electronic bibliographic databases need to do so quickly. University librarians often provide traditional, face-to-face library workshops and online tutorials to help students become proficient in using library services and conducting bibliographic searches. DNP students, especially those who have been away from the academic setting for some time, should seriously think about participating in these learning activities to ensure that their level of library literacy meets the demands of doctoral study. Although research consistently has shown that nursing students tend to use learning resources that are easily accessible and familiar to them (Barnett-Ellis & Restauri, 2006; Dee & Stanley, 2005), DNP students need to move beyond what is easy and familiar to locate the cross-disciplinary information that informs their practice and scholarship.

The DNP's involvement in EBNP is likely to proceed along two distinct dimensions. One dimension relates to the requirement to continuously update one's own practice. Nurturing the habit of regularly conducting keyword searches in one's area of expertise, getting linked to relevant Rich Site Summary feeds, and serving as a sentinel reader of research in one's area of expertise are strategies DNPs can employ to ensure timely access to evidence that is pertinent to their areas of practice. McMaster University's Health Information Research Unit (accessible at http://plus.mcmaster.ca/np) provides access to current best evidence to support evidence-based decision making for nursing practice. To become a sentinel reviewer for McMaster University's evidence-based nursing initiative, contact them directly by email at MOREebn@mcmaster.ca. A second dimension for DNP involvement in evidence-based practice has more to do with promoting and facilitating its use within healthcare organizations.

The movement toward EBNP within an organization is more likely to occur in organizations that value the use of knowledge and provide resources to access that knowledge (Rosswurm & Larrabee, 1999). Although evidence-based practice is rapidly becoming an expectation for nurses at all levels of practice, this expectation may be an unrealistic one. Research has shown that staff nurses tend to undervalue research, rely heavily on informal sources to inform practice-related decisions, and are poorly equipped to access and critically appraise research literature (Pavikoff, Tanner, & Pierce, 2005; Spenceley, O'Leary, Chizawsky, Ross, & Estabrooks, 2008). Moreover, staff nurses who know about evidence that supports a change in practice are not at liberty to implement practice changes that supersede institutional policies. In contrast, DNPs are well equipped for evidence-based practice. Moreover, DNPs with clinical concentrations that prepare them to work in clinical nurse specialist and administrative roles are likely to be hired into positions of authority where they can build human capital and bring about changes in policy to promote the use of evidence-based practice within an organization. Mentoring staff nurses through the design and implementation of EBP projects is a much-needed service. Stupnyckj, Smolarek, Reeves, McKeith, and Magnan (in press) speak cogently to the importance of having knowledgeable and capable mentors available to help sustain commitment to initiating and completing a clinically relevant EBP project.

The DNP and Scholarship

Scholarship is a way of thinking and being in the world. The term *scholarship* refers to the character, qualities, activities, and attainments of a scholar or a learned person (Scholarship, 1993). Doctoral education in nursing, whether research or practice focused, prepares graduates for a scholarly approach to the discipline of nursing (AACN, 2006). However, it is important to recognize that scholarship is developed, not awarded. Earning the DNP or PhD degree is a noteworthy accomplishment; it is not a mark of scholarship. Ideally the work of earning a doctoral degree and exposure to and close interaction with scholars from nursing and other fields will set into motion certain habits of thought, a questioning attitude, and a disciplined approach to work that might eventually lead to the full bloom of scholarship. As budding scholars, DNP hopefuls might want to think carefully about scholarship, what it means, how it might be developed over the course of one's career, and, most important, what skills of scholarship are required to succeed in doctoral study and beyond.

There is no agreed-upon definition of scholarship. However, the literature consistently points to three recurring themes: (1) breadth and depth of knowledge within a defined area, (2) innovation and creativity, and (3) exposure of the scholarly product to public scrutiny and peer review (AACN, 1999; Kitson, 1999/2006; Morahan & Fleetwood, 2008). The AACN defines scholarship in nursing as "those activities that systematically advance the teaching, research, and practice of nursing through rigorous inquiry that (1) is significant to the profession, (2) is creative, (3) can be documented, (4) can be replicated or elaborated, and (5) can be peer reviewed through various methods" (AACN, 1999, p. 3).

Developing one's self as a scholar takes time and dedication. Typically it takes decades of scholarly productivity before one is recognized as a scholar in one's field. Acquiring the skills of scholarship often begins, unavoidably, during doctoral study. Kitson (2006) has identified four skills of scholarship deemed to be relevant for nursing research and practice that seem to coalesce around the following:

1. being able to find and understand what has gone before (literature searching, comprehension, critical appraisal, interpretation);

2. reviewing the published literature in a fair and unbiased way, accurately reflecting the state of the field, showing judgment and the ability to integrate and synthesize a diverse body of knowledge;

3. the ability to communicate ideas effectively, cogently, coherently, and concisely through the written word (using proper grammar, syntax, punctuation, and spelling) and orally;

4. the ability to think logically and clearly and knowing how to present the pros and cons of an argument in a balanced way. (2006, p. 541)

The first skill listed was already discussed in this chapter under the section titled "Research Capabilities for Evidence-Based Practice." The fourth skill seems to be somewhat self-explanatory and is probably learned best within the context of participating in doctoral-level seminars. The second and third skills seem worthy of some additional comments because doctoral students seem to have difficulty getting a good start on developing these skills.

Developing scholarship in the area of "reviewing the published literature in a fair and unbiased way, accurately reflecting the state of the field, showing judgment and the ability to integrate and synthesize a diverse body of work" (Kitson, 2006, p. 541) can be particularly difficult to master if the mind is not open to alternative views. In other words, the problem of introducing bias is one that novice readers must overcome when reading scholarly publications. The challenge in reading scholarly publications is to first attempt to understand what the author is trying to say from the author's point of view rather than disputing what the author says in an off-handed way because it does not concur with one's own point of view. A second problem that must be overcome is believing everything in print. Doctoral students may feel reluctant to dispute what is written, especially if the author has a recognized, famous name. However, it is important to recognize that doctoral faculty often assign specific readings for the very reason that the author's ideas, as presented, are indefensible. This is one way faculty help students learn how to critically appraise the literature.

In reviewing the published literature, it is important to recognize that it is reviewed one manuscript at time. Thus, learning how to read articles published in professional journals is a foundational skill that must be mastered before taking on the challenge of integrating and synthesizing a diverse body of literature. Given the vast amount of reading required of doctoral students, it would seem that some rules of engagement should be in place beyond the old standby of just reading for ideas. One thing that must be understood is that articles published in professional journals are basically of two types, research and nonresearch, and each requires a distinct approach. **Box 4-2** lists some tips for reading nonresearch articles.

BOX 4-2

Tips for Reading Nonresearch Articles

1. Read with a pen and highlighter in hand. There are some important seminal works in the nursing literature, but there are no sacred documents. Highlighting key points and writing in the margins is not sinful, and it can help with information retention.

2. Avoid the sickness of highlighter mania. Highlight sparingly so that important ideas and key points can be found easily when the document is revisited, for example, during class discussion or when writing a literature review.

3. Inspect the article critically before reading. This critical inspection should include looking at the title and the subheadings in the body of the article. The title should give a general idea of the topic being addressed, and the subheadings should relate to the title and provide some early insight into how the author is approaching the topic or building an argument. Then look at the credentials and affiliations of the author to determine whether the author is likely to be an authoritative source of information.

4. Read the abstract. Abstracts of nonresearch articles vary in length and degree of helpfulness. Some may actually state the purpose of the article and provide a conclusion or summary statement.

5. Read the introductory paragraphs to locate the purpose or thesis of the article. The purpose will jump off the page when it is stated as *the purpose of this article is*. More subtle statements of purpose might be written, such as *to more fully understand*. A thesis is an argument that the author wants to challenge or defend. Theses often are prefaced by the words *but* and *however*. When the thesis is located, it helps to write in the margin *purpose* or *thesis* and then look again at the subheadings in the article. The subheadings should provide insight and anticipation about the approach the author is taking to achieve the purpose or defend the thesis.

6. When reading the remainder of the article, use a highlighter or preferably an ink pen to number and comment on key points that relate directly to the purpose or thesis.

7. Finally, read the conclusion critically. Try to determine to what extent the author's conclusion is supported by key points made in the article. It is equally important to determine whether the conclusion goes beyond what can be supported by the key points made in the body of the article.

8. Conclude your reading by writing a brief synopsis (I put this on the front page of the article) using bullet points and sentence fragments. This final step, while tedious, should not take more than 5 minutes, and it really helps lock into memory what was read. Generally, the synopsis uses a format such as the following:

   - The author proposes/argues that . . . [state purpose or thesis].
   - The author's position is supported by . . . [bullet points for two or three strong key points].
   - Weak and contradictory points of support include . . . [bullet points for two or three points].
   - The author's conclusion is reasonable [supported by the key points] or unreasonable [goes beyond what has been reported].
   - Sometimes an additional note is added if it is immediately apparent that current work agrees or disagrees with the work of another author. In this case, I make a note such as *compare to Smith, 2004*.

Research reports generally follow a standard format with relatively standard subheadings, such as an introduction, review of literature, methods (including sample, setting, instrumentation, measurement, etc.), results, discussion, and conclusion.

Reading research reports is not the same as critiquing research. When reading research, it helps to understand thoroughly what should be included in each major section of the research report. For example, the introduction section should identify a knowledge gap and a statement of purpose. The knowledge gap is, as it implies, an area of knowledge that is missing or only partially understood. The knowledge gap is usually identifiable by statements such as *little is known about*, or *the extent to which . . . something occurs . . . is poorly understood*. The purpose statement is often identified by the words *the purpose of this study is*. Also, there should be a logical relationship between the knowledge gap and the purpose such that if the purpose of the research is fulfilled, the knowledge gap will be closed or narrowed. A full discussion of the details of reading research reports is beyond the scope of this chapter. However, Macnee and McCabe (2008) have published an excellent book on research utilization that states explicitly what readers should expect to find in each section of a research report. Although the book was designed for undergraduate students, I found it to be a useful starting point when teaching DNP students how to read and interpret research reports.

Kitson notes that one skill of scholarship (the third skill previously listed) is "the ability to communicate ideas effectively, cogently, coherently, and concisely through the written word (using proper grammar, syntax, punctuation, and spelling)" (2006, p. 541). In acquiring this skill of scholarship, smart DNP students learn quickly that academic success depends on mastering the parenthetical elements first. Doctoral-level faculty tend to be highly critical of poor punctuation and grammar, get unnerved when referenced works are cited improperly, and some go absolutely bonkers when a reference list is incomplete or poorly punctuated. To achieve some consistency in the production of scholarly papers (which, in this case, means every paper written for a class), many schools of nursing endorse following guidelines set forth in the *Publication Manual of the American Psychological Association* (APA, 2010). Every doctoral student should possess a current copy of the APA manual. Abridged and online versions of the APA manual are available but should be avoided because they often do not provide full or correct rules for referencing materials (especially electronic sources), and they are definitely not the rules being used by the faculty.

After purchasing the APA manual (or whichever style manual is endorsed by your school), it is important to learn how to work with the manual. Buying lunch for a colleague who knows the APA manual well in exchange for some APA pointers is money well spent. Trying to figure out how to use the APA manual the night before a paper is due is a recipe for disaster.

Learning to communicate ideas effectively, cogently, and concisely in writing is a skill that comes with practice. However, even the most practiced and highly skilled authors ask colleagues to review their manuscripts before submitting them for publication in peer-reviewed journals. Doctoral students are well advised to follow this lead. Having a colleague, such as another doctoral student, read a scholarly paper for grammar, punctuation, APA format, clarity of thought, and conciseness before turning it in for grading can save embarrassment and grade points. The choice of colleague is important. It is best to choose a trusted colleague who has writing skills that are equal to or greater than your own. A friend or family member who is unwilling to provide an honest critique, including negative feedback, is never a good choice.

Some DNP students, especially those with poor writing skills, become bitter about the amount of scholarly writing required. Typically the argument hinges on the notion that the DNP is, after all, a clinical degree, or the faculty expectations are too high. Unfortunately, curriculum standards are not going to change to accommodate students who do not produce doctoral-level work. Fortunately, most universities have a writing center where tutors are available to help students learn how to develop their ideas and express them in writing. Students who have weak writing skills but a strong commitment to completing their doctoral studies should avail themselves of these services.

One additional challenge that DNP students must learn to deal with is the experience of feeling marginalized—socially and professionally. Doctoral study is demanding and transformative. Involvement in doctoral study and the effort invested in acquiring the skills of scholarship will change one's habits of thought, introduce new language into one's vocabulary, and stimulate the acquisition of new behaviors. These changes inevitably find their way into the students' personal and professional lives. Family and spouses, no matter how supportive, will grow tired of hearing about what's happening at school and may become frustrated when the demands of school and scholarship seem to constantly interfere with family time. Professional colleagues may question the student's motives for pursuing the DNP. Even long-standing colleagues may choose to distance themselves when the DNP student starts to act and talk differently. As a result, the DNP student may start to feel marginalized, misunderstood, and cut off from valued sources of support at a time when support is needed most. That is the time to turn to fellow doctoral students for support. Collateral support from fellow doctoral students often is the only source of support that seems to genuinely ease the discomfort that comes from feeling marginalized and misunderstood.

The DNP Scholarly Project

Students can gain entry into a DNP program without knowing in advance what will be the focus of their final DNP project, but nobody graduates without completing a final scholarly project. Although academicians tend to agree that all students must complete a final project, there is disagreement about what it should be called and what it should contain. In the DNP essentials document (AACN, 2006) it is referred to as the final DNP project, and others refer to it as a capstone project (Lenz, 2005). By whatever name, DNP students need to appreciate that the final project is not just one more paper. Instead, it is a scholarly project that demonstrates synthesis of course content, including research and theory. Moran, Burson, & Conrad (2014) have dedicated an entire book to the DNP scholarly project. DNP hopefuls may find it helpful as they try to navigate their way through this aspect of their DNP education. Still, DNP applicants need to understand that there is no uniform agreement about the content and form of the DNP final project (Kirkpatrick & Weaver, 2013). As a result requirements for the final project vary widely across programs. Therefore, one should carefully investigate the program requirements for the final project.

The focus of the final DNP project will depend, in part, on the candidate's point of entry into the doctoral program of study. Students with master's degrees who are already functioning as APRNs may choose to focus on a practice or policy issue pertinent to their area of specialization. Postbaccalaureate students will be required to complete a clinical residency. In this case the capstone project is likely to be an end product emerging from and completed during the course of the clinical residency. It has been suggested that projects emanating from the clinical residency might focus on such things as "the development of a program of intervention, or an analysis of health care policy, or a discussion of patient care provided" (Lenz, 2005, p. 4). In the final analysis, the focus of the final project may be less important than the rigor of the project. The final project should be of sufficient rigor that it meets program requirements and warrants recognition as doctoral-level work.

Success in completing the final DNP project depends, in part, on knowing exactly what is required. Universities routinely establish guidelines for the completion of scholarly projects. Guidelines for scholarly projects may vary across academic units (e.g., psychology versus nursing) and within departments, depending on the degree being sought—bachelor's, master's, PhD, or DNP. Typically a doctoral student handbook provides detailed information about departmental expectations regarding the final project, approvals needed to initiate and complete the project, and important information about style, formatting, and deadlines. DNP students need to get their hands on this important document early, study it thoroughly, and refer to it often through the course of their program.

CHOOSING A TOPIC

Choosing a topic for the final DNP project can be difficult. It is best to choose something that captures one's intellectual interests in a sustainable way. Passion for a topic seems to be important. However, do not worry if absolute passion and motivation for the topic seem to be insufficient. Passion and motivation tend to be somewhat fickle. Expect both to wax and wane then gain momentum once again as the project nears completion. Do worry if passion for the subject matter seems to be driven by strong emotions (e.g., anger, frustration) or value conflicts (e.g., social injustice) rather than intellectual curiosity. The quest for knowledge and understanding requires some degree of impartiality and scientific objectivity. The prospects of maintaining objectivity and finishing the capstone project on time are dismal if encounters with the literature, the study subjects, or the data trigger strong emotions. Although it is possible to acknowledge, clarify, and bracket strongly held feelings and beliefs to achieve an impartial, balanced view of one's subject matter, this often requires special guidance and instruction, which may not be available or sufficient. Therefore, DNP students are well advised to discuss with their chairpersons any concerns they have about their ability to maintain an objective, impartial view of their topic.

An early decision regarding the topic for the final DNP project is better than a later decision—maybe! Students who enter the DNP program with a topic in mind or who latch on to a topic early in the program have the distinct advantage of using course work efficiently to enlarge and refine their understanding of the subject matter. On the other hand, there is a risk of cutting one's self off from exciting, new ideas encountered as one proceeds through the program.

Whether the choice of topic for the final project is made early or late, the student's original view of the final project, undoubtedly, will get modified along the way. Often refinements are needed to clarify what questions are being raised, to set boundaries on the scope of the project, and to ensure that the data collected will yield valid and reliable information pertinent to the questions being asked. Typically the student's committee will recommend modifications and refinements before the student launches the project. These recommendations often mean more work for the student, but they also mean that the committee is doing its job.

DNP students should never commit to a final project that is too large to finish within a reasonable time frame. Committee members, especially the chairperson, should help the student determine what is a reasonable time frame. In more structured settings, for example, when the capstone project is completed during the course of the clinical residency, specific indicators of semester-to-semester progress are likely to be identified in advance and detailed in writing in the doctoral student handbook.

Securing approval for capstone projects that require review by an internal review board (IRB) can be a time-consuming process. IRBs and human subjects committees are known for their thoroughness, not their speed. Often proposed projects need to be reviewed by several IRBs, for example, the university-level IRB and the human subjects committee of the hospital or institution where data will be collected. Typically it is best to proceed in an orderly fashion by first getting approval from the university-level IRB before submitting the project proposal to a hospital or outside institution. During my own doctoral-level study, I was advised to allot one full semester (4 months) to the IRB approval process. This proved to be sound advice.

CHOOSING A COMMITTEE

Typically a committee of faculty collaborators is assembled to mentor the student through the final DNP project. Bringing together the right group of people is important to the success of the project. Getting the right person to chair the committee is absolutely critical. It is nice if the chairperson of the committee likes the student. It is more important that the chairperson has at least a passable interest in the student's topic. It is better if he or she has theoretical, methodological, or content expertise, but it is absolutely essential that he or she knows how to get the student through the final project on time.

Students should choose their chairperson first. When the chairperson understands the nature of the student's project and agrees to chair the project, he or she can provide direction and facilitate decision making about additional areas of expertise needed to ensure a well-rounded committee. The committee should be configured so it lends strength to the project. If, for example, the planned project focuses on conducting a depth analysis of healthcare policy related to access to health care, then at least one committee member should have expertise in the area of healthcare policy. Students need to establish and maintain productive working relationships with committee members. Similarly, committee members need to establish and maintain productive working relationships with one another. If the chairperson suggests that a certain faculty member may not be a good choice for committee membership, the wise student will accept this suggestion at face value and widen the search until a more suitable, mutually agreed upon, committee candidate is found. It is always good practice to check with the committee chairperson first before inviting someone to join the committee.

GETTING THE DNP SCHOLARLY PROJECT PUBLISHED

There are many reasons to write for publication. One well-recognized reason is to advance nursing knowledge by disseminating the results of nursing research. Other reasons include advancing professional practice and the quality of nursing care by publishing exemplars of excellence in nursing care or the results of quality improvement initiatives. In addition, reporting new and interesting observations in the literature is one way of influencing professional opinion by drawing attention to, stimulating dialogue about, and shifting perspectives on pesky clinical problems or troublesome professional issues. More personal reasons for publishing include establishing one's self as an expert within a specialized area of practice or building a portfolio of scholarship that includes publication in peer-reviewed journals, a requirement for nursing academicians living under the publish or perish edict of university tenure systems. Whatever reason motivates one to write for publication, rest assured that the work of writing will stimulate brain activity (Johnson, 2008). Good writing brings the added benefits of cultivating clear thinking, discipline, analytical ability, the emergence of logically coherent arguments, and a deep sense of accomplishment (Fahy, 2008; Johnson, 2008).

In this chapter the DNP final project is referred to as a scholarly project. Scholarship is open to public scrutiny, and it is debatable, adaptable, and subject to improvement. Conferences and peer-reviewed journals are the venues most commonly used to showcase one's scholarship. Disseminating findings from the DNP scholarly project at conferences and in peer-reviewed journals is a mark of good scholarship. DNP students should think seriously about using both venues to showcase their scholarly work. Presenting at professional conferences brings with it the distinct advantage of meeting and networking with professional colleagues who share similar interests. Publishing in peer-reviewed journals has the advantage of reaching a wider audience.

Presenting a poster at a conference is one way to disseminate knowledge from the DNP scholarly project. Preparing an effective poster presentation requires time, creativity, and clarity of thought. Christenbery and Latham (2013) provide excellent recommendations for producing an effective scholarly poster. Importantly, a poster presentation should not be viewed as an end unto itself. It should be understood as a stepping stone toward developing a publishable scholarly manuscript.

Scholarly writing for publication is a skill that is developed over time, but the pace at which this skill is developed can be accelerated. Mentoring and critical feedback can help accelerate the pace of developing one's capacity for scholarly writing. Some DNP schools are now offering courses to help students develop their capacity for scholarly writing (Shirey, 2013). Clearly, getting a manuscript published in a peer-reviewed journal requires good scholarly writing, but journal choice and following author guidelines are equally important. The focus of a manuscript submitted for publication in a refereed journal must match the mission of the journal. Also, the presentation and style of the manuscript must exactly match the journal's guidelines for authors. Nothing is more aggravating for journal editors than disregard for journal format or mission, or both (Froman, 2008).

By the time DNP students come to the end of their program of study, they should have a good idea about which professional peer-reviewed journals publish work similar to their own. These are the journals that should be targeted for publication. The manuscript can be submitted to only one journal at a time. It is recommended that the would-be author choose from among two or three of these journals, then review the journal mission, access the journal's author guidelines, and decide which journal seems to be most appropriate. Author guidelines should be kept close at hand throughout the production of the manuscript, but don't start writing yet! Although most journals accept unsolicited manuscripts, a query letter to the editor can be extremely beneficial because it helps the editor decide whether a proposed manuscript is in keeping with the mission of the journal, avoids having a manuscript rejected because the journal has recently accepted a manuscript of similar content and focus, and helps the author synthesize manuscript ideas within one or two short paragraphs. Well-written query letters are difficult to produce, but they are well worth the effort. A number of online resources are available to guide new writers through the do's and don'ts of crafting an effective query letter. See, for example, the recommendations of John Hewitt (2014).

HUMAN SUBJECTS CONCERNS

Federal guidelines define research as "a systematic investigation, including research development, testing and evaluation, designed to develop or contribute to generalizable knowledge" and go on to note that "some demonstration and service programs may include research activities" (U. S. Department of Health and Human Services, 2009). The *Belmont Report* specifically states that "if there is any element of research in an activity, that activity should undergo review for protection of human subjects" (U.S. Department of Health and Human Services, 1979, p. 4). The interpretation of these guidelines continues to evolve. It has been argued, for example, that data collected outside the confines of standard practice and presented at a public meeting or in a publication should require the same IRB approval and informed consent as data collected for research purposes (Glatstein, 2001). Thus, data-based quality improvement initiatives that involve human subjects may be subjected to the same level of scrutiny as research that involves human subjects (Newhouse, Pettit, Poe, & Rocco, 2006).

DNP students who are interested in publishing the results of data-based projects that involve human subjects should anticipate that journal editors will ask them to explicitly disclose whether IRB approval was obtained. Also, journal editors will ask whether an informed investigational consent explaining, in clear language, the purpose, possible risks, and benefits of the study was signed by all participating subjects. Often this information must be included within the body of the manuscript. Any attempt to deceive the journal on these points is considered evidence of ethical misconduct.

WHOSE WORK IS GETTING PUBLISHED?

Decisions about authorship may seem straightforward but can become complex very quickly. This is especially true when generating publications from the final DNP project. At first blush it seems reasonable to think about the capstone project as the student's work alone. However, it is important to remember that doctoral projects, whether a dissertation or a final DNP project, are mentored, collaborative projects. Typically the collaborators—faculty chairperson and committee members—provide guidance and input into the conceptualization and design of the project and devote considerable time and effort in directing and redirecting the project, facilitating the interpretation of results, and editing the final report. Thus, each collaborator may have a substantial claim to some of the intellectual property reflected in the final DNP project. To avoid contention, it is wise to discuss the topic of authorship early in the development of a project (King, McGuire, Longman, & Carroll-Johnson, 1997). This discussion should address important issues such as who will be included as authors, the order of authorship, who will be acknowledged, and an agreement to revisit these points of concern as publication draws near. A final agreement on author inclusion should be stated in writing to dispel erroneous assumptions that could lead to embarrassment and erosion of professional relationships down the road (King et al., 1997).

Relying on standards or guidelines to direct decision making about authorship is highly recommended (King et al., 1997). A dependable and frequently cited formal statement of criteria for authorship comes from the International Committee of Medical Journal Editors:

> Authorship credit should be based on 1) substantial contributions to conception and design, acquisition of data, or analysis and interpretation of data; 2) drafting the article or revising it critically for important intellectual content; and 3) final approval of the version to be published. Authors should meet conditions 1, 2, and 3. (International Committee of Medical Journal Editors [ICMJE], 2013, p. 2) .

The preceding statement helps clarify what is meant by *substantial contribution*. To further avoid problems of loose authorship and questions regarding the order of authorship, journals routinely ask for written certification from all authors whose names appear on the byline of an article. In addition, journals increasingly require each author to specify the nature of their contribution to the published product. In some journals a brief description of the functional role of each author is appended to the end of the published piece (for example, see recent publications from the *Journal of Advanced Nursing*). In the final analysis, all persons designated as authors should qualify for authorship, and all those who qualify should be listed (ICMJE, 2013).

The faculty member who chairs the student's committee often will initiate discussions about authorship and help negotiate the finer points, such as what constitutes a substantial contribution worthy of authorship versus minor contributions worthy of acknowledgment. However, if the chairperson does not take the lead, it is in the student's own best interest to launch the discussion. Moving to publication as sole author on a manuscript without consulting one's collaborators is bad form at best and scientific misconduct at worst, especially if the intellectual work of collaborators is presented as though it were the student's own work (Grinnell, 1997). On the other hand, DNP graduates should not naïvely weight the contributions of collaborators more heavily than their own by giving away first authorship. Students have a right to list their name as first author when they publish major findings of their final DNP project. Moreover, the APA explicitly endorses listing the student as principal author "of any multiauthored papers substantially based on their dissertation" (APA, 2010, p. 19).

New authors may find it especially helpful to read Baggs's (2008) excellent editorial, which speaks clearly and succinctly about issues of authorship, acknowledgement, duplicate publication, self-plagiarism, and salami slicing (i.e., trying to slice too many publications out of one piece of research).

PEER REVIEW

Peer review is one way of ensuring that what is being printed in the literature is relevant, innovative, and nonredundant. Double-blind peer review is a long-standing tradition in nursing. When double blinded, the manuscript under review moves, through the editor, from an unidentified writer to a similarly unidentified reviewer (hence, double blind) (Walker, 2004). The peer-review process can be highly politicized and may even squelch creativity. However, it is unlikely that peer-review processes will change between now and the time that current DNP students submit their manuscripts for publication, so it is probably best for students to adopt a healthy attitude toward peer review. To begin with, it helps if new authors try to think about reviewers as colleagues.

Rarely is a manuscript accepted as is, without revision. Authors may not like what reviewers say about their manuscripts, but constructive criticism from objective reviewers with relevant expertise can be used to clarify thinking and sharpen writing skills (Fahy, 2008). Therefore, recommendations for revision with resubmission should be viewed optimistically, especially if the reviewers have provided substantive feedback. Reviewer feedback almost always tells the author exactly what needs to be done to the manuscript to increase the chances of getting it published. All reviewer comments must be addressed. Addressing reviewer comments does not mean the author agrees with every critique or recommendation. It does mean that the author should provide rationales for reviewer recommendations that have not been followed. Editors do not look favorably upon authors who ignore reviewer comments (Froman, 2008). Multiple revisions and resubmissions may be needed before a manuscript is finally accepted for publication. Enduring what might seem like an overabundance of help from peer-review colleagues requires a special kind of perseverance, but don't give up! If the reviewers were not interested in seeing the manuscript in print, they would not persist in providing collegial feedback.

DEALING WITH REJECTION

Outright rejection is a hard blow to the ego, but rejection should not lead to dejection. It is important to remember that it is the work that is being rejected, not the author. One of the leading causes for rejection of a manuscript is a mismatch between the journal's mission and the focus of the manuscript (Froman, 2008). Also the choice of journal can influence the likelihood of rejection. Highly competitive, top-tier journals, such as *Advances in Nursing Science, Nursing Research*, and *Research in Nursing and Health*, tend to have higher rejection rates than specialty journals, such as *Clinical Nurse Specialist, Journal of Advanced Nursing, Heart & Lung*, and *Dimensions in Critical Care Nursing*.

Scholarship and Research Beyond Graduation

Scholarship and scholarly productivity are work-related expectations of university faculty. New DNP graduates who interview for faculty appointments at university schools of nursing need to come away from those interviews with a full understanding of the scholarship expectations of their potential employers. It is important, for example, to know what counts as scholarship, expectations regarding scholarly productivity, and the level of support provided for faculty scholarship. Historically publication of research findings in peer-reviewed journals has been the gold standard of faculty scholarship. However, since the publication of Boyer's (1990) seminal work, *Scholarship Reconsidered: Priorities of the Professoriate*, many schools of nursing have broadened the definition of scholarship, especially as it relates to the scholarship of clinical faculty (see, for example, Jones & Van Ort, 2001). Boyer's (1990) conceptualization of scholarship includes four categories: discovery, integration, application, and teaching. The scholarship of discovery generates new and unique knowledge. The scholarship of integration refers to the synthesis of knowledge across fields. The scholarship of application focuses on using new knowledge to solve social problems. Finally, the scholarship of teaching takes into account the relationship between teaching and learning and upholds the importance of using creative approaches to bridge the gap between what the teacher knows and what the student learns.

Job security at universities and decisions about tenure and promotion are based on scholarly productivity. Therefore, it is important for DNP graduates to know whether potential employers define scholarship exclusively as research publications or along a number of categories, such as those described by Boyer (1990). In university settings, expectations for scholarly productivity are typically stated in quantifiable terms; for example, one to two publications per year or two to four paper presentations at local, regional, or national professional conferences. It is important that DNP graduates who are seeking faculty appointments understand that a continuous, identifiable, year-to-year record of scholarly productivity is expected. The volume of scholarly work produced may fluctuate from year to year, but long dry spells should be avoided. Partnering with other faculty to coauthor a publication, copresent at a conference, or redesign a course can help carry new faculty members through dry spells.

Partnering often brings with it the unexpected benefits of stimulating creativity and reinvigorating interest and excitement about one's own area of scholarship.

Making time for scholarship is a huge problem. University faculty carry heavy workloads that include course preparation and evaluation, teaching, service to the school and university, and student advisement and counseling. Learning to make time for scholarship can be very challenging, especially for new faculty members. Often workload documents specify that a percentage of time (for example, 10% or 20%) is allotted for faculty scholarship. However, it is up to the faculty member to protect this time. In other words, if 4 hours per week are allotted for scholarship, then a 4-hour block of time should be scheduled in one's personal calendar as time protected for scholarship. Self-discipline is required to ensure that the time protected for scholarship is, in fact, used for the intended purpose and not frittered away on other activities. Creating a protected work space for scholarship is equally important. It is difficult to be productive when one's work space is constantly invaded by phone calls and drop-in visits from faculty and students. Posting an office schedule, closing the office door, and turning the phone off are some strategies that can be used to protect the work space from these distractions.

DNP graduates who take positions in clinical service settings may find that their employers have no clearly stipulated expectations for scholarship and scholarly productivity. In fact, research has shown that nurse executives have a poor and inconsistent understanding of DNP capabilities (Nichols, O'Connor, & Dunn, 2014). In these situations the DNP needs be highly self-directed when it comes to clarifying his or her value orientations toward scholarship, choosing an area for scholarship that will advance the profession, determining how his or her scholarship will be developed, negotiating release time for scholarship, and garnering recognition for scholarly productivity in annual performance evaluations. Currently there are no widely recognized models of scholarship for clinical practice. In medicine, Morahan and Fleetwood (2008) have proposed a conceptual model of scholarship in which practice activities, such as teaching students, teaching patients, providing services, and conducting research, are linked to scholarship activities, such as teaching others how to teach students; teaching procedures to other clinicians; informing others how to design, implement, and evaluate programs; and informing others of research findings by presenting results at conferences and publishing papers. DNP graduates might use a similar strategy to conceptualize linkages between their own practice-related activities and areas of scholarship. Alternatively, DNPs who work in clinical service settings might consider adapting Boyer's (1990) four dimensions of scholarship—discovery, integration, application, and teaching—to organize their thinking about scholarship in practice. For example, APRNs who work at the Detroit Medical Center demonstrated the scholarship of teaching when they developed, tested, and disseminated a teaching program designed specifically to help staff nurses learn how to use the Braden Scale correctly to assess a patient's level of risk for developing pressure ulcers (Maklebust et al., 2005).

Getting caught in the practice trap is a barrier to scholarship for all practitioners. DNPs will know they are caught in the practice trap if all their work time is dedicated to clinical practice. To advance the profession, it is imperative that DNPs make time in their work schedules (and time at home) for scholarship. Dialogue and up-front negotiation with potential employers will be needed to ensure adequate release time and financial support for involvement in scholarly activities. In exchange for release time and financial support, DNP employers should expect to see tangible results, such as presentations (not merely attendance) at conferences or publications in professional peer-reviewed journals.

Mentored Scholarship

There is an assumption in nursing that mentoring is critical to career success, especially if one chooses to develop one's self as a productive scholar after earning the doctoral degree (Morse, 2006; Roy & Linendoll, 2006). Mentors typically are defined as individuals with advanced experience and knowledge who are committed to providing support—career building and psychosocial—to less experienced, more junior individuals who are referred to as protégés or mentees (Maas et al., 2006; Yonge, Billay, Myrick, & Luhanga, 2007). A number of mentoring models are portrayed in the literature. One model depicts mentoring as a long-standing, dyadic relationship between a mentor and a protégé that begins during doctoral study and proceeds throughout the span of one's career. Another model depicts mentoring as an activity orchestrated within the hierarchical structure of an organization; for example, when a senior faculty member is assigned to mentor a junior faculty member. Other, more contemporary, models suggest that mentoring may come from multiple sources and that the exchange between the mentor and the protégé emerges from what is needed at some point in time (Broome, 2003; de Janasz & Sullivan, 2004). Parse (2002), for example, speaks of mentoring moments that emerge as individuals engage in a dialogue about a scholarly project or career development. From Parse's (2002) perspective, mentoring moments are characterized by choice rather than a long-standing relationship. Accordingly, the mentor chooses to offer wise counsel for the moment and the project, whereas the protégé chooses to accept mentoring from someone who espouses value orientations similar to his or her own. Higgins (2000) has suggested that the amount and type of help provided (i.e., career versus psychosocial) can be used to conceptualize mentoring and that mentors can range from acting merely as an ally (someone who helps only if and when help is needed) to friend (someone who provides high amounts of psychosocial support) to sponsor (someone who provides high amounts of career support) to true mentor (someone who provides high amounts of both career and psychosocial support).

The literature on mentoring consistently identifies the mentor as the helper and the protégé as the one being helped; however, it has been suggested that "the best mentoring relationships include mutual benefits and positive attitudes between the mentor who enjoys guiding and supporting the protégé and the protégé who seeks to model the behaviors and achievements of the mentor" (Maas et al., 2006, p. 184). The chairperson of the DNP student's capstone project may be the first person to take an active interest in guiding the DNP's scholarly development. The relationship between the capstone advisor and the DNP student often resembles what Higgins (2000) describes as a sponsored mentorship in which the mentor (advisor) provides a high amount of project mentoring to ensure that the protégé (doctoral student) succeeds in meeting curriculum requirements for the capstone project. Thus, the relationship between the chairperson and the doctoral student might be more appropriately understood as a time-limited, project-specific, advisor–advisee relationship. There is no way of predicting whether this type of sponsored mentorship will transition to a true mentoring relationship that extends beyond the duration of the capstone project. There is always the risk that expectations of either the mentor or the protégé will not be met, especially when one considers how extensive these expectations can be. Maas and colleagues (2006) noted that:

> protégés expect mentors to be role models and to have the expertise, interest, and demeanor needed to guide and support protégés in seizing and using opportunities to develop a successful career. Mentors seek protégés who are motivated for success and leadership, and are a good match with the mentor in terms of career interests and a mutually beneficial relationship. (Maas et al., 2006, pp. 183–184)

After graduation, finding a mentor—whether a true mentor, an ally, a sponsor, or a cadre of mentors—to guide, support, and inspire the development of one's scholarship can be challenging. The DNP graduate may long for a true mentor, but until one is found it might be best to make good use of whatever qualified help is available. As Dave Thomas, the founder of Wendy's, stated, "Instead of waiting for someone to take you under his [sic] wing, go out and find a good wing to climb under" (Phillips-Jones, 2001, p. 1). This may require learning how to network effectively in the hallways, at meetings, by email, and at professional conferences.

The search for a mentor and mentoring can be made easier if the DNP graduate (protégé) proactively identifies areas where mentoring is wanted and needed. This search should be guided by a clear understanding that mentoring often occurs in phases (Broome, 2003). What is needed in the early part of one's DNP career will not be equal to what is needed in the later part of one's DNP career. New DNP graduates, for example, may find that situation-specific mentoring from multiple mentors is sufficient to help them negotiate job interviews, get their scholarly project published, overcome self-doubt, redefine their professional identity, and become comfortable using their new title. Often it is within the context of engaging in mentoring moments that relationships take shape; values, ideas, and aspirations are exchanged; and the ground is made fertile for developing an enduring relationship between the mentor and the protégé.

Mentored Research

It has been established that the DNP is not a research-focused degree. Nevertheless, results from a survey of DNP students ($N = 69$) have shown that nearly one-third of the students surveyed anticipated being involved in research after graduation (Loomis, Willard, & Cohen, 2006). It is unclear from the survey report whether the anticipated postgraduation research involvement is limited to evidence-based practice or extends to actual involvement in knowledge-generating research. Although it is recognized that the DNP is not a research degree, no universal law prohibits DNPs from conducting knowledge-generating research. However, DNP graduates who are interested in conducting research may find it helpful to work with a PhD-prepared nurse who can bring research and statistical expertise to the project. If the DNP is interested in serving as the sole principal investigator on the project, then a research consultant or mentor might be brought on board. Research consultants and mentors can provide "advice regarding research-related questions and issues, proposal development, funding sources, and manuscript development" (Whittemore, 2007, p. 235). Typically a consultant is paid, whereas a mentor is not. Alternatively, the DNP may choose to work more collaboratively with a PhD-prepared nurse as a coinvestigator on a project. In a collaborative effort there is shared accountability for the outcome. My own experience in collaborating with APRNs on research projects has been personally and professionally enriching and has led to a number of coauthored publications in peer-reviewed journals (see, for example, Magnan & Maklebust, 2008a, 2008b, 2009a, 2009b; Magnan & Reynolds, 2006; Magnan, Reynolds, & Galvin, 2005; Reynolds & Magnan, 2005). These authors identified trust as the most important feature of a collaborative relationship. APRNs need to trust that their important research ideas will not be stolen by a PhD-prepared nurse. In addition, it seems to be very important to APRNs that PhD-prepared nurses understand nursing practice and respect the clinical expertise of APRNs. DNP graduates might recognize from this personal account that effective, productive collaborations with a PhD-prepared nurse need to be based on trust and mutual respect.

Building a Network for Research and Scholarship

A network is a circuit through which things flow: ideas, energy, dialogue, information, favors, and so on. Networking involves proactive involvement in activities to develop and maintain personal and professional relationships with others for the purpose of mutual benefit in their work or career (Forret & Dougherty, 2001). Thus, one common purpose of networking is career advancement, which may extend from finding a first job to finding a new job with higher pay and status. Networking also plays an important role in building professional identity and reputation (Rojas-Guyler, Murnan, & Cottrell, 2007). The more extensive the network, the more people there are who know about your skills, initiative, areas of interest, scholarly pursuits, and reputation. Other purposes of networking include identifying and cultivating mentoring relationships and meeting research collaborators (de Janasz & Forret, 2008).

Opportunities for networking are almost limitless. Networking can be done in person, over the phone, via the Internet, and through professional organizations. Professional conferences are great venues for networking. However, it is important to use conference time wisely; planning ahead helps. Plan to attend conference symposia and breakout sessions where the topic being presented is likely to attract an audience with interests similar to your own. Little networking occurs during the actual presentation, so plan to linger afterwards to meet the presenter, especially if he or she is a known expert in your area of interest. Traveling to the next session with a newly found colleague is a good way of extending your network. If you are the presenter, be prepared to graciously engage members of the audience who stay afterwards to talk about your presentation.

For networking purposes, the wise use of conference time must include taking full advantage of all conference-hosted social events, especially if food is being served! Nonfood events may include guided tours of historical sites or morning walks. Food events usually include a continental breakfast, a box lunch, and, at some conferences, a posh evening event complete with chamber music, a shrimp bar, a cash bar, and several serpentine tables stacked with hors d'oeuvres and desserts. These food events provide opportunities to network in a relaxed social setting while sharing a bite to eat. The conference-hosted evening event is a must attend for all serious networkers. Often more formal evening wear is required and, because these are usually stand-up events (no seating available), sensible shoes are a must. It is extremely difficult to work a room and network effectively if your feet are killing you. Do not carry a handbag to an evening event. The hands must be kept free to handle tiny food plates, but more important, the hands must be free to shake hands. Do take business cards but keep them in a pocket or an over-the-shoulder bag so they are accessible but out of the way.

Networking often begins with a succinct introductory icebreaker followed by an introduction. Painfully shy people may want to rehearse responses to questions such as, Where do you work?, What are your areas of interest?, and Are you working on any exciting projects? However, learning how to lead a conversation by asking questions of others is more important to networking than reporting on one's own accomplishments (Puetz, 2007).

The biggest barrier to networking is avoiding it altogether. Introverted individuals with low self-esteem may find it especially difficult to engage in networking activities (Forret & Dougherty, 2001). However, training with opportunities for practice and feedback can help individuals increase their confidence and comfort with networking skills (de Janasz & Forret, 2008). Setting a goal to make at least two or three new contacts at a conference can help motivate one in the right direction. Other mistakes in networking include leaving business cards at home, asking others for too much too soon, failing to follow-up with new contacts, and not having clearly identified career-related goals (Agre, 2002; Nickleston, 2008; Puetz, 2007).

Building a network of support to advance scholarship and research requires some up-front self-reflection. It is important to come to terms with what you are about and what your scholarship and research interests are. The following advice is especially relevant: "Don't follow fashion. Don't imagine that the world compels you to work on certain topics or talk a certain way. First things first: once you can explain what you care about, then you can build a community of people who also care about that. That's what networking is for" (Agre, 2002, p. 4). It is important for DNP graduates to recognize that they are pioneering a new role in the profession. The frontiers for DNP scholarship and involvement in research that will advance the discipline and profession of nursing are wide open, so find out what you really care about then gather your resources, rally all your faculties, marshal all your energies, and focus all your capacities upon mastery in your chosen area of scholarship and research.

SUMMARY

- The utility of a theory comes from the organization it provides for thinking, observing, and interpreting what is observed.
- Acquire skills needed to apply middle-range theory to practice.
- A foundation in research ethics, the fundamentals of research methodology, core statistical principles, and the critical appraisal of research literature is needed to achieve some of the DNP competencies.
- DNP graduates will play a pivotal role in nursing's research enterprise, particularly at the juncture of providing leadership for evidence-based practice.
- Doctoral study provides opportunities to start developing skills of scholarship, especially skills related to reviewing the literature and writing cogently, clearly, and concisely.
- Publishing findings from the final DNP project is a mark of good scholarship. Acknowledging contributions of collaborators is a mark of ethical conduct.
- Make good use of mentors and mentoring moments to advance career, scholarship, and research goals.
- Build a network of support to advance scholarship and research goals beyond graduation.

REFLECTION QUESTIONS

1. Does theory add anything to daily practice? In what ways might you use theory in practice?

2. Should DNP graduates avoid engaging in research undertaken to generate new knowledge?

3. How important is it to foster a mentoring relationship to advance your scholarship or research?

4. What qualities would you find most helpful in a mentor?

5. Do you think networking will help you grow as a scholar? If so, have you started networking with others who have similar interests?

REFERENCES

Agre, P. (2002). Networking on the network: A guide to professional skills for PhD students. Retrieved from http://vlsicad.ucsd.edu/Research/Advice/network.html

Ajzen, I., & Madden, T. J. (1986). Prediction of goal-directed behavior: Attitudes, intentions, and perceived behavioral control. *Journal of Experimental Social Psychology, 22,* 453–474.

American Association of Colleges of Nursing. (1999). *Defining scholarship for the discipline of nursing.* Washington, DC: Author.

American Association of Colleges of Nursing. (2006). *Essentials of doctoral education for advanced nursing practice.* Retrieved from www.aacn.nche.edu/publications/position/DNPEssentials.pdf

American Nurses Association. (2003). *Nursing's social policy statement* (2nd ed.). Silver Spring, MD: Author.

American Psychological Association. (2010). *Publication manual of the American Psychological Association* (6th ed.). Washington, DC: Author.

Baggs, J. G. (2008). Issues and rules for authors concerning authorship versus acknowledgements, dual publication, self plagiarism, and salami publishing. *Research in Nursing & Health, 31*(4), 295–297.

Bandura, A. (1977). Self-efficacy: Toward a unifying theory of behavioral change. *Psychological Review, 84*(2), 191–215.

Bandura, A. (1997). *Self-efficacy: The exercise of control.* New York, NY: W. H. Freeman.

Barnett-Ellis, P., & Restauri, S. (2006). Nursing student library usage patterns in online courses: Findings and recommendations. *Internet Reference Services Quarterly, 11*(4), 117–138.

Boyer, E. L. (1990). *Scholarship reconsidered: Priorities of the professoriate.* Princeton, NJ: Carnegie Foundation for the Advancement of Teaching.

Broome, M. E. (2003). Mentoring: To everything a season. *Nursing Outlook, 51*(6), 249–250.

Burns, N., & Grove, S. K. (2005). *The practice of nursing research: Conduct, critique, and utilization* (5th ed.). St. Louis, MO: Elsevier Saunders.

Christenbery, T. L., & Latham, T. G. (2013). Creating effective scholarly posters: A guide for DNP students. *Journal of the American Association of Nurse Practitioners, 25*, 16–23.

Cox, C. L. (1982). An interaction model of client health behavior: Theoretical prescription for nursing. *Advances in Nursing Science, 5*(1), 41–56.

de Janasz, S. C., & Forret, M. L. (2008). Learning the art of networking: A critical skill for enhancing social capital and career success. *Journal of Management Education, 32*(5), 629–650.

de Janasz, S. C., & Sullivan, S. E. (2004). Multiple mentoring in academe: Developing the professorial network. *Journal of Vocational Behavior, 64*(2), 263–283.

Dee, C., & Stanley, E. E. (2005). Information-seeking behavior of nursing students and clinical nurses: Implications for health sciences librarians. *Journal of Medical Librarians Association, 93*(2), 213–222.

DiCenso, A., Guyatt, G., & Ciliska, D. (2005). *Evidence-based nursing: A guide to clinical practice.* St. Louis, MO: Elsevier Mosby.

Donaldson, S. K. (1995). Nursing science for nursing practice. In A. Omery, C. E. Kasper, & G. G. Page (Eds.), *In search of nursing science* (pp. 3–12). Thousand Oaks, CA: Sage.

Donaldson, S. K., & Crowley, D. M. (1978). The discipline of nursing. *Nursing Outlook, 26*(2), 113–120.

Fahy, K. (2008). Writing for publication: The basics. *Women and Birth, 21*(2), 86–91.

Fawcett, J. (2005). *Contemporary nursing knowledge: Analysis and evaluation of nursing models and theories.* Philadelphia, PA: F. A. Davis.

Forret, M. L., & Dougherty, T. W. (2001). Correlates of networking behavior for managerial and professional employees. *Group & Organization Management, 26*(3), 283–311.

Froman, R. D. (2008). Hitting the bull's eye rather than shooting yourself between the eyes. *Research in Nursing & Health, 31*(5), 399–401.

Glatstein, E. (2001). What is research? *International Journal of Radiation Oncology, Biology, Physics, 5*(2), 288–290.

Grinnell, F. (1997). Truth, fairness, and the definition of scientific misconduct. *Journal of Laboratory and Clinical Medicine, 129*(2), 189–192.

Hewitt, J. (2014). How to write a query letter. Retrieved from http://www.poewar.com/how-to-write-a-query-letter/

Higgins, M. (2000). The more, the merrier? Multiple developmental relationships and work satisfaction. *Journal of Management Development, 19*(4), 277–296.

International Committee of Medical Journal Editors. (2013). *Uniform requirements for manuscripts submitted to biomedical journals: Writing and editing for biomedical publications.* Retrieved from http://www.icmje.org/icmje-recommendations.pdf

Jacobs, M. K., & Huether, S. E. (1978). Nursing science: The theory-practice linkage. *Advances in Nursing Science, 1*(1), 63–73.

Johnson, T. M. (2008). Tips on how to write a paper. *Journal of the American Academy of Dermatology, 59*(6), 1064–1069.

Jones, E. G., & Van Ort, S. (2001). Facilitating scholarship among clinical faculty. *Journal of Professional Nursing, 17*(3), 141–146.

Kerlinger, F. N. (1973). *Foundations of behavioral research* (2nd ed.). New York, NY: Holt Rinehart & Winston.

King, C. R., McGuire, D., Longman, A., & Carroll-Johnson, R. M. (1997). Peer review, authorship, ethics, and conflict of interest. *Image, 29*(2), 163–167.

Kirkpatrick, J. M., & Weaver, T. (2013). The doctor of nursing practice capstone project: Consensus or confusion? *Journal of Nursing Education, 52*(8), 435–441.

Kitson, A. (2006). The relevance of scholarship for nursing research and practice. *Journal of Advanced Nursing, 55*(5), 541–545. (Reprinted from *Journal of Advanced Nursing, 29*(4), 773–775, by A. Kitson, 1999)

Lenz, E. R. (1998a). The role of middle-range theory for nursing research and practice: Part 1. Nursing research. *Nursing Leadership Forum, 3*(1), 24–33.

Lenz, E. R. (1998b). The role of middle-range theory for nursing research and practice: Part 2. Nursing practice. *Nursing Leadership Forum, 3*(2), 62–66.

Lenz, E. R. (2005). The practice doctorate in nursing: An idea whose time has come. *Online Journal of Issues in Nursing, 10*(3), Manuscript 1. Retrieved from http://www .nursingworld.org/MainMenuCategories/ANAMarketplace/ANAPeriodicals/OJIN /TableofContents/Volume102005/No3Sept05/tpc28_116025.html

Lenz, E. R., Pugh, L. C., Milligan, R. A., Gift, A., & Suppe, F. (1997). The middle-range theory of unpleasant symptoms: An update. *Advances in Nursing Science, 19*(3), 14–27.

Lenz, E. R., Suppe, F., Gift, A. G., Pugh, L. C., & Milligan, R. A. (1995). Collaborative development of middle-range theory: Toward a theory of unpleasant symptoms. *Advances in Nursing Science, 17*(3), 1–13.

Loomis, J. A., Willard, B., & Cohen, J. (2006, December). Difficult professional choices: Deciding between the PhD and DNP in nursing. *OJIN: The Online Journal of Issues in Nursing, 12.* Retrieved from http://www.doctorsofnursingpractice.org/UserFiles/File /Loomis2006.pdf

Maas, M. L., Strumpf, N. E., Beck, C., Jennings, D., Messecar, D., & Swanson, E. (2006). Mentoring geriatric nurse scientists, educators, clinicians, and leaders in the John A. Hartford Foundation Centers for Geriatric Nursing Excellence. *Nursing Outlook, 54*(4), 183–188.

Macnee, C. L., & McCabe, S. (2008). *Understanding nursing research: Using research in evidence-based practice* (2nd ed.). Philadelphia, PA: Lippincott Williams & Wilkins.

Magnan, M. A., & Maklebust, J. (2008a). Multi-site web-based training in use of the Braden Scale for predicting pressure sore risk. *Advances in Skin & Wound Care, 21*(3), 124–133.

Magnan, M. A., & Maklebust, J. (2008b). The effect of web-based Braden Scale training on the reliability and precision of Braden Scale pressure ulcer risk assessments. *Journal of Wound, Ostomy and Continence Nursing, 35*(2), 199–208.

Magnan, M. A., & Maklebust, J. (2009a). The effect of web-based Braden Scale training on the reliability of Braden subscale ratings. *Journal of Wound, Ostomy and Continence Nursing, 36*(1), 51–59.

Magnan, M. A., & Maklebust, J. (2009b). The nursing process and pressure ulcer prevention: Making the connection. *Advances in Skin & Wound Care, 22*(2), 83–92.

Magnan, M. A., & Reynolds, K. E. (2006). Barriers to addressing sexuality across five areas of specialization. *Clinical Nurse Specialist, 20*(6), 285–292.

Magnan, M. A., Reynolds, K., & Galvin, L. (2005). Barriers to addressing patient sexuality in nursing practice. *Medical-Surgical Nursing, 14*(5), 282–289.

Magyar, D., Whitney, J. D., & Brown, M. A. (2006). Advancing practice inquiry: Research foundations of the practice doctorate in nursing. *Nursing Outlook, 54*(3), 139–151.

Maklebust, J., Sieggreen, M. Y., Sidor, D., Gerlach, M. A., Bauer, C., & Anderson, C. (2005). Computer-based testing of the Braden Scale for predicting pressure sore risk. *Ostomy Wound Management, 51*(4), 40–42, 44, 46.

McDiarmid, S. (1998). Continuing nursing education: What resources do bedside nurses use? *Journal of Continuing Education in Nursing, 29*(6), 267–273.

Melnyk, B., & Fineout-Overholt, E. (2005). *Evidence-based practice in nursing and healthcare: A guide to best practice.* Philadelphia, PA: Lippincott Williams & Wilkins.

Mishel, M. H. (1990). Reconceptualization of the Uncertainty in Illness theory. *Image: Journal of Nursing Scholarship, 22*(4), 256–262.

Morahan, P. S., & Fleetwood, J. (2008). The double helix of activity and scholarship: Building a medical education career with limited resources. *Medical Education, 42*(1), 34–44.

Moran, K., Burson, R., & Conrad, D. (Eds.). (2014). *The doctor of nursing practice scholarly project: A framework for success.* Burlington, MA: Jones & Bartlett Learning.

Morse, J. M. (2006). Deconstructing the mantra of mentorship in conversation with Phyllis Noerager Stern. *Health Care for Women International, 27*(6), 548–558.

Newhouse, R. P., Pettit, J. C., Poe, S., & Rocco, L. (2006). The slippery slope: Differentiating between quality improvement and research. *Journal of Nursing Administration, 36*(4), 211–219.

Nichols, C., O'Connor, N., & Dunn, D. (2014). Exploring early and future use of DNP prepared nurses within healthcare organizations. *Journal of Nursing Administration, 44*(2), 74–78.

Nickleston, P. (2008, April). 7 networking mistakes to avoid. *Dynamic Chiropractic, 29*(19). Retrieved from http://www.dynamicchiropractic.com/mpacms/dc/article.php?id=53149

Olson, J., & Hanchett, E. (1997). Nurse-expressed empathy, patient outcomes, and development of a middle-range theory. *Image: Journal of Nursing Scholarship, 29*(1), 71–76.

Parse, R. R. (2002). Mentoring moments. *Nursing Science Quarterly, 15*(2), 97.

Pavikoff, D., Tanner, A., & Pierce, S. T. (2005). Readiness of U.S. nurses for evidence-based practice: Many don't understand or value research and have had little or no training to help them find evidence on which to base their practice. *American Journal of Nursing, 105*(9), 40–51.

Peterson, S. J., & Bredow, T. S. (2004). *Middle range theories: Application to nursing research.* Philadelphia, PA: Lippincott Williams & Wilkins.

Phillips-Jones, L. (2001). *The new mentors and protégés: How to succeed with the new mentoring partnerships.* Grass Valley, CA: Coalition of Counseling Centers.

Prochaska, J. O., & DiClemente, C. C. (1983). Stages and processes of self-change of smoking: Toward an integrative model of change. *Journal of Consulting and Clinical Psychology, 51*(3), 390–395.

Puetz, B. E. (2007). Networking. *Public Health Nursing, 24*(6), 577–579.

Reynolds, K., & Magnan, M. A. (2005). Nurses' attitudes and beliefs toward human sexuality: Collaborative research promoting evidence-based practice. *Clinical Nurse Specialist, 19*(5), 255–260.

Rice, V. H. (2000). *Handbook of stress, coping, and health: Implications for nursing research, theory, and practice.* Thousand Oaks, CA: Sage.

Rojas-Guyler, L., Murnan, J., & Cottrell, R. R. (2007). Networking for career-long success: A powerful strategy for health education professionals. *Health Promotion Practice, 8*(3), 229–233. Retrieved from http://hpp.sagepub.com/cgi/content/abstract/8/3/229

Rosenstock, I. M. (1990). The health belief model: Explaining health behavior through expectancies. In K. Glanz, F. M. Lewis, & B. K. Rimer (Eds.), *Health behavior and health education: Theory research and practice* (pp. 39–62). San Francisco, CA: Jossey-Bass.

Rosswurm, M., & Larrabee, J. (1999). A model for change to evidence-based practice. *Image: Journal of Nursing Scholarship, 31*(4), 317–322.

Roy, C., & Linendoll, N. M. (2006). Deriving international consensus on mentorship in doctoral education. *Journal of Research in Nursing, 11*(4), 345–353.

Sackett, D., Rosenberg, W., Gray, J., Haynes, R., & Richardson, W. (1996). Evidence based medicine: What it is and what it isn't. *British Medical Journal, 312*(7023), 71–72.

Scholarship. (1993). In *Merriam-Webster's collegiate dictionary* (10th ed.). (1993). Springfield, MA: Merriam-Webster.

Shirey, M. R. (2013). Building scholarly writing capacity in the doctor of nursing practice program. *Journal of Professional Nursing, 29*(3), 137–147.

Spenceley, S. M., O'Leary, K. A., Chizawsky, L. L., Ross, A. J., & Estabrooks, C. A. (2008). Sources of information used by nurses to inform practice: An integrative review. *International Journal of Nursing Studies, 45*(6), 954–970.

Stetler, C. B., & DiMaggio, G. (1991). Research utilization among clinical nurse specialists. *Clinical Nurse Specialist, 5*(3), 151–155.

Stupnyckyj, C., Smolarek, S., Reeves, C., McKeith, J., & Magnan, M. (in press). Using EBP to change transfusion policy and practice. *American Journal of Nursing.*

Titmus, C. (1999). Concepts and practices of education and adult education: Obstacles to lifelong learning. *International Journal of Lifelong Education, 18*(5), 343–354.

U.S. Department of Health and Human Services. (1979). *Belmont report.* Retrieved from http://www.hhs.gov/ohrp/humansubjects/guidance/belmont.html

U.S. Department of Health and Human Services. (2009). Code of Federal Regulations, Department of Health and Human Services, Title 45 Part 46.102(d). Retrieved fromwww.hhs.gov/ohrp/humansubjects/guidance/45cfr46.html#46.102

Walker, K. (2004). 'Double b(l)ind': Peer-review and the politics of scholarship. *Nursing Philosophy, 5*(2), 135–146.

Weaver, K., & Olson, J. K. (2006). Understanding paradigms used for nursing research. *Journal of Advanced Nursing, 53*(11), 459–469.

Whittemore, R. (2007). Top 10 tips for beginning a program of research. *Research in Nursing & Health, 30*(3), 235–237.

Yonge, O., Billay, D., Myrick, F., & Luhanga, F. (2007). Preceptorship and mentorship: Not merely a matter of semantics. *International Journal of Nursing Education Scholarship, 4*(1), Article 19. Retrieved from http://www.bepress.com/ijnes/vol4/iss1/art19

CHAPTER 5

DNP Involvement in Healthcare Policy and Advocacy

Marlene H. Mullin

Our nation currently faces many challenges. In 2013 46 million Americans of all ages (14.8%) were uninsured at the time of the National Health Interview Survey conducted by the Centers for Disease Control and Prevention's National Center for Health Statistics (2013). According to the U.S. Department of Housing and Urban Development, an estimated 610,042 persons are homeless on any given night in the United States, with 109,132 being chronically homeless (U.S. Department of Housing and Urban Development, 2013). Disparities in health care, education, food distribution, and housing demand the attention of the doctor of nursing practice (DNP) graduate.

Although the enormity of these problems may seem daunting and may cast doubts on how one can make a difference, DNP graduates possess the tools to make changes in our society. Knowledge and education are powerful instruments; DNP graduates possess both. DNP graduates also possess practical experience, leadership skills, and knowledge regarding research and evidence-based practice, which allows them to be powerful advocates for healthcare policies. Utilizing the gifts of knowledge, education, practice experience, leadership skills, and research to their full potential for the betterment of society is a challenge that all DNPs must undertake. Due to our nation's many challenges, it is imperative that DNP graduates become involved in shaping healthcare policy and promoting advocacy. DNP graduates are prepared to meet these challenges.

Nursing's Social Policy Statement (American Nurses Association [ANA], 2003) clearly states the nursing profession's commitment to society and the people who are served. Nursing's relationship with society is "based on an ethic of trust and the principle of justice" (Ballou, 2000, p. 178). Involvement in healthcare policy and advocacy that addresses issues of social justice and equity in health care are vital roles that all DNP graduates must assume to fulfill our responsibility to society (American Association of Colleges of Nursing [AACN], 2006).

It is also important for DNP graduates to remember that political decisions and social policy initiatives have an impact on the practice of nursing. DNP graduates need to attain a place at the table where policy decisions are made to have a say in the policies that govern nursing. DNP graduates are prepared to assume a leadership role in influencing and shaping policies that affect nursing practice.

This chapter provides a brief overview of the history of nursing's involvement in healthcare policy and advocacy. Specific strategies for becoming informed and involved in healthcare policy and advocacy are outlined. An interview with a nursing policy expert is also included in the chapter. Nancy M. George is the director of the DNP program and an associate professor at Wayne State University College of Nursing. Her valuable insights on nurses and health policy are shared in this interview.

Curriculum Standards

Essential V of the *Essentials of Doctoral Education for Advanced Nursing Practice* (AACN, 2006) provides specific curriculum standards for the DNP graduate related to healthcare policy and advocacy under the title Healthcare Policy for Advocacy in Health Care. Essential V states that DNP programs prepare graduates for the following activities related to healthcare policy and advocacy:

> DNP graduates are prepared to design, influence, and implement healthcare policies that frame health care financing, practice regulation, access, safety, quality and efficacy (IOM, 2001). Moreover, the DNP graduate is able to design, implement, and advocate for healthcare policy that addresses issues of social justice and equity in health care. The powerful practice experiences of the DNP graduate can become potent influencers in policy formation. Additionally, the DNP graduate integrates these practice experiences with two additional skill sets: the ability to analyze the policy process and the ability to engage in politically competent action. (O'Grady, 2004)

The DNP graduate has the capacity to engage proactively in the development and implementation of healthcare policy at all levels, including institutional, local, state, regional, federal, and international levels. DNP graduates, as leaders in the practice arena, provide a critical interface among practice, research, and policy. Preparing graduates with the essential competencies to assume a leadership role in the development of healthcare policy requires that students have opportunities to contrast the major contextual factors and policy triggers that influence healthcare policy making at the various levels.

The DNP program prepares the graduate to do the following:

1. Critically analyze health policy proposals, health policies, and related issues from the perspective of consumers, nursing, other health professions, and other stakeholders in policy and public forums.

2. Demonstrate leadership in the development and implementation of institutional, local, state, federal, and/or international health policy.

3. Influence policy makers through active participation on committees, boards, or task forces at the institutional, local, state, regional, national, and/or international levels to improve healthcare delivery and outcomes.

4. Educate others, including policy makers at all levels, regarding nursing, health policy, and patient care outcomes.

5. Advocate for the nursing profession within the policy and healthcare communities.

6. Develop, evaluate, and provide leadership for healthcare policy that shapes healthcare financing, regulation, and delivery.

7. Advocate for social justice, equity, and ethical policies within all healthcare arenas. (AACN, 2006, pp. 13–14)

Historical Perspective

The modern nursing movement was started by Florence Nightingale in 1860 when she opened the first nurse training program at St. Thomas Hospital in England (Lewenson, 2007). "This landmark event signaled to the world that nurses required schooling for the work they did" (2007, p. 23). Nightingale's concept that nurses should be trained, supervised, and managed by nurses themselves was adopted by many nurse training programs during this period. She believed that nursing and medicine should be separate disciplines. Most important, Nightingale believed nursing should organize and control itself. Nightingale's ambitious letter writing to influential people enabled her to obtain support for changes in healthcare and nursing education. She ultimately was able to garner worldwide support for her visionary ideas about sanitation, nursing education, and the separation of nursing from medicine.

In the United States the modern nursing movement began with the opening of many Nightingale-influenced nurse training schools in 1873 (Lewenson, 2007). This also signaled the changing role of women in society. The nursing profession provided one of the first opportunities for women to work outside the home and financially support themselves. However, due to the fact that nursing's roots were in the church and military, patriarchal control existed (2007). To overcome this issue, political action was necessary by nurses, and women in general, to obtain control over their education, work, and lives.

Between 1873 and 1893 many more nurse training schools opened, with the number rising to more than 1,129 by 1910 (Burgess, 1928). During this time nursing was not regulated by any professional nursing group, which resulted in significant misuse of nurses. In fact, physicians and pharmacists controlled much of nursing practice, particularly in the private duty sector (Lewenson, 2007). Ultimately, this mistreatment and lack of control and regulation were the impetus for early nursing leaders to form professional nursing organizations (Lewenson, 2007).

The first professional nursing organizations were formed between 1893 and 1912. Although these organizations were originally formed to address the misuse and lack of representation for nurses, members ultimately became involved in social and political reforms that affected health issues in society. The first professional nursing organizations included what are now known as the National League for Nursing (NLN) and the ANA. The NLN originated in 1893, and its goal was to bring "uniformity in nursing curricula and standards of nursing practice" (Lewenson, 2007, p. 24). Nursing leaders of the NLN favored and encouraged collective action, which demonstrated the political and progressive nature of this group.

Nationally, nurse training programs were encouraged to form alumnae associations to bring nurses together at the state level and ultimately at the national level (Lewenson, 2007). The ANA originally was developed to unite the various alumnae groups that had been formed by nurse training programs across the country. All alumnae associations were encouraged to be involved in political action and social reform. Sophia Palmer, founding editor of the *American Journal of Nursing* (*AJN*), was one of the nursing leaders who spearheaded this effort. Palmer used the *AJN*, which was first published in 1900, to stimulate discussion among nurses about policy and political issues. The *AJN* also encouraged collective action on the part of nurses to influence legislation that affected the profession and the health of the public (Lewenson, 2007). The publication of the *AJN* was an important early political strategy undertaken by the ANA and the NLN to increase communication among nurses. Of interest, the *AJN* was originally funded by members of these two organizations (Lewenson, 2007).

One very important issue that was addressed by members of the ANA and discussed in the *AJN* was the registering of nurses. Significant political action and organization among nurses were taken to obtain recognition of nursing as a profession. The first state nurse registration act was passed in 1903, originally in the states of North Carolina, New York, New Jersey, and Virginia. This resulted in protecting the title *nurse* by law (Lewenson, 2007). Other states soon began to register nurses.

During this time frame, the Spanish-American War erupted. Nurse leaders attempted to control which nurses were chosen to serve in the war. They were unsuccessful in their efforts against Anita Newcomb McGee, a physician and socialite from Washington. Much to the dismay of nursing leaders, McGee ultimately served as the leader and therefore chose which nurses served in the war. It was believed by many nursing leaders that this unfortunate outcome had occurred due to a lack of formal organization of nurses. Lessons were learned from this incident, and the need for political action to control and organize nursing was recognized more than ever (Lewenson, 2007).

Subsequently, two other nursing organizations were developed: the National Association of Colored Graduate Nurses (NACGN) and the National Organization for Public Health Nursing (NOPHN). NACGN arose out of the fact that African American nurses were initially barred from membership in the ANA as a result of discrimination. The NACGN was organized in 1908. Its focus included issues of discrimination, education, standards of practice, and nursing registration (Lewenson, 2007).

The nursing leaders of the ANA and the NLN formed the NOPHN in 1912 to address substandard nursing practices in public health nursing. Public health nursing needs significantly increased in the beginning of the 20th century due to the overwhelming public health problems that occurred in the United States as a result of urbanization, industrialization, and immigration (Lewenson, 2007). NOPHN leaders recognized the importance of forming coalitions with other healthcare professionals and laypeople to form a larger political base to advocate for changes to improve the health of the public (Lewenson, 2007).

The formation and organization of formal nursing organizations led to the involvement of nurses in other political issues, such as the campaign for suffrage. It was recognized that the ability to vote would enable nurses to have a voice in the laws that regulated practice, education, and health (Lewenson, 2007). Letters from the National American Woman Suffrage Association that requested support and articles about suffrage were published in the *AJN*. Initially nurses were hesitant to participate in the suffrage movement due to fear that it would negatively influence efforts to obtain state nursing registration. In fact, at the 11th annual ANA convention in 1908, members opposed a resolution for the organization to support suffrage (Lewenson, 2007). Four years later nursing leaders were successful in obtaining support from the nursing profession for women's suffrage. Political action to support women's suffrage was continued by the nursing profession until the 19th Amendment, which gave women the right to vote, was passed in the summer of 1920.

Finally, no history of nursing's involvement in political activities would be complete without mentioning two significant nurses who had an impact on public healthcare policy during this early period of the nursing profession. Lillian Wald and her colleague Mary Brewster opened the Henry Street Nurses' Settlement in 1893 in New York City. This was, in essence, the first nurse-run clinic in the United States (Fitzpatrick, 1975). Wald and her staff lived in this community and provided nursing care, health education, social services, and cultural experiences to clients who were seen in the clinic. The clinic gained world recognition for its success in addressing public health issues (Lewenson, 2007). Utilizing her knowledge and political savvy, Wald was able to influence and make many changes that affected the health of the residents and their community. She was influential in establishing the first park in New York City, which promoted children playing in a safe environment rather than in the streets (Lewenson, 2007). Wald is also credited with advocating for the first school nurse after noting that many children missed school due to medical problems. Although the board of health initially hired a physician to examine the children, Wald ultimately was successful in convincing them to hire a public health nurse as well. Wald considered these nurses to be the first school nurses in the world. They were hired in 1902; amazingly, their salary was $30,000 (Lewenson, 2007).

Another nurse, Margaret Sanger, revolutionized healthcare practice as a result of her political activism. Sanger led the struggle for legalizing birth control in the early 20th century. Sanger, a visiting nurse, was passionate that women should have control over their own bodies, specifically their reproductive functions. She was very politically savvy and sought support not only from nursing but from other organized groups of women, labor organizers, and philosophers (Lewenson, 2007). She met government resistance when she attempted to publish information about health issues such as syphilis. Sanger ultimately fled the United States in 1914 after being criminally convicted of writing an article that supported women separating procreation from the sexual act (Lewenson, 2007). She returned to the United States in 1915 following the death of her daughter. Ultimately the government dropped the charges against Sanger due to public pressure. Sanger's efforts to provide birth control and health information to mothers continued when she opened a clinic in 1916 in New York City. Once again her efforts were met with resistance, and she again faced arrest, prosecution, and imprisonment. Although Sanger was not successful, her efforts ultimately resulted in changes in the interpretation of the law, which influenced the founding of the Planned Parenthood organization (Lewenson, 2007).

Nursing's rich and fruitful political activism history in the 19th and early 20th centuries unfortunately did not continue in the mid-20th century when the feminist movement began in the United States. Initially, nursing's involvement in this movement was basically nonexistent (Chinn & Wheeler, 1985). Although nursing was a female-dominated profession, nurses failed to become actively involved in the fight for equal rights for women until the 1970s. Two notable nursing leaders, Wilma Scott Heide and JoAnn Ashley, led the profession in recognizing the value of the feminist movement for the nursing profession. It became obvious to nurses that it was imperative to become involved in political activities that addressed the inequalities faced by women overall. It was also clear that nursing needed to assume a leadership role to promote changes in health care for the betterment of society. Nursing's support for the feminist movement was fully realized when the ANA supported the Equal Rights Amendment in the early 1970s (Lewenson, 2007). Two other pivotal events also occurred during this time. The National Organization for Women was organized, and the Nurses Coalition for Action in Politics was established. The Nurses Coalition for Action in Politics was the first political action committee (PAC) for the nursing profession (Lewenson, 2007).

Although the political activities of nursing have continued from the late 20th century to the present, they have not been as vigorous as those of early nursing leaders. "Too often nurses are not included in policy decisions, not involved in policy making, or just not recognized at all" (Gordon, as cited in Lewenson, 2007, p. 31). It is obvious that much work is still needed by nursing to realize its full potential of influencing health care through healthcare policy. Lewenson says, "Nurses will learn that their extensive knowledge base and experience lend themselves to political activism" (2007, p. 31). Early nursing leaders, such as Florence Nightingale, used the professional education of nurses to facilitate their political activism. Nursing has this opportunity once more with the advent of the DNP degree.

Involvement in political activities has always been an integral part of the nursing role. Due to their expanded scopes of practice, it has been necessary for nurses to be involved in such issues as expanding nurse practice acts and obtaining third-party reimbursement and prescriptive authority. The shortage of physicians in primary care, and medical residents in many areas, has increased the demand and need for expanded roles in nursing. For this reason, more than ever, nurses need to be involved in political activities.

Of concern, the majority of political activities by nurses have focused on areas that expand and promote their practice (Oden, Price, Alteneder, Boardley, & Ubokudom, 2000). Given the dominance of medicine, this is not surprising; nevertheless, nursing involvement in healthcare policy and advocacy to benefit the general population is imperative. DNP graduates are well prepared, as a result of their education and experience, for involvement in healthcare policy and advocacy. DNP graduates can serve as leaders in influencing and shaping healthcare policies and advocating for healthcare issues. In addition, DNP graduates can influence and shape policies that impact the practice of nursing.

The next section of this chapter discusses avenues for becoming informed and involved in political activities. Whether the DNP graduate chooses to be knowledge-able only about current political issues or chooses to run for public office, some level of involvement is vital. DNP graduates are in the unique position to influence the future of health care through an array of positions and activities. It is also important to recognize that political activism may contribute to the long-term success and viability of DNP graduates in the healthcare arena.

Tips for Becoming Informed and Involved

Although the ideal method for learning to be politically savvy is through mentoring, role-modeling, and practice, there are many catalysts for becoming informed about and involved in politics. Due to our nation's current healthcare environment, there are a multitude of causes and issues that demand the attention of DNP graduates. It is the responsibility of all DNP graduates to become informed and involved to influence and shape healthcare policies and advocate for patients and the nursing profession.

A good way to start is to first determine your areas of interest; find something you care about or find something new to care about. Next, determine the amount of time and energy you have to devote to political activism. Finally, be passionate and get started by being informed and involved!

Sources of Information

There are many outstanding sources for obtaining information in our technologically advanced society. In addition to written materials, the Internet provides a wealth of information regarding healthcare policy and advocacy issues. Multimedia resources such as television and radio are also good sources for obtaining information. More in-depth information may be obtained through courses and continuing education offerings.

PROFESSIONAL JOURNALS

Many professional nursing journals contain policy and political updates. Other sources for this information include medical journals and other healthcare professional journals. The names of nursing journals that frequently contain policy and political information may be found in **Box 5-1**.

INTERNET

The Internet provides endless access to information regarding public policies, healthcare policies, government information, academic information, and government officials. In addition, many nursing associations provide specific information for nurses through the Internet. For example, the ANA website offers the *Online Journal of Issues in Nursing*, and the NLN's website has a section titled Governmental Affairs.

To start a search, there are several terms that are helpful for locating information on the Internet. These terms include *administration, economics, law, management,*

BOX 5-1

Healthcare Policy- and Advocacy-Related Journals

- The *American Journal of Nursing*, since 1900, has provided editorials, articles, and commentaries on political issues that affect nursing (monthly).

- The *Journal of Professional Nursing*, the official journal of the American Association of Colleges of Nursing (AACN), provides information on public policy (bimonthly).

- *Nursing Economic$* provides a "Capitol Commentary" that examines current healthcare policy issues (bimonthly).

- The *Journal of Nursing Scholarship*, the official publication of Sigma Theta Tau International Honor Society of Nursing, provides articles regarding healthcare policy and systems (quarterly).

- *Policy, Politics & Nursing Practice* provides information regarding legislation that affects nursing practice, case studies in policy and political action, interviews with policy makers and policy experts, and articles on trends and issues (quarterly).

- Other journals with articles regarding healthcare policy, health law, and ethics include *Yale Journal of Health Policy, Law, and Ethics*; *Journal of the American Medical Association*; *The New England Journal of Medicine*; *American Journal of Public Health*; *American Political Science Review*; *Health Affairs*; *Health Services Research*; *Journal of Health Politics, Policy and Law*; and *Journal of Public Health Policy*.

---

policy, and *statistics* preceded by the terms *health* or *medical*. These terms usually result in the successful location of healthcare policy data. Tips for narrowing the search include enclosing the terms in quotation marks and utilizing conjunctions (i.e., and, or, and not). The use of a website's internal search engine is also highly recommended to refine the search. In addition, Google frequently provides an excellent beginning search and a vast array of information.

Box 5-2 lists several excellent websites for initiating a search. Take a moment to explore these websites for learning purposes and volunteer activities. Frequently, information regarding the advocacy and legislative programs for associations is available through their websites.

TEXTBOOKS

Several excellent textbooks are available for DNP graduates to increase their knowledge regarding politics and healthcare policy. The textbooks listed in **Box 5-3** provide a start for the DNP graduate to become more informed and politically savvy, and **Box 5-4** provides a list of some multimedia resources.

BOX 5-2

Healthcare Policy- and Advocacy-Related Websites

- Government-related websites:

  U.S. Department of Health and Human Services (http://www.hhs.gov/)

  World Health Organization (http://www.who.int/en)

  U.S. Government Printing Office (http://www.access.gpo.gov)

- Legislative websites:

  Legislation & Votes (http://clerk.house.gov/legislative/legvotes.aspx)

  U.S. House of Representatives (http://www.house.gov)

  U.S. Senate (http://www.senate.gov)

- Academic websites:

  Duke Center for Health Policy & Inequalities Research (U.S. Health Policy Gateway) (http://ushealthpolicygateway.wordpress.com)

  Muskie School of Public Service (http://muskie.usm.maine.edu/cutler)

  National Health Policy Forum (http://www.nhpf.org)

- Professional nursing association websites:

  American Association of Colleges of Nursing (http://www.aacn.nche.edu)

  American Nurses Association (http://nursingworld.org)

  National League for Nursing (http://www.nln.org)

- Specialty association websites:

  American Association of Critical-Care Nurses (www.aacn.org)

  American Association of Nurse Practitioners (http://www.aanp.org)

- Healthcare professional association websites:

  American Cancer Society (http://www.cancer.org)

  American Heart Association (http://www.americanheart.org)

  National Multiple Sclerosis Society (http://www.nationalmssociety.org /government-affairs-and-advocacy/index.aspx)

COURSES AND CONTINUING EDUCATION

Many nursing associations offer courses specifically regarding healthcare policy and legislative issues. For example, the American Association of Nurse Practitioners (AANP) offers a Health Policy Conference yearly. AANP also offers a Health Policy Fellowship for nurse practitioners who are interested in a more extensive program. For more information, go to their website at http://www.aanp.org. Check national, state, and specialty nursing organization websites for information regarding healthcare policy meetings and conferences. For DNPs who are interested in a

BOX 5-3

Healthcare Policy- and Advocacy-Related Textbooks

- Bodenheimer, T. S., & Grumbach, K. (2012). *Understanding health policy: A clinical approach* (6th ed.). New York, NY: McGraw Hill.

  Provides a good overview of the basic principles of healthcare policy and how the healthcare system works.

- DeLaney, A. (2002). *Politics for dummies* (2nd ed.). New York, NY: John Wiley & Sons.

  Good book for a review of politics for both novices and those who are familiar with the political arena.

- Mason, D. J., Leavitt, J. K., & Chaffee, M. W. (2012). *Policy & politics in nursing and health care* (6th ed.). St. Louis, MO: Elsevier Saunders.

  Excellent textbook that provides a vast amount of information regarding nursing's history and progress in policy and politics.

- MoveOn. (2004). *MoveOn's 50 ways to love your country: How to find your political voice and become a catalyst for change.* Novato, CA: New World Library.

  Excellent resource for DNP graduates who want to make changes but don't know how.

- Weissert, C., & Weissert, W. (2012). *Governing health: The politics of health policy* (4th ed.). Baltimore, MD: Johns Hopkins University Press.

  Provides an excellent review of the politics of healthcare policy making.

BOX 5-4

Other Multimedia Resources

- Newspapers are a good source of information regarding international, national, state, and local politics and public policy issues. Two examples of newspapers that provide a significant amount of information on healthcare policy issues include the *Wall Street Journal* (http://www.wsj.com) and the *New York Times* (http://www.nytimes.com).

- Network and cable television programs are a good source of information regarding political activities and public policy. C-SPAN and CNN are two networks that provide a vast amount of political information. C-SPAN broadcasts live government events.

- National Public Radio (NPR) (http://www.npr.org) and C-SPAN radio (http://www.c-span.org) are both excellent sources for public and political issues. DNP graduates can also listen to these radio stations through the Internet. Many talk shows that address political issues are also available on radio.

more in-depth program, the Robert Wood Johnson Foundation (RWJF) offers a Health Policy Fellowship Program. This yearlong fellowship brings healthcare professionals to Washington, DC, to experience an immersion in national healthcare policy, primarily through working assignments in Congress (Michnich, 2007). For more information regarding the RWJF Health Policy Fellowship Program, go to their website at http://www.healthpolicyfellows.org.

Avenues for DNP Involvement in Healthcare Policy and Advocacy

Many outstanding opportunities exist for the DNP to be involved in shaping healthcare policy and advocating for patients. Membership and involvement in professional nursing organizations is an excellent source for initial involvement. The DNP graduate may also choose to use the workplace environment as well as educational and research-based endeavors to become involved in healthcare policy and advocacy. Some DNP graduates may choose to become more actively involved by seeking election for a public office.

Professional Nursing Organizations

Membership and participation in national, state, local, and specialty professional nursing organizations are critical for DNP graduates. Unity is vital for nurses if they wish to be successful in addressing problems in health care and in the nursing profession. Membership in these organizations provides nurses with a voice when healthcare issues are being discussed and changes are being proposed at all levels in healthcare policies. These associations frequently provide legislative and public policy updates to members via newsletters or the Internet. Leavitt, Chaffee, and Vance noted that "many professional nursing associations offer opportunities for volunteer services that lead to rich educational, mentoring and networking experiences" (2007, p. 42).

DNP graduates who are members of the AANP may choose to be involved with or contribute to the AANP Political Action Committee (AANP-PAC). The AANP-PAC "supports candidates who believe in the purposes, principles and mission of AANP" (AANP, 2014). In addition, AANP's legislative team "represents nurse practitioners (NPs) and their patients on critical issues related to licensure, access to care, patient safety, health care reform, reimbursement, and other concerns at all policy levels" (AANP, 2014). Involvement by NPs in legislative activities is greatly encouraged, and the AANP provides a great avenue for participation. AANP's website offers excellent information regarding federal and state legislation and regulation. Their website also has an outstanding Policy Toolkit covering such topics as NP Policy Essentials, Advocacy, and Current Issues & Analysis, which provides a wealth of information on how to become involved in legislative issues and activities.

The AANP Advocacy Center (www.capwiz.com/aanp/home) offers the ability to impact healthcare policy by allowing members to directly inform federal representatives about issues that are important to their practice and patients. AANP also offers a Health Policy Fellowship for those NPs interested in a more in-depth program. State NP organizations also provide vast opportunities for legislative involvement and activities.

DNP graduates who are members of the ANA may volunteer to participate in the Nurses Strategic Action Team (N-STAT) or the American Nurses Association Political Action Committee (ANA-PAC). N-STAT members act by being alerted by the ANA about critical healthcare issues and personally contacting their members of Congress and writing letters to them (Leavitt et al., 2007). The ANA-PAC, which is the one of the top healthcare PACs in the United States, speaks for all 2.7 million registered nurses (Malone & Chaffee, 2007). The ANA-PAC is involved in direct and grassroots lobbying and "endorsing and supporting those candidates who have a record of supporting ANA policy interests or who have expressed positions that are consistent with ANA policy interests" (ANA, 2014). In addition, the ANA-PAC makes monetary contributions to candidates. PACs also exist in specialty, state, and local nursing professional associations. Their activities are similar to those of national associations. Many opportunities exist for involvement by DNP graduates in the political arms of these associations. "ANA-PAC is committed to increasing the number of RNs in public office at every level of government" (Malone & Chaffee, 2007, p. 772). The leadership skills and knowledge of DNP graduates make them excellent candidates for public offices. Visibility by involvement in these activities is vital for DNP graduates. Again, all it takes is interest, time, and energy!

Please see the ideas in **Box 5-5** for how to become involved in professional nursing organizations and how to contact and communicate with legislators.

Workplace Involvement

The leadership skills of DNP graduates make them highly qualified for influencing and facilitating changes in the workplace environment. DNP graduates can serve as advocates to change and improve the policies and procedures that affect patients and nursing practice in their places of employment. DNP graduates can also serve as catalysts to implement new policies based on their vast knowledge and understanding of research and evidence-based practices. **Box 5-6** lists some examples of how DNPs can become involved in the workplace.

Involvement Through Education

The role of the DNP in education goes beyond the academic setting. One of the key ways to be a patient advocate is to develop and provide evidence-based, culturally relevant, and culturally sensitive patient education material. With our culturally

BOX 5-5

Ideas for Involvement in Professional Nursing Organizations

- Support your national, state, specialty, and local nursing professional associations by joining them as a member.
- Be visible by attending association meetings.
- Volunteer to be on a PAC or other committees, task forces, or boards that are involved in healthcare policy, advocacy, or nursing practice issues.
- Volunteer to join a coalition.
- Volunteer to campaign for PAC-endorsed candidates.
- Offer to contact and write letters or emails to political officials regarding issues that influence healthcare policies and nursing practice and promote patient advocacy. Traditional letters and emails are highly effective tools to let public officials know what you think. To find the postal or email address or phone number of your lawmaker, go to the websites for the Senate (http://www .senate.gov/general/contact_information/senators_cfm.cfm) and the House of Representatives (http://www.house.gov/representatives/find/).
- Speak with legislators and policy makers. As citizens of the United States, we have access to policy makers like no place else in the world. Tips for speaking effectively with politicians may be found on the websites of many professional nursing associations. In addition, when speaking to politicians, be sure to explain and promote the role of the DNP because many of them are not familiar with this new degree in nursing.
- Some general rules for writing, emailing, or speaking with your legislators include keeping your tone positive, being brief, staying focused on the subject, identifying the issue or specific bill being discussed, and, finally, presenting your position and giving a sound rationale.

BOX 5-6

Examples of Workplace Involvement

- Serve in leadership positions on policy and procedure committees.
- Serve in leadership positions on other committees or task forces that affect patient care and nursing practice.
- Serve in leadership positions when the workplace is undergoing reviews from accrediting agencies (e.g., The Joint Commission).
- Serve in leadership positions when the workplace is seeking Magnet status.
- Serve as a role model and mentor to staff members when changes are being implemented.

diversified nation, this is more important than ever. This is also one way to assist in correcting healthcare disparities. Health promotion and advocacy through patient education continues to be a major focus for nursing, as reflected in *Nursing's Social Policy Statement* (ANA, 2003). DNP graduates, as a result of their education and clinical expertise, are highly qualified to serve as leaders in developing and disseminating patient education material. There are also a multitude of ways for DNPs to be patient advocates through educational endeavors that involve public speaking and writing. Use your writing and speaking engagements for health promotion and advocacy for patients and families and to educate the public about DNP graduates and nursing. Please refer to **Box 5-7** for some examples of how to become involved through education.

BOX 5-7

Examples of Involvement Through Education

- Design education programs for staff members and other healthcare professionals.
- Serve as a leader in developing evidence-based, culturally relevant, and culturally sensitive patient education material.
- Serve as a leader in staff and patient education committees at the workplace.
- Facilitate evidence-based journal clubs that address cultural issues and health promotion and other topics that promote quality patient care.
- Facilitate staff education programs regarding different learning methods.
- Serve as a role model and mentor to staff regarding patient education.
- Facilitate patient support groups in your area of specialization that are culturally relevant and culturally sensitive.
- Seek opportunities to provide health education to the public via interviews on television or radio shows. Share your expertise!
- Volunteer to write health articles for your local newspapers. Newspaper editors are always looking for experts to write articles regarding health topics!
- Volunteer to speak at support group meetings (e.g., cancer and multiple sclerosis support groups) regarding health topics. Support groups are always looking for speakers, particularly nurses, to provide health information to their participants.
- Volunteer to speak at community group meetings (e.g., Rotary International) regarding health topics. Community groups are always looking for speakers, particularly nurses, to provide health information to their members.

BOX 5-8

Examples of Involvement Through Research

- Present research to support policy and procedure changes in the workplace.
- Present research to initiate or support health or social policy initiatives at the local, state, or national level.
- Conduct research on topics that will advocate for patients and influence health and social policies. Publishing the research in a refereed journal is vital to increase the credibility of the study and disseminate the results to others.
- Facilitate evidence-based journal clubs for staff to promote evidence-based practice.
- Serve on institutional review boards to support nursing research and advocate for patients.

Involvement Through Research

Diers and Price state that "research may be a tool to carve policy, if it is in the right hands and is carefully sharpened and skillfully applied" (2007, p. 195). DNP graduates are knowledgeable regarding research and evidence-based practice. This knowledge can be applied to influence and initiate public, social, and healthcare policies and to advocate for patients. DNP graduates possess the knowledge to use research and evidence-based practices to influence the decision making of policy makers. In addition, DNP graduates may choose to be involved in research studies that influence organizational, healthcare, and social policies. *Nursing's Social Policy Statement* (ANA, 2003) serves as a guide for nursing research efforts related to healthcare policy and advocacy. There is a wealth of opportunities for DNP graduates to use research to shape health and social policy and promote advocacy. Please refer to **Box 5-8** for examples of involvement through research.

Other Avenues for Involvement

Nursing is one of the most trusted professions in our nation (Feldman & Lewenson, 2000). DNP graduates can capitalize on this trust by becoming involved in many other political activities to advocate for patients and shape healthcare and social policies. As stated earlier, "ANA-PAC is committed to increasing the number of RNs in public offices at every level of government" (Malone & Chaffee, 2007, p. 772). The leadership skills and knowledge of DNP graduates make them excellent candidates for public offices, where they can gain visibility to educate politicians and the public regarding this new role and degree in nursing. To get started, first become familiar with the public policy and healthcare policy issues that are currently under consideration at all levels of the government. Pay specific attention to issues of interest at the desired level of involvement. Remember, all it takes to become involved is interest, time, and energy! **Box 5-9** provides some ideas for becoming involved through other avenues.

BOX 5-9

Examples of Other Avenues for Involvement

- Vote! Exercise your right to vote on issues that promote advocacy and affect healthcare policies. Be aware of issues and vote in elections at all levels—local, state, and national.

- Volunteer to be on a local, state, or national committee, board, or task force. It is not necessary to be only on health-related committees. Consider other areas of interest for involvement.

- Familiarize yourself with the elected officials that represent you at all levels of government. Communicate with them. Educate them about DNP graduates. Share your expertise and perspectives regarding healthcare and nursing issues. Write letters that indicate your viewpoint and desired outcomes. See Box 5-2 for information about how to contact, write to, and speak with your legislators.

- Volunteer to campaign for elected officials who are supportive of health and nursing issues.

- Choose a political party affiliation. This is essential to obtain support for a political appointment.

- Seek opportunities for appointments. Most nurse and specialty associations offer appointment information. Another source for information is the League of Women Voters.

- Contact elected and appointed leaders, such as the governor and chief nurse executives, regarding involvement with task forces, boards, committees, and opportunities for appointments.

- Seek election for office. To start, consider running for a local office, such as becoming a member of the school board or city council.

- Volunteer to be interviewed for newspapers, journals, and television and radio broadcasts regarding advocacy and healthcare policy issues. Use these opportunities to promote and educate the public about DNP graduates and nursing.

- Respond to editorials and articles published in newspapers and journals regarding advocacy, healthcare policy, and nursing practice issues.

Interview with Nancy M. George

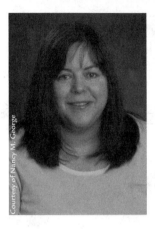

NANCY M. GEORGE, PHD, RN, FNP-BC, is the director of the DNP Program and an associate professor (clinical) of nursing at Wayne State University College of Nursing. Dr. George is also president of the Michigan Council of Nurse Practitioners and chairperson of the Michigan APRN Coalition. She received her BS in biological sciences from Michigan Technological University, her diploma in nursing from Bronson School of Nursing, and her MSN and PhD from the University of Michigan. Her interest in policy was nurtured in her nurse practitioner and doctoral studies. Dr. George was recently elected a fellow of the American Association of Nurse Practitioners.

Dr. George, please describe specifically how you became involved in health and social policy activities.

My interest in policy and politics began in a bipartisan household with political discussions over the dinner table. My mother ran for township clerk as a Democrat in a Republican-dominated township. My mother demonstrated that it is always important to be involved in the policy process and stay true to your beliefs. She instilled in me the importance of voting and staying informed about the decisions that are being made for me at the local, state, and national levels. When I was in the Peace Corps in Kenya, I learned firsthand the importance of a free and elected government and the impact it can have on people. I believe that these activities influenced my thinking when it comes to nursing and nurse practitioner practice environments. I had several influential nurse practitioner mentors when I was new in my career who got me involved with our state nursing organization. That was the start of being involved and staying involved in the health and social policy issues that impact nursing.

Dr. George, please describe specific health and social policies you have initiated, influenced, and so forth.

I have been involved in the past two attempts to get nurse practitioners (NPs) prescriptive authority in Michigan. I helped draft language, attended hearings, testified, and met with legislators. In our current attempt to gain autonomous plenary authority, I have been actively involved in drafting the prescriptive authority language and bringing the statutes in Michigan in line with the APRN [advanced-practice registered nurse] Consensus Model language supported by the National Council of State Boards of Nursing (NCSBN) and many other professional organizations. I currently am the chairperson of the APRN Coalition as we continue to move forward the agenda of SB 2 that was passed in the Michigan Senate in November 2013. SB 2 is currently awaiting a hearing before the Michigan House of Representatives Health Policy Committee. I work tirelessly to bring the APRN groups (NPs, CNSs [clinical nurse specialists], CNMs [certified nurse–midwife]) together.

Moving forward our main charges have been to have a consistent message, have a united front, and work hard to bring the Michigan regulatory environment into the 21st century. These duties include producing brochures and pamphlets with my APRN colleagues and meeting with legislators, regulators, and other influential healthcare groups in Michigan. While these activities have, I believe, had the most direct impact on policy, my role as a nurse educator has had a significant impact on future and current NPs. I believe if I can influence five students who were not previously active in the policy activities that impact their profession, then I have succeeded in assisting my chosen profession.

Dr. George, what do you view as the role of the nursing profession in advocacy and influencing and shaping healthcare and social policies?

I think that nursing gets a reputation of not being politically active, but I think our history tells a different story. Nurses have always been politically active . . . we only have to look at the work of Florence Nightingale, Lavinia Dock, Margaret Sanger, Dorothea Dix, and many others to see the influence that nursing has had on health and healthcare policy. I believe that there are many of us that continue to work on the health issues that impact our patients/clients on a daily basis. Some of us are more visible in our activities. If you believe that part of nursing's role is to advocate for patients/clients, then how can we not view being active in healthcare policy as an aspect of advocacy? Good healthcare policy allows for good patient care. So nurses need to be involved, even if that means their only activity is voting in every election. We need a strong nursing voice in healthcare policy for the patients, and we can't have that if we don't have nurses interested and involved in healthcare policy.

Dr. George, what activities do you recommend for DNPs to become involved in to influence and shape healthcare and social policies?

The first activity is to be informed. Use your talents of understanding and disseminating complex information to inform and shape healthcare policy. Use your passion for nursing and the people that we care for to direct you to the healthcare and social policies that you could influence. Policy is the penultimate way to roll all the skills you have learned or are learning as a DNP into an action plan. Taking the advocacy for patients to the next level and making a difference on a broader scale is vital. So the real question is where do you start . . . join your professional organizations. Find out what needs these organization have; there is usually more work than can be completed by a few individuals. Work on policy or political campaigns. Many NPs, CNSs, and CNMs are working on the passage of SB 2, including meeting with legislators, some of them for the first time, so don't be afraid to step into an area in which you are unfamiliar. Think about running for office. There are too few nurses in the legislature, and individuals with little health and nursing knowledge are making decisions that impact your professional lives. Think about becoming influential providers in the systems you work in . . . ever thought of being chief nursing officer or chief executive officer? As the healthcare arena changes, DNPs can be at the forefront of our new healthcare system . . . nurse owned and run hospitals, anyone? Be involved, because if you aren't driving the bus, someone else will, and you will just be along for the ride.

Dr. George, what do you view is the role of the DNP in advocacy and influencing and shaping healthcare and social policies?

DNPs have the ultimate skills at being the movers and shakers of healthcare and social policy. DNPs have the educational background that prepares them for making a difference. The advent of the IOM [Institute of Medicine] report on the future of nursing and many other reports have put APRNs in the forefront of health care. DNPs should have read these documents and could use them to support the need for change in our healthcare system that will improve the outcomes for all. Skills in communication, research, policy, clinical practice, and leadership are geared to prepare DNP leaders for the future of nursing and advanced-practice nursing. As a DNP you will have the skills necessary to make some of the changes that need to be made.

Dr. George, how do you foresee DNPs impacting the future of health care through their role in advocacy and healthcare and social policy activities?

I believe that as more DNPs are in the clinical arena using research to make the needed evidence-based clinical changes, they will become leaders of the emerging new healthcare system. As the DNP numbers increase, there will be more individuals with the credentials, communication skills, and knowledge to be leaders in advocating for changes to the healthcare and social systems that impact so many Americans. Further, legislators, policy makers, and regulators will have nursing professionals who can provide accurate evidence-based information regarding the quality outcomes of health care that are so needed to improve our healthcare system. Perhaps most important is that with increased policy activity, many of these DNPs will actually decide to run for office. The horizons are bright for the DNP who becomes active in the policy arena.

Case Scenario: DNP Involvement in Healthcare Policy and Advocacy

Dr. K. is a DNP graduate who is employed as an adult nurse practitioner specializing in the care of cardiac surgery patients at a large teaching hospital. Additionally, Dr. K. has a special interest in homelessness. For the past several years Dr. K. has volunteered at a local shelter once a month. The shelter where she volunteers is a nonprofit program that focuses on providing shelter, education, and counseling to rehabilitate homeless individuals. Participation in the program is on a voluntary basis. Candidates for the program undergo intense intake interviews before being accepted. Individuals who are accepted into the program must be drug free and willing to undergo random drug testing. The program is very structured and rigorous; therefore, only those individuals who truly want to change are accepted. A major focus of the program is to provide participants with assistance in acquiring employment and permanent housing. Thirty individuals are accepted into the program every 60 days. Participants receive meals, shelter, education, and counseling for a maximum of 60 days. Funding for the program is provided by government agencies (60%) and private contributions (40%).

Dr. K. provides health education to participants; therefore, she generally becomes well acquainted with each of them. During the years that Dr. K. has been volunteering at the shelter, she has noticed that many individuals repeat the program. Several of the returnees have told Dr. K. that they believe they would have been successful the first time they were enrolled if they had been given more time. Dr. K. shares these discussions and her concerns with Ms. T., the program director. Ms. T. indicates that the program has a recidivism rate of approximately 20% yearly. Dr. K. suggests that perhaps the length of the program should be individualized because some participants need more time and others need less. Ms. T. indicates that to her knowledge no clear guidelines exist regarding the optimal length of programs to rehabilitate homeless individuals. She states that the 60-day stay is based on networking with programs that have similar goals and objectives. Dr. K. is concerned that there are no clear guidelines regarding the length of a program. Dr. K. offers to perform a search to find out if there is any new information regarding rehabilitating homeless individuals. Ms. T. is skeptical but agrees to have Dr. K. investigate the matter.

Dr. K. starts the search to determine if there is any evidence-based information regarding the rehabilitation of homeless people. First, Dr. K. does an extensive review of the literature at the hospital library where she is employed. Next, she does an Internet search using the terms *homelessness* and *rehabilitation*. Dr. K. then decides to go to the websites of various government agencies, such as the U.S. Department of Health and Human Services, to investigate rehabilitation of homeless people. Although there is not a great deal of information regarding the subject, she is successful in locating several research articles regarding homelessness rehabilitation. One of the articles is a research study performed by one of the professors at the local university. Dr. K. contacts the professor, Dr. S., who provides her with additional research articles regarding rehabilitating homeless individuals. Ultimately, Dr. K.'s search uncovers several articles that provide evidence-based practice information about rehabilitating homeless people. Three specific articles discuss individualizing the length of the program to decrease recidivism rates.

Dr. K. shares her findings with Ms. T. She also provides Ms. T. with the names and phone numbers of the programs that are discussed in the research articles. Ms. T. agrees to review the information and contact the other programs. Several weeks later Ms. T. approaches Dr. K. and asks for her assistance in developing a plan to individualize the length of the program for participants. A formal plan is developed, including specific intake criteria and methods for evaluating the ongoing progress of participants. Ms. T. seeks Dr. K.'s assistance in presenting this information to the shelter's board of directors. The board of directors is very impressed with Dr. K.'s and Ms. T.'s presentation, which includes information regarding research and evidence-based practice. As stakeholders in the program, they are very interested in decreasing the recidivism rate to rehabilitate new homeless individuals rather than work with repeat participants. From the stakeholder's perspective, this will make the program more efficacious and cost effective. Additionally, if participants do not require the entire 60-day stay, cost savings may be realized. The board of directors overwhelmingly approves the plan to individualize the length of stay for shelter participants starting with a 1-year trial. The policy and procedures for the program are temporarily revised.

The new program is implemented with careful monitoring over the next year. Dr. K. continues volunteering at the shelter and hears many positive remarks from participants regarding the individualization of the program. Some remarks include "I feel like I have more control" and "I think I am ready to go out on my own." Dr. K. notices that there are fewer repeat participants, and this is verified when Ms. T. tells her the recidivism rate is down to 10%. The board of directors is very pleased with the results and approves continuation of the individualized program. The policy and procedures for the program are permanently revised.

Dr. K. decides to conduct a research study with Dr. S. (PhD) regarding homeless individuals who participate in the program. The focus of the study is on factors that contribute to the participants' success or failure with the program. Funding for the study is obtained from the U.S. Department of Health and Human Services. This information will be used by the shelter to assist and support future participants.

This case study demonstrates the role of the DNP as an advocate and influencer of policy. It demonstrates the DNP's utilization of research and evidence-based practice to affect access to care and quality of care, shape policy, implement change, and influence healthcare financing. Finally, it demonstrates collaboration between a DNP and a PhD in conducting clinical research.

SUMMARY

- *Nursing's Social Policy Statement* clearly states the nursing profession's commitment to society and the people who are served (ANA, 2003).
- Involvement in advocacy and healthcare policy is a natural extension of nursing's responsibilities and activities.
- Essential V of the *Essentials of Doctoral Education for Advanced Nursing Practice* provides specific curriculum standards for DNP programs related to healthcare policy and advocacy.
- DNP graduates possess the knowledge and education, as well as leadership skills and practice experience, to be powerful advocates for patients and to shape healthcare policy.
- Nursing has a rich and fruitful history of political activism, beginning with Florence Nightingale in 1860 and continuing through the present. However, it is evident that nursing still has much work to do to realize its full potential of influencing health care through policy.
- Tips for DNP graduates who are getting started in advocacy and healthcare policy include determining areas of interest, determining the amount of time and energy available to devote to political activism, and becoming informed and involved.
- There are multiple sources for DNP graduates to become informed regarding advocacy and healthcare policy, including professional journals, Internet searches, textbooks, policy courses, newspapers, and television and radio programs.
- Avenues for involvement by DNP graduates in advocacy and shaping healthcare policy include membership in professional nursing organizations, workplace involvement, educational endeavors, and research endeavors.
- Nursing is one of the most trusted professions in our nation (Feldman & Lewenson, 2000). DNP graduates can capitalize on this trust by becoming involved in political activities that advocate for patients and shape healthcare policies. DNP graduates are excellent candidates for public offices because of their knowledge and leadership skills.

REFLECTION QUESTIONS

1. Do you believe it is important for DNP graduates to be involved in advocacy and shaping healthcare policy? Why or why not?
2. What do you see as the role of DNP graduates in advocacy and shaping healthcare policy?

3. Do you see yourself assuming a leadership role in advocacy and healthcare policy? If yes, how? If not, why?

4. What are your areas of interest regarding advocacy and healthcare policy?

5. What are some specific ways you have advocated for patients? Recall specific instances where you made a difference for a patient or family through advocacy.

6. What are some specific policies you have designed, influenced, or implemented? Be sure to include institutional policies, community policies, and so forth.

7. Do you think it is important to be a member of professional nursing organizations? If yes, what organizations do you belong to? If no, what organizations could enhance your interests and allow you to become more politically involved?

8. What do you believe is the role of education and research in advocacy and healthcare policy?

9. Are you active in workplace committees, such as education and research committees? If not, in what ways do you think you can become involved in education and research in your workplace?

10. Would you be comfortable seeking election for a public office? Why or why not?

EDITOR'S NOTE

The author of this chapter is an excellent example of a DNP graduate in a healthcare policy role. Dr. Marlene Mullin has been on the Board of Directors for Hope Warming Center in Michigan since March 2010. Dr. Mullin has also volunteered to provide health care, meals, clothes, and so forth to the homeless population since 2005. Dr. Mullin is immediate past president of the Metro Detroit Chapter of MICNP (Michigan Council of Nurse Practitioners) and is currently chairperson of the chapter's Legislative Committee. The Metro Detroit Chapter of MICNP is the largest chapter in Michigan, which has 535 members. She assumed the presidency in January 2012. As president of the Metro Chapter, she oversaw all activities of the chapter in collaboration with the other board members, which included the president elect, secretary, treasurer, and education coordinator. The Detroit Metro chapter also provides monthly educational sessions and participates in fundraisers for various healthcare organizations. Dr. Mullin was the 2014 recipient of the MICNP President's Leadership Award. Dr. Mullin has also been a member of the APRN Coalition since 2009, which has been actively lobbying to make legislative changes for APRNs in Michigan. The proposed legislative changes include adding a definition of APRNs to the public health code, granting the Board of Nursing the authority to issue an APRN license, creating an APRN task force as a subcommittee of the Board of Nursing, adding APRNs to the list of licensed healthcare providers who are able to prescribe medications independently, including schedule II through V controlled drugs, and the ability to prescribe physical therapy and speech therapy. To date, the bill supporting these proposed changes has passed in the Michigan Senate and is currently awaiting review by the state House of Representatives' Health Policy Committee. Dr. Mullin continues to meet personally with Michigan state senators and representatives to garner support for the bill. Dr. Mullin is indeed a DNP graduate affecting practice through active involvement in healthcare policy and advocacy, and I am proud to call her my colleague.

REFERENCES

American Association of Colleges of Nursing. (2006). *Essentials of doctoral education for advanced nursing practice.* Retrieved from http://www.aacn.nche.edu/publications/position/DNPEssentials.pdf

American Association of Nurse Practitioners. (2014). Political Action Committee (AANP-PAC). Retrieved from http:www.aanp.org/legislation-regulation/federal-legislation/pac

American Nurses Association. (2003). *Nursing's social policy statement* (2nd ed.). Washington, DC: Author.

American Nurses Association. (2014). ANA-PAC. Retrieved from http:/www.nursingworld.org/anapac

Ballou, K. A. (2000). A historical-philosophical analysis of the professional nurse obligation to participate in sociopolitical activities. *Policy, Politics, & Nursing Practice, 1*(3), 172–184.

Burgess, M. A. (1928). *Nurses, patients, and pocketbooks.* New York, NY: Committee on the Grading of Nursing Schools.

Centers for Disease Control and Prevention, National Center for Health Statistics. (2013). *Health insurance coverage: Early release of estimates from the national health interview survey, 2013.* Hyattsville, MD: Author.

Chinn, P. L., & Wheeler, C. E. (1985). Feminism and nursing: Can nursing afford to remain aloof from the women's movement? *Nursing Outlook, 33*(2), 74–76.

Diers, D., & Price, L. (2007). Research as a political and policy tool. In D. J. Mason, J. K. Leavitt, & M. W. Chaffee (Eds.), *Policy & politics in nursing and health care* (5th ed., pp. 195–207). St. Louis, MO: Elsevier Saunders.

Feldman, H. R., & Lewenson, S. B. (2000). *Nurses in the political arena: The public face of nursing.* New York, NY: Springer.

Fitzpatrick, L. (1975). *The National Organization for Public Health Nursing, 1912–1952: Development of a practice field.* New York, NY: National League for Nursing Press.

Institute of Medicine. (2001). *Crossing the quality chasm: A new health system for the 21st century.* Washington, DC: National Academies Press.

Leavitt, J. K., Chaffee, M. W., & Vance, C. (2007). Learning the ropes of policy, politics, and advocacy. In D. J. Mason, J. K. Leavitt, & M. W. Chaffee (Eds.), *Policy & politics in nursing and health care* (5th ed., pp. 34–52). St. Louis, MO: Elsevier Saunders.

Lewenson, S. B. (2007). A historical perspective on policy, politics, and nursing. In D. J. Mason, J. K. Leavitt, & M. W. Chaffee (Eds.), *Policy & politics in nursing and health care* (5th ed., pp. 21–33). St. Louis, MO: Elsevier Saunders.

Malone, P. S., & Chaffee, M. W. (2007). Interest groups: Powerful political catalysts in health care. In D. J. Mason, J. K. Leavitt, & M. W. Chaffee (Eds.), *Policy & politics in nursing and health care* (5th ed., pp. 766–777). St. Louis, MO: Elsevier Saunders.

Michnich, M. (2007). The Robert Wood Johnson health policy fellowship. In D. J. Mason, J. K. Leavitt, & M. W. Chaffee (Eds.), *Policy & politics in nursing and health care* (5th ed., pp. 52–57). St. Louis, MO: Elsevier Saunders.

Oden, L. S., Price, J. H., Alteneder, R., Boardley, D., & Ubokudom, S. E. (2000). Public policy involvement by nurse practitioners. *Journal of Community Health, 25*(2), 139–155.

O'Grady, E. (2004). Advanced practice nursing and health policy. In J. Stanley (Ed.), *Advanced practice nursing emphasizing common roles* (2nd ed., pp. 374–394). Philadelphia, PA: F. A. Davis.

U.S. Department of Housing and Urban Development. (2013). *The 2013 annual homeless assessment report to Congress.* Washington, DC: U.S. Government Printing Office.

CHAPTER 6

The DNP Graduate as Educator

Karen McBroom Butler

A clinical doctorate provides graduates with enhanced knowledge to improve nursing practice and patient outcomes; advanced competencies for extremely complex clinical, faculty, and leadership roles; enhanced leadership skills; and parity with other professions (American Association of Colleges of Nursing [AACN], 2004a). All these functions are essential for educators. However, despite preparation with the practice doctorate—doctor of nursing practice (DNP)—the role of the nurse educator is not emphasized or recognized as fully as other roles for the degree.

The *AACN Position Statement on the Practice Doctorate in Nursing* (AACN, 2004a) states that the practice doctorate should be the graduate degree for advanced nursing practice, including but not limited to the four current advanced-practice roles: clinical nurse specialist, nurse anesthetist, nurse–midwife, and nurse practitioner. An additional recommendation is that practice doctorate programs, as in research-focused doctorate programs, offer additional course work and practicums that would prepare graduates to fill the role of nurse educator (AACN, 2004a).

The traditional view is that nurses who are prepared with a research doctorate (PhD, DNS, DSN, or DNSc) should be nurse educators and function in faculty roles, particularly in research-intensive institutions. Certainly their role is extremely valuable to both nursing education and to the generation of new knowledge. However, there is a history of valuing individuals with professional doctorates in nursing education as well. Many schools of nursing employ faculty with a professional education doctorate (EdD), which is different from the PhD in education. These individuals play an important role in collegiate nursing education (Hathaway, Jacob, Stegbauer, Thompson, & Graff, 2006).

The DNP prepares nurses with advanced skills and specialized knowledge in an identified area of nursing practice, including translation of science into clinical practice. This preparation is important for the educator role. In addition, the discipline of education, which encompasses a completely separate body of knowledge and competence, is important. Graduates of research-focused and practice-focused doctoral programs may need additional preparation in teaching methodologies, curriculum design and development, and program evaluation if those areas of preparation have not been addressed in the students' original programs of study (AACN, 2006b). With preparation in teaching methodologies and curriculum design, graduates of both practice- and research-focused programs can function effectively as nursing faculty members. More important, together they contribute alternate, complementary approaches and expertise to the educator role. The pairing of professional and academic degrees within a discipline is common practice in academics, both inside and outside of health sciences (Hathaway et al., 2006).

This chapter provides a case for the DNP graduate in a nurse educator role and explains how nursing can be influenced and strengthened as a result. Specific case scenarios describing DNP graduates in educator roles are included to illustrate how they can effectively contribute to the traditional education, research and scholarship, practice, and service roles in nursing education.

Curriculum Standards

The *Essentials of Doctoral Education for Advanced Nursing Practice* (AACN, 2006b) discusses curriculum standards but does not speak directly to the role of nurse educator (**Box 6-1**). However, there is content inherent to nursing education and advanced nursing practice, which is broadly defined by the AACN as "any form of nursing

---

BOX 6-1

Curriculum Standards: Essentials of Doctoral Education for Advanced Nursing Practice

- Scientific underpinnings for practice
- Organizational and systems leadership for quality improvement and systems thinking
- Clinical scholarship and analytical methods for evidence-based practice
- Information systems and technology and patient care technology for the improvement and transformation of health care
- Healthcare policy for advocacy in health care
- Clinical scholarship and analytical methods for evidence-based practice
- Clinical prevention and population health for improving the nation's health
- Advanced nursing practice

Source: Data from the American Association of Colleges of Nursing (AACN). (2006). Essentials of doctoral education for advanced nursing practice. Retrieved from http://www.aacn.nche.edu/publications/position

intervention that influences health care outcomes for individuals or populations, including the direct care of individual patients, management of care for individuals or populations, administration of nursing and health care organizations, and the development and implementation of health policy" (2004a, p. 2).

DNP Essentials and National Initiatives

Certainly nurse educators who are experts in advanced nursing practice are needed and timely, given the initiatives by the Institute of Medicine (Greiner & Knebel, 2003; Institute of Medicine [IOM], 2011) and the National Research Council (2005). These reports call for nursing education that prepares individuals for interdisciplinary practice, information systems, quality improvement, and patient safety expertise. Not only are these essential skills for DNP graduates; they are also important skills for nurse educators to teach and role-model for students.

In the introduction to the *Essentials of Doctoral Education for Advanced Nursing Practice* (AACN, 2006b), additional IOM recommendations are referenced that include promotion of health care that is safe, effective, client centered, timely, efficient, and equitable; it also recommends education of healthcare professionals that includes delivery of patient-centered care while working on interdisciplinary teams and an emphasis on evidence-based practice, quality improvement, and informatics. The best-prepared senior nurses should be in key leadership positions and should participate in executive-level positions. DNP-prepared educators serve as key leaders in nursing and as such are positioned to make a powerful impact on health care that incorporates the IOM recommendations. Such an impact could be made through education of students, professional role-modeling, scholarship, and clinical practice opportunities.

DNP Essentials and the Educator Role

Although the *Essentials of Doctoral Education for Advanced Nursing Practice* (AACN, 2006b) do not speak directly to the educator role, there are competencies in every essential that are important and relevant to nurse educators. The introduction to the essentials document contains a section titled "DNP Graduates and Academic Roles," which states that DNP graduates "will seek to fill roles as educators and will use their considerable practice expertise to educate the next generation of nurses" (AACN, 2006b, p. 7). The major focus of DNP programs, as in other practice disciplines, will be practice specialization. Those who desire to hold an educator role should have additional preparation in pedagogy to enhance their ability to teach the science of the profession they practice and teach. Some of this formal course work may occur within the context of the DNP program (AACN, 2006b).

The Nursing Faculty Shortage

When considering the role a DNP graduate may assume as a nursing faculty member, it is important to examine the context in which the conversation takes place. This is particularly pertinent now when we are facing a national shortage of registered nurses.

Exacerbating the overall nursing shortage is the increasing deficit of full-time master's and doctorate-prepared nursing faculty members.

The Shortage of Nurses and Nursing Faculty

A national conversation about the DNP graduate as nurse educator is both essential and timely. Literature in professional journals and publications, and the popular press, is full of stories about the dwindling supply and increased demand for registered nurses.

The U.S. Bureau of Labor Statistics' employment projections (2012) report that registered nursing will be the top occupation for job growth through 2020. The projections indicate the need for 495,500 replacements in the nursing workforce, bringing the total number of job openings to 1.2 million by 2020. Buerhaus, Auerbach, and Staiger (2009) suggest that despite some easing of the nursing shortage due to the recent economic recession, the U.S. nursing shortage is projected to be 260,000 registered nurses by 2025. This projection represents twice as large a nursing shortage as we have seen in previous decades and can largely be attributed to an aging nursing workforce. The authors further suggest that until nursing educational capacity is increased, such shortages will be unavoidable.

There is no lack of literature on the nursing shortage; in fact, the current and future shortage of registered nurses has been reported extensively (AACN, 2013c; Aiken, Clark, Sloane, Sochalski, & Silber, 2002; Berliner & Ginzberg, 2002; Buerhaus, Potter, Staiger, & Auerbach, 2009; Buerhaus, Staiger, & Auerbach, 2000; Goodin, 2003; Greiner & Knebel, 2003). Only recently has more attention been given to a critical factor in resolving the problem: the availability of adequate numbers of appropriately educated, highly qualified nursing faculty to teach students. Indeed, this shortage of faculty in nursing programs may negatively affect the number of qualified applicants accepted to both basic and advanced-practice nursing education programs. Difficulty in filling nursing faculty positions may be the most crucial factor affecting the future supply of nurses (Brendtro & Hegge, 2000).

History of the Nursing Faculty Shortage

Nursing educational institutions have always had a shortage of doctorate-prepared faculty, partly due to this academic norm occurring later in nursing than other professions. A substantial decrease in nursing school enrollments in the 1980s led to a decrease in faculty positions (Brendtro & Hegge, 2000). As early as the 1980s concerns were being expressed about nursing faculty shortages (Fitzpatrick & Heller, 1980). One study (Zebelman & Olswang, 1989) found that students in doctoral programs became more focused on research than on faculty roles and preparation as they progressed through their programs; these authors voiced concern that this approach might have a negative impact on the supply of doctorate-prepared nursing faculty. Likewise, Princeton (1992) looked at the development and status of graduate nursing education for teachers and argued that the numbers of graduate programs should be increased to deal with the faculty shortage. De Tornyay (1989) wrote that the environment of graduate programs discouraged students from seeking teaching positions. The 1980s predictions of a faculty shortage became a reality as opportunities for those with PhDs in nursing extended beyond educational institutions (Mullinix, 1990). The National Sample Survey of Registered Nurses estimated that in 1992, 1996, and 2000 the proportion of nurses with nursing doctorates who were employed in schools of nursing with baccalaureate and higher degrees showed steady declines, falling from 68% in 1992 to 49% in 2000 (Division of Nursing, 2001).

Faculty Shortage Impacts on Student Enrollment

The AACN reports that 79,659 qualified nursing school applicants were turned away from baccalaureate and graduate programs in 2012 because of the insufficient number of faculty, clinical sites, classroom space, and clinical preceptors, as well as budget concerns and restraints. Nearly two-thirds of the nursing schools that responded to this survey identified the faculty shortage as a primary reason for not accepting all qualified applicants into entry-level nursing programs (AACN, 2013a). The AACN estimates that the national nurse faculty vacancy rate is 8.3% in baccalaureate and graduate programs, with almost 87% of the vacancies being faculty positions requiring or preferring a doctoral degree (AACN, 2013d). The problem is not limited to university nursing programs. A National League for Nursing report (2006) found that the total average faculty vacancy rate was 5.6% in associate's degree programs and 7.9% in bachelor's degree and higher programs.

In a Southern Regional Education Board survey of 491 institutions in 16 states, researchers found more than 425 unfilled faculty positions, and 86 institutions reported they did not have enough faculty to cover the offered undergraduate and graduate programs. The data also revealed that 144 faculty members retired in that academic year, and more than 550 resignations had been received in the current academic year or were expected in the coming 2 years. In terms of educational preparation, most of the 6,322 nurse educators had master's degrees in nursing (Southern Regional Education Board, 2003).

Related Factors

There are additional factors that contribute to the nursing faculty shortage. For example, the average age of faculty members is increasing, thus reducing the number of productive years nurse educators can teach (AACN, 2013c). The average ages of doctorate-prepared faculty holding the ranks of professor, associate professor, and assistant professor were 61.3, 57.7, and 51.5 years, respectively. A complicating issue is that nurses enter academia later in their careers (AACN, 2013b). Data suggest there is an oncoming wave of faculty member retirements. Some researchers project that for individuals who were faculty members in 2001, between 200 and 300 will be eligible for retirement annually from 2003 through 2012. The average age of nursing faculty at retirement is 62.5 years (Berlin & Sechrist, 2002).

Higher compensation in the clinical arena is becoming more available and increasingly attractive to current and potential faculty members. Average salaries for clinical nursing positions have risen more than those for nursing faculty positions, probably because most universities are constrained in their ability to increase faculty salaries (AACN, 2005; Brendtro & Hegge, 2000). In fall 2004 the median salaries for teaching faculty with doctoral degrees, in the ranks of associate and assistant professors, were $77,605 and $73,333, respectively; those with master's degrees had median salaries of $62,778 and $58,567, respectively (Berlin, Wilsey, & Bednash, 2005). In comparison, the 2004–2005 median salaries for nurse anesthetists, heads of nursing (executive and management) and nursing directors were $121,698, $157,754, and $104,191, respectively (Berlin et al., 2005). The American Academy of Nurse Practitioners reports that the average salary of nurse practitioners, across all settings and specialty areas, is $94,050 (AACN, 2013c), contrasted with master's-prepared faculty serving as associate professors, who earn an annual average salary of $80,690 (AACN, 2013b).

Although the number of doctoral programs increased from 54 in 1992 to 93 in 2004 (Berlin, Bednash, & Alsheimer, 1993; Berlin et al., 2005), this did not result in an increase in graduates. In 2012 the AACN found that 13,311 qualified applicants were turned away from master's programs, and more than 1,348 qualified applicants were turned away from doctoral programs. The primary reason given for these numbers was a shortage of faculty (AACN, 2013c). The ultimate consequence is further reductions in doctorate-prepared nurse educators who are available for faculty positions. An adverse effect of the faculty shortage is an increase in faculty workload, with the added likelihood of stress, burnout, and attrition. Researchers report faculty members' ages are increasing steadily, shortening the length of time to likely retirement and a loss of younger faculty (AACN, 2005; Berlin & Sechrist, 2002). The use of part-time or less-qualified faculty members or assigning faculty members to teach outside their areas of specialization may result in lower-quality programs. Schools may hire more master's-prepared clinical experts with little or no preparation for teaching (Brendtro & Hegge, 2000). Princeton described this type of "on-the-job training" as a costly "hit-and-miss situation" (1992, p. 35). Other issues related to the nursing faculty shortage include a decline in the percentage of younger faculty (Berlin & Sechrist, 2002), tuition and loan burden for graduate study (Peterson's Colleges of Nursing Database, 2002), workload and role expectations (Brendtro & Hegge, 2000), and alternate career choices (AACN, 2013c).

The nursing faculty shortage cannot be viewed separately from the overall nursing shortage, but the implications of decreasing numbers of faculty members are twofold—both are of equal importance. First, it is essential to have faculty members with the knowledge and skills needed for good teaching; there is a pressing need for scholars and researchers in education (Tanner, 1999). Second, institutions must have nursing faculty members with the requisite education and skills to be researchers to continue to generate and advance the scientific knowledge base for nursing (Hinshaw, 2001). DNP graduates possess the educational preparation and experience to have a positive, significant impact on the nursing faculty shortage.

DNP Graduates Can Fill the Nursing Faculty Gap

The AACN (2006b) states that DNP graduates will seek to fill roles as educators and use their wealth of practice expertise to educate the next generation of nurses. With additional work in pedagogy, DNP graduates are uniquely qualified to help fill the nursing faculty gap.

Nursing Leadership and the Shortage

Many strategies have been proposed to address the overall nursing and nursing faculty shortage. Among these are federal and state funding initiatives; strategic partnerships with private corporations; national media campaigns (AACN, 2013c); career progression initiatives to reach out to students early; moving nursing graduates through graduate studies more rapidly; identifying a range of options beyond entry-level roles of faculty, researcher, and administrator; and fostering competitive salaries and improved work environments (AACN, 2001). Berlin and Sechrist (2002) state that nurse educators must rapidly arrive at both short- and long-term solutions that may require examination of some of the sacrosanct traditions of nursing education and an unbiased scrutiny of faculty work environments. They suggest a streamlined educational process and consideration for adopting a broader-based view of educational preparation for faculty status.

National and state nurse leaders and deans of schools of nursing, along with nursing faculty members and others, have a great opportunity to work in collaborative leadership to affect the nursing faculty shortage. Heifetz (1994) writes of working together as partners in shared leadership to face current issues, create a new paradigm, and stimulate action to create a desired future. If ever there was a time for nursing leaders in education to work together to create a preferred future, this is certainly the era.

Strategic Leadership: DNP-Prepared Educators

The DNP degree offers education that prepares graduates for leadership roles at the highest level, with clinical expertise and the knowledge and skills necessary to translate research findings into practice. These are all areas that can be used to build a successful career in nursing education. Depending on a specific curriculum, graduates may need additional preparation in pedagogy. This is not different than graduates of many PhD programs. According to the National League for Nursing (2002), all nurse educators need core knowledge and skills that entail the ability to enhance learning, advance the total development and professional socialization of students, design appropriate learning experiences, and evaluate learning outcomes.

Inclusion of educational content in DNP curricula is one way to address the nursing faculty shortage. A recent survey of Pennsylvania schools with DNP programs revealed that at least one of them included education as a specialty area (Dunbar-Jacob, Nativio, & Khalil, 2013). This is a strategy that nursing leaders in education could adopt to address the deficit in pedagogy in both DNP and PhD curricula. This research also revealed that the second most common placement for DNP graduates was in academics (32.5%). This finding further indicates the need for revisions in curricula to include content that will enable these graduates to be successful educators.

Although the original stated intent of the DNP degree did not include the preparation of nurse educators, there is evidence in the literature that this is occurring, and certainly it is timely. Danzey, Fitzpatrick, Garbutt, Rafferty, and Zychowicz (2011) reported that some DNP programs offer specialty content in education or educational leadership and that doing so gives experienced master's-prepared nurses formal preparation in educational theory and methodology. These authors report that graduates of such programs are prepared to develop, implement, and evaluate nursing curricula and actively participate in educational scholarship.

Another strategy that has been cited to reverse the nursing faculty shortage includes career progression initiatives that move nurses through graduate school more quickly. The AACN (1999) recommended that education be compressed to become more attractive. The AACN's *Essentials of Doctoral Education for Advanced Nursing Practice* (2006b) recommends that DNP programs be 3 calendar years (36 months of full-time study, including summers) or 4 academic years. This recommendation is for those programs that offer a BSN-to-DNP option, and it is much more stream-lined than the time and expense necessary to obtain the two previously required degrees (master's and doctorate). It also gives the student a doctoral education with an appropriate number of academic credits. For those who already have a master's degree, the time to completion of a DNP program would be even shorter and less expensive.

A third proposed strategy to reduce the nursing faculty shortage is to encourage students to return to graduate school at an earlier age. This is a paradigm change; no longer is it feasible to recommend that students work for years in clinical settings to gain experience between degrees. Undergraduate students should be encouraged to return to master's programs early after graduation; master's students should be encouraged to obtain doctorates earlier in their careers as well (Anderson, 2000). Because the DNP degree will, in many cases, replace master's degree programs that prepare nurses for advanced nursing practice, it follows that students will be entering DNP programs at an earlier age than students in prior doctoral programs, with the additional benefit of students being doctorate prepared in 3 years. Not only could these efforts increase the number of younger nurses with advanced degrees, but faculty members would enter the workforce at earlier ages, thus increasing the amount of time they have available for productive academic careers.

A fourth proposed strategy to reduce the nursing faculty shortage is the devel-opment of more flexible degree programs. Distributed learning and online courses would increase the availability of graduate education to those who may not live near a school that offers doctoral programs. Accelerated career pathways, such as BSN to DNP, may entice those who have a limited number of years and money to invest in graduate education. Current clinically focused, master's-prepared faculty members should be encouraged to pursue a DNP degree. Such new programs make graduate opportunities available to those who do not wish to be researchers and are interested in clinical leadership and expertise, often in educational settings (Marion et al., 2003).

Another way to stretch available resources is to adequately prepare faculty mem-bers to use technology (Boyden, 2000). DNP graduates will begin preparation for this role as addressed in the AACN's *Essentials of Doctoral Education for Advanced Nursing Practice* (2006b). The use of information technology will be incorporated into DNP curricula and will set the stage for additional work with teaching technology.

A New Paradigm

With decreasing numbers of nursing faculty has come more responsibility for those left behind. Traditionally faculty roles have been threefold: education, research, and service. Perhaps it is time to reexamine those roles and, at least in some cases, separate them to create more realistic work expectations (Brendtro & Hegge, 2000).

For example, a faculty member who is an expert in teaching may be allowed to teach most of the time with less research effort; a researcher may be able to devote the majority of his or her time to concentrate on generating new knowledge; and a DNP graduate may be given the opportunity to teach, function in clinical practice leadership roles, or work as a member of a research team in partnership with research-focused colleagues to translate findings into practice. This is being done by some schools of nursing already; yet for others—particularly parent institutions in which schools of nursing reside—the paradigm shift is pending.

To promote such a paradigm shift, it is important to think outside the box about those who may be able to fulfill faculty roles and obligations. The creative use of diversely prepared faculty members is a good option; the strengths of the individual and his or her educational preparation should be capitalized upon. It may take a real paradigm change for nursing educators to accept that there are those without PhDs in nursing who can successfully teach student nurses. Nurse leaders need to work together to establish a place and a role for these professionals and to incorporate them effectively into nursing education.

Sebastian and Delaney (2013) state that utilizing nurse faculty composed of experts in direct and indirect nursing practice and research are essential to preparing future clinicians and systems change agents. An example is a faculty with some members involved in clinical scholarship and others engaged in funded research who strategically partner to advance science (Sebastian & Delaney, 2013). In addition, incorporating DNP-prepared nursing faculty into the existing faculty ranks not only increases the numbers of doctorate-prepared faculty, but it also allows for parity with other university departments and disciplines. In doing so, there is the potential for increasing educational capacity (Dunbar-Jacob et al., 2013).

Undergraduate Education

DNP graduates are prepared to teach at the undergraduate level. Fitzpatrick states that "expert clinicians are needed to teach clinicians" (2002, p. 57). Further, she proposes that nursing faculty members who teach at the basic (and advanced practice) level principally need expert clinical skills paired with skills in teaching; therefore, the best preparation for teaching these clinicians is the clinical doctorate (Fitzpatrick, 2002). After all, one can best teach what one knows well.

Baccalaureate nursing students love clinical practice. It is the foremost reason they come to nursing school, and it is their primary framework for nursing. DNP-prepared educators can make a real difference in the education of these young nurses, both in the classroom and in clinical settings. Because DNP graduates are expert clinicians, they can clearly explain and demonstrate clinical phenomena. In addition, they can write realistic case studies and simulation scenarios (both low and high fidelity) and have the expertise and experience to answer difficult, complex clinical questions.

DNP graduates are excellent nursing role models for undergraduate students, both in advanced nursing practice utilizing expert clinical skills and as doctorate-prepared educators who are dedicated to nursing practice. National scholars recognized this potential when they wrote *Advancing the Nation's Health Needs: NIH Research Training Programs* (Committee for Monitoring the Nation's Changing Needs for Biomedical, Behavioral, and Clinical Personnel, 2005). The authors state that "the need for doctorally-prepared practitioners and clinical faculty would be met if nursing could develop a new nonresearch clinical doctorate, similar to the MD and PharmD in medicine and dentistry" (p. 74).

DNP graduates are performing scholarly work related to undergraduate education. A recent study that identified peer-reviewed, published scholarly articles authored by DNP graduates (Broome, Riner & Allam, 2013) found that educational topics, such as student satisfaction and self-confidence after simulation (Alfes, 2011) and active learning via classroom participation systems (Smith and Rosenkoetter, 2009), are being explored. Not only are DNP graduates successfully teaching in undergraduate programs; they are also participating in scholarship designed to advance the knowledge related to their work as educators.

Graduate Education

DNP graduates are prepared to teach at the graduate level. Particularly for faculty members who teach in clinically focused graduate programs, clinical teaching necessitates advanced clinical knowledge and enhanced practice skills. DNP graduates are master teachers in clinical practice and are role models for advanced nursing practice. DNP graduates bring strengths to graduate education, including a clinical and health systems depth of understanding, increased knowledge of quality and safety, expertise in team practice, and the use of evidence-based practice in care delivery (Dunbar-Jacob et al., 2013). These faculty also model advanced-practice education and can foster a methodological expansion to scholarship in nursing by emphasizing utilization of evidence (Dunbar-Jacob et al., 2013).

The AACN's *Essentials of Doctoral Education for Advanced Nursing Practice* (2006b) states that faculty members who teach in DNP programs should have diverse backgrounds and scholarly perspectives in the specialty areas for which they are preparing graduates. Broad faculty expertise is needed, which includes doctorate-prepared, research-focused faculty and doctorate-prepared, practice-focused faculty with expertise to support the educational program. Collaboration among DNP-prepared faculty and those with research expertise represents an opportunity for innovation, which will only be beneficial to the profession.

In addition, there is a need for a group of faculty members who are actively engaged in practice as part of their faculty roles, because active practice provides the same type of applied clinical learning environments for DNP students that active research programs provide for PhD students (AACN, 2006b). Faculty members should have current experience by participating in clinical practice or monitoring current nursing practice to prepare students to enter the complex world of health care (Sperhac & Goodwin, 2003). Faculty practice provides a learning environment that models rapid translation of new knowledge into practice and evaluates practice-based models of care (AACN, 2006b). Additionally, the development and implementation of scholarship programs that represent knowledge development from original research for some faculty members and application of research in practice for others is recommended (AACN, 2006b).

Diverse Opportunities

There are many opportunities for DNP graduates to pursue and fulfill academic roles. These are not restricted to research-intensive institutions. There are regional universities, community colleges, and other institutions that offer nursing education programs. All of these venues are in need of doctorate-prepared nursing faculty. The possibilities are there for those who choose to pursue them, and nursing will be better for the inclusion of educational diversity among its faculty ranks. **Box 6-2** lists tips for DNP graduates who are interested in pursuing a career in academia. Case scenario 3 (later in this chapter) illustrates the successful career of a DNP-prepared faculty member who teaches at both the undergraduate and graduate levels at a regional state university.

Promotion and Tenure

Conversations about DNP graduates in faculty roles generally involve discussions about promotion and tenure. Although criteria for promotion and tenure are determined mostly by individual institutions, there are some commonalities. Strategies used by someone with a clinically focused doctorate to achieve promotion and tenure may be somewhat different than those used by someone with a research-focused doctorate, but it is possible to attain both promotion and tenure, even at research-intensive institutions (see case scenarios 1 and 2 for illustrative examples).

University promotion and tenure policies should accommodate newer forms of scholarship for DNP-prepared faculty (Bellini, McCauley, & Cusson, 2012). It is important for such faculty to have opportunities for development related to each of the three traditional missions typically identified for tenure (teaching, research and scholarship, and service) (Sebastian & Delaney, 2013). This adds additional emphasis for the need to include educational theory and methods in DNP programs for those who wish to join the academy. At the least, universities should offer a teaching certificate or continuing education opportunities for both PhD and DNP graduates who wish to further their knowledge in this area.

BOX 6-2

Tips for DNP Graduates Who Are Interested in Pursuing a Career in Academia

- Do your homework! The requirements for faculty roles are different at every institution. What is expected of the faculty? What are the options and specifications for attaining promotion and tenure? What is the emphasis? Is it a community college with the primary goal of educating students or a research-intensive university that values grant funding and scholarly productivity? Is it a mix of these things? If so, where would you fit into the mix?

- Know what your interests and talents are (teaching, implementation of evidence-based clinical practices, faculty practice, partnering with researchers, etc.). Match your interests with the priorities and strengths of the institution.

- If you are primarily interested in education, are there other nurse educators at the institution who will support you in this role? Is there support for continuing work in curriculum development, implementation and evaluation, teaching strategies, and student outcomes evaluation?

- If you are interested in teaching undergraduates, what is the school's NCLEX pass rate for the past 5 years? If you are interested in teaching at the graduate level, what programs are available, and how many of the students are successful in attaining certification in their specialties?

- If you are interested in faculty clinical practice, are clinical sites that fit your expertise associated with the institution? Are the sites willing to consider a joint appointment?

- If you are interested in partnering with researchers, is there a researcher or a research team with interests similar to yours? Are they willing to discuss partnering opportunities and support you in your role, including assistance with meeting the criteria for promotion and tenure? Remember, academic scholarship should include the application of knowledge, and you are an expert in this area.

- Market what you can do! DNP preparation and roles are relatively new, and many parent institutions do not understand the competencies that a DNP-prepared faculty member brings to the role. Be specific about what you can offer, and provide this information in writing when you apply for a faculty position.

- Don't give up! There are many opportunities for DNP-prepared faculty members to serve and flourish. Finding the right fit is essential and will create a path for a successful, satisfying career in academia.

Promising findings from a study conducted by Nicholes and Dyer (2012) indicate that it may be feasible for DNP-prepared faculty to become eligible for tenure. Although this has been the case in some settings, attainment of tenure for DNP graduates still requires a paradigm change for many. Nicholes and Dyer's exploratory study surveyed PhD-prepared faculty and deans identified from AACN's DNP program list. The questions related to feasibility, benefits, concerns, and challenges in the tenure process for DNP-prepared faculty who wish to become eligible for tenure. In addition to the finding that achievement of tenure may be possible, the benefit of recruitment and retention of qualified faculty was cited. The concerns included lack of training for the DNP to be successful in producing scholarly research. Other researchers, however, have found that DNP graduates are successfully engaging in scholarly research and publishing their findings (Broome et al., 2013). Challenges identified from the Nicholes and Dyer study include reevaluating the criteria traditionally used in awarding tenure to DNP-prepared faculty.

Practice Doctorates: A Case for Tenure

Promotion and tenure are primarily institutional decisions, for both eligibility and standards. The AACN (2004b) voices confidence that a DNP-prepared faculty member will compete favorably with faculty members who hold other practice doctorates in tenure and promotion decisions. This is the case in law, education, physical therapy, pharmacy, public policy and administration, public health, and other disciplines (AACN, 2004b). It is common for institutions to have policies that enable those with professional doctorates to attain tenure (Hathaway et al., 2006).

There are institutions of higher learning in which different types of tenure lines are available, such as a regular title series (the traditional, research-based format) and alternate options, such as clinical or special title series, in which requirements for tenure may be based more on clinical practice or teaching excellence. It is important for DNP graduates to be fully cognizant of the opportunities and requirements at a particular institution before accepting employment.

The AACN's *Essentials of Doctoral Education for Advanced Nursing Practice* (AACN, 2006b) lists indicators of productive programs of nursing practice scholarship, many of which may be used toward promotion and tenure in various settings. These include

> extramural grants in support of practice innovations; peer reviewed publications and presentations; practice-oriented grant review activities; editorial review activities; state, regional, national, and international professional activities related to one's practice area; policy involvement; and development and dissemination of practice improvement products such as reports, guidelines, protocols and toolkits. (AACN, 2006b, p. 21)

The DNP graduate is educationally prepared with the relevant knowledge and skills to accomplish these indicators and thereby should be considered for tenure-track positions at academic institutions that host schools of nursing. Inclusion of these skills in written communications when applying for academic positions may be helpful both to the applicant and the employer.

Hathaway et al. (2006) argue that having the ability to earn a practice doctorate will enhance many nursing faculty members' scholarly productivity and have a positive impact on their ability to earn tenure. Many schools employ master's-prepared nursing faculty members who are important to the educational mission and are devoted to clinical practice. These faculty members may not wish to pursue research doctorates, or, if they do, they may not use their research preparation, thereby limiting their scholarly productivity and the ability to earn tenure. This is supported by data showing that only 11% of doctorate-prepared nurses are working in research-intensive institutions (AACN, 2006a; Health Resources and Services Administration, 2004). Earning a practice doctorate, such as a DNP, will provide knowledge and skills to faculty members who are clinically focused and contribute to their ability to earn tenure (Hathaway et al., 2006).

The Scholarship of Application

Scholarship application has been described by Boyer (1990). Although the generation of new scientific knowledge and scholarly publication are appropriate performance criteria for research faculty, Boyer argues that application of knowledge through professional practice should also be valued. This definition of scholarship legitimizes nonresearch endeavors by emphasizing that application of knowledge engages scholars who must determine how knowledge can be applied to problems, how it can be helpful to stakeholders outside the institution, and how social or clinical problems can create an agenda for future research. New understanding can come from application of knowledge. When this occurs, theory and practice interact, and each renews the other. According to Boyer, the logical conclusion is that if the institution values clinical practice, the scholarship of application must be considered in tenure decisions.

Graduates from DNP programs are practicing scholarship, working collaboratively with their research colleagues and other professions, and publishing their work. A recent article investigated publication practices of DNP graduates in the scholarly nursing literature. The researchers looked at published studies over a 7-year period that had at least one author with a DNP degree. Of the 300 articles identified, 175 met the inclusion criteria. In 75% of the studies a DNP-prepared individual was the first author. Most commonly found were clinical investigations, followed by practice-focused patient and healthcare provider studies. The number of peer-reviewed and published studies increased over time (Broome et al., 2013).

Almost half of the authors were from multiple settings (practice and academia) or held a joint appointment in academia and a healthcare agency. Coauthors from other disciplines were found in 34 of the articles. This study clearly shows that DNP-prepared nurses are contributing to the body of nursing knowledge and practicing interprofessional collaboration that is consistent with the DNP essentials and the scholarship of application.

A Valuable Partnership: Research and Clinical Experts

One creative approach involves having DNP graduates partner with researchers, either individually or as part of a research team. Researchers are skilled in the generation of new knowledge, and DNP graduates are prepared to translate this new knowledge into practice and evaluate outcomes (thereby generating new research questions). This is a perfect marriage of interest, education, and talents, and it also puts the theory–research–practice loop that has been advocated for many years into active practice (Fawcett, 2005; Fawcett, Watson, Neuman, Walker, & Fitzpatrick, 2001; Hathaway et al., 2006; Neuman & Fawcett, 2001). Although PhD and DNP programs have distinct outcomes, Melnyk states that graduates must work together and with interprofessional colleagues to effectively and efficiently translate evidence-based interventions supported by research findings into clinical settings. The ultimate goal is to improve patient outcomes and quality of care (Melnyk, 2013).

Hinshaw (2001) states that there must be nursing faculty with the requisite education and skills to be researchers to continue the generation and advancement of the scientific knowledge base for nursing. This author contends that there must also be nursing faculty with the requisite education and skills to be expert clinicians to apply new knowledge and evaluate outcomes. Through the development of such teams of faculty, the scientific knowledge base for nursing can be generated, applied, refined, and advanced. Examples of such partnering opportunities are illustrated in the first two case scenarios at the end of this chapter.

Conclusion

Education is a part of every nurse's role, whether we are educating our patients, their families, our colleagues, or students. This chapter has made a case for why DNP graduates are uniquely prepared to function as nursing faculty in diverse settings and how this fits into the current context of nursing education, the nursing faculty shortage, and the current, complex healthcare system. The creative use of diversely prepared faculty is essential and will capitalize on the strengths of individuals and their educational preparation while bringing alternate, complementary approaches and expertise to the role.

It may take a real paradigm change for those in nursing education to accept that there are those without research-focused doctorates in nursing who can successfully teach nursing students at all levels and fulfill the roles necessary to attain promotion and tenure. Nurse leaders must work together to establish a place and a role for these DNP-prepared professionals and to incorporate them effectively into nursing education.

Case Scenarios: The DNP Graduate as Nurse Educator

It is useful for DNP students and graduates who are interested in pursuing nursing faculty roles to see illustrative examples of those who have been successful in this quest. The following three case scenarios are examples of how three DNP graduates are working to successfully fulfill nursing faculty roles, both in research-intensive and regional state universities.

Case Scenario 1: A DNP Graduate in a Tenured Faculty Role in a Research-Intensive State University

Dr. B. is a 2006 DNP graduate who is a nursing faculty member at a large public research-intensive land grant university in the southeastern United States. Prior to graduation from her DNP program, she was an undergraduate course coordinator, lecturer, and clinical instructor (nontenure track) in a nationally ranked college of nursing for 5 years. Upon graduation, her rank was changed to assistant professor, special title series (tenure track). Her additional new responsibilities at that time included teaching leadership in the school's DNP program and serving as a faculty associate in the university's Tobacco Policy Research Program (TPRP). Following a rigorous 6-year peer evaluation process focused on teaching excellence, clinical practice, scholarship, and service, she was promoted to associate professor with tenure.

Dr. B. is well prepared and suited for her responsibilities. In practice prior to teaching she held several high-level nursing administrative positions in the medical center. Therefore, not only is she well versed in the leadership literature from her DNP curriculum, but she also has actual practice experience in leadership roles, which enhances her ability to teach the content and illustrate its use. Dr. B. has taken advantage of continuing education opportunities and has used peer review to hone her teaching skills.

In addition, she functions as a leader in the College of Nursing as chairperson for several committees and as an undergraduate course coordinator, and she leads in the broader university setting by serving on committees and partnering with faculty from other departments for specific scholarly projects. Dr. B. also advises DNP students and chairs their doctoral committees. She serves as a leader in the community by donating her time and expertise to various health-related interest groups. She is a reviewer for nine professional journals and has served on statewide, regional, and national professional committees. Leadership in the form of serving the College of Nursing, the university, the profession, and the community satisfies the traditionally held tenure requirement for service.

Dr. B.'s baccalaureate students are intensely interested in her practice doctorate; clinical nursing is their primary framework for nursing. They love that when they ask clinically oriented questions she has the expertise to answer them and can illustrate the answer with real-life clinical experiences. They are fascinated that she has a doctorate focused on clinical nursing practice, and they strive to learn more about this option. Through her, they are able to see a role model who loves clinical nursing as they do and who also has the professional accomplishment of obtaining a doctoral degree. Dr. B. received an Outstanding Undergraduate Faculty Award in 2006 and a Teacher Who Made a Difference Award in 2011.

Dr. B.'s DNP students are interested in why she chose a DNP for her terminal degree and enjoy hearing what she has been able to accomplish since completion of the program. Many of them are interested in faculty roles themselves and consult with her about the possibilities that are inherent in teaching. She serves as a role model for them both in terms of working as a nursing leader and a nursing educator with DNP preparation.

Dr. B. has a great interest in health promotion for college students based on almost 20 years of working with them. Her DNP capstone project involved the creation and publication of an evidence-based tool kit to prevent meningococcal meningitis in college students, which is still used in student health services.

Upon completion of her DNP program, she joined the TPRP, knowing that both tobacco use and exposure to secondhand smoke are significant threats to health, including the health of college students. The mission of the TPRP is to reduce tobacco use and exposure to secondhand smoke through research, education, and policy development. The TPRP is made up of professionals with diverse backgrounds and degrees, including PhDs with expertise in research, biostatistics, health administration, public health, social work and counseling, and clinical expertise, among others. Dr. B. has been mentored by and partners with the other members and participates in program planning, implementation, and evaluation; writing grants, abstracts, and manuscripts; and presenting work at professional meetings. She has a particular interest in tobacco use prevention and tobacco dependence treatment, and she works on programming in this area. One example of these efforts includes helping to design cessation programs for hospital employees, patients, and visitors prior to the medical campus becoming entirely smoke free. This accomplishment laid the groundwork for a totally smoke-free campus.

An additional area of interest lies in educating nursing students to assist their patients with tobacco use prevention and tobacco dependence treatment. She designed, implemented, and evaluated a tailored, evidence-based curriculum to educate nursing students to assist patients through the use of national, evidence-based guidelines. The findings of this research project were published in a national refereed journal, and her work has been incorporated into the undergraduate curriculum.

Since her 2006 graduation, Dr. B. has had many other scholarly accomplishments. She works with community partners to reduce the health and economic burden of tobacco use in rural populations. Dr. B. was the principal investigator (PI) on a research study using community engagement strategies with local health department personnel, cooperative extension agents, and other community members to develop evidence-based interventions to motivate rural smokers to consider quitting. She was nominated by her colleagues for a national Community Engagement Award in 2011. She is also the co-PI on a grant funded by the Centers for Disease Control and Prevention through the Kentucky Department of Public Health to address tobacco prevention and cessation issues. More recently, she serves as a coinvestigator (Co-I) on a study by the National Institutes of Health entitled *FRESH: Freedom from Radon and Secondhand Smoke Exposure in the Home*. Her scholarly work has been peer reviewed and presented in local, state, national, and international venues, and it has been published in a variety of refereed professional journals including *Nicotine and Tobacco Research, Nursing Clinics of North America, Journal of Nursing Education, Nursing Leadership Forum, Worldviews on Evidence-based Nursing, Family and Community Health, Public Health Nursing, Preventive Medicine*, and *Policy, Politics & Nursing Practice*.

Since she completed the DNP program, Dr. B. has had 17 manuscripts published (11 are first authored) and two textbook chapters. Dr. B. has also had 41 abstracts peer reviewed and accepted for publication or presentation at regional, national, and international professional meetings, 30 of which are first authored. She is an active member of five professional societies in which she has served in leadership roles on committees and as an abstract reviewer for state, regional, and national meetings.

In 2013 Dr. B. was promoted to associate professor with tenure following a rigorous review trajectory that included teaching excellence, scholarship, and service. Following promotion she was awarded full graduate status at a research-intensive university.

Recognition of excellence in teaching; scholarly achievements; nomination for a national Community Engagement Award; and evidence of university, professional, and public service were the basis of Dr. B.'s achievement of promotion and tenure. Her DNP education prepared her well and laid the foundation for all these accomplishments.

Case Scenario 2: A DNP Graduate in a Tenured Faculty Role That Includes Clinical Practice in a Research-Intensive State University

Dr. H. P. is a 2006 DNP graduate who is a nursing faculty member at a large public research-intensive land grant university in the southeastern United States. Prior to graduation from her DNP program, she was an assistant clinical professor without tenure in a nationally ranked college of nursing and taught in the undergraduate program where she coordinated a high-acuity nursing course and provided clinical instruction. She first became involved in graduate education by teaching physical assessment in a master's program. Upon graduation with her DNP degree, she was promoted to assistant professor, special title series (tenure track). Following a rigorous 6-year peer evaluation process focused on teaching excellence, clinical practice, scholarship, and service, Dr. H. P. was promoted to associate professor with tenure.

Dr. H. P. now serves as the coordinator of the DNP program Acute Care Nurse Practitioner (ACNP) track, where she provides leadership over program and curricular matters. In addition to her administrative role, she coordinates other core DNP and master's-level courses. Dr. H. P. assumes full faculty membership on multiple university academic and governance committees while maintaining an active practice as an acute care nurse practitioner intensivist in a private hospital setting. Through her practice she manages the care of critically ill adult and geriatric patients within an interdisciplinary practice environment. Faculty practice allows Dr. H. P. to maintain advanced-practice registered nurse (APRN) certification, which is a requirement of her track coordinator administrative role and supports her effectiveness in faculty teaching in the ACNP program.

Dr. H. P. participates in research as a PI and Co-I for both sponsored and nonsponsored research. Her research has included an outcomes evaluation study of the APRN intensivist role, which she helped to implement. She was the PI for a funded translational research project designed to explore the relationship among inflammation, cardiac function, and weaning from mechanical ventilation. She is also a Co-I with other researchers who are examining heart rate variability in mechanically ventilated adults, and in another study, using retrospective chart review, to evaluate characteristics of mechanically ventilated patients. She regularly collaborates with her PhD research colleagues to provide leadership and clinical expertise.

Dr. H. P. functions as a leader in the College of Nursing and the broader university by serving on program and governance committees. Dr. H. P. assumes regional and national leadership roles by serving as a grant reviewer for organizations such as the Health Resources and Services Administration (HRSA), Sigma Theta Tau, and the American Association of Critical-Care Nurses. She is a textbook author and editor and reviews manuscripts for numerous professional nursing journals.

She serves on the Undergraduate Education Committee of the Society of Critical Care Medicine. She is an active member of the Acute Care Advanced Practice Special Interest Group of the National Organization of Nurse Practitioner Faculties.

Dr. H. P. is a role model for undergraduate and graduate students who respect her expertise and her willingness to mentor them. Her students have presented and won awards at local, regional, and national professional conferences. They are interested in why she decided to obtain a practice doctorate and how she uses it in her professional role. She is a role model who loves clinical nursing as they do and also has the professional accomplishment of obtaining a terminal degree. Dr. H. P. works with undergraduate research interns, involving them in clinical and practice-related research in collaboration with her PhD mentor and coinvestigator. She is excited to mentor undergraduate students in this role, and they are fortunate to benefit from her expertise. Dr. H. P. also works with DNP and PhD students as they conceptualize and develop their practice inquiry and dissertation work. Students want to work with Dr. H. P. because of her practice and research expertise. She hosts visiting scholars who are interested in conducting research in critically ill patients at her clinical practice site.

Dr. H. P. has created a collaborative model between herself as a DNP-prepared nurse and her mentor, who is PhD prepared. In addition, her DNP preparation has enabled her to provide the leadership needed to build a collaborative program in the acute care hospital setting. Her work will have a significant impact on clinical practice, focusing on mechanically ventilated patients and interdisciplinary collaborative practice.

Dr. H. P. is often called on to consult in the research and development of medical equipment and to serve as an expert witness in litigation cases across the nation. These examples are evidence of national recognition for her practice expertise and influence.

Since her 2006 graduation, Dr. H. P. has maintained active scholarship, serving as editor, author, and presenter. She has presented at regional, national, and international venues on topics that include critical care, oral health, inflammation, cardiovascular function, liberation from mechanical ventilation, the intensivist role, and most recently interprofessional education (IPE). This level of scholarship assisted Dr. H. P. to achieve promotion and tenure.

Dr. H. P. is well prepared for the responsibilities required of an associate professor with tenure while maintaining an active clinical practice. She continues to be involved in creative endeavors. Recently she was recognized as a leader in IPE and has been involved in the development of innovative programs to train DNP and physician assistant students, resident physicians, and pharmacists to be effective leaders and members of interdisciplinary teams for patient-centered, collaborative care and quality improvement. She has been nominated for a national faculty scholar award to develop graduate-level IPE. Her DNP education has provided her with the foundation to create and drive change in education and clinical practice. She is a strong role model as a DNP-prepared advanced-practice nurse educator, leader, and healthcare provider.

Case Scenario 3: A DNP Graduate in a Tenured Faculty Role at a Regional State University

Dr. P. is employed as a nursing faculty member at a regional state university in the southeastern United States, which has both baccalaureate and graduate nursing programs. Prior to achieving the DNP degree, Dr. P. served as assistant faculty in a nontenure-track position, teaching mental health nursing at the baccalaureate level. After graduation with her DNP degree in 2006, Dr. P. was promoted to a tenure-track position, and her responsibilities were expanded to include a position as graduate faculty. She now teaches nursing research at the master's level and will be teaching evidence-based practice in the university's newly developed DNP program.

Dr. P.'s prior nursing experience included clinical work in medical–surgical areas, home care, and hospice care. After achieving a master's degree in psychiatric and mental health nursing and earning accreditation through the American Nurses Credentialing Center as a clinical nurse specialist, she worked at a large state hospital where her duties included staff supervision and support, clinical case management, and staff education. Although she has a full-time teaching position, she continues to work at the hospital several hours each week to develop curricula for and lead clients in psychoeducational groups.

The combination of her extensive nursing experience and the education she received in the DNP program has provided Dr. P. with a solid basis for teaching both undergraduate and graduate students. She believes the DNP emphasis on evidence-based practice has been especially helpful in her teaching and in clinical practice; she also has an increased ability to evaluate and discuss current healthcare issues with students. Because they have heard different views of the practice doctorate, Dr. P.'s students are interested in discussing the program with her. In addition, she has been able to demonstrate the value of the DNP degree to other faculty and to emphasize to them the benefits of having faculty members with both clinically based and research-based doctoral degrees. It is significant that the university recently began a DNP program (in which Dr. P. will also be teaching).

Since her graduation, Dr. P.'s article describing her capstone project has been published by a peer-reviewed psychiatric nursing journal. Her other recent scholarly activities include development and presentation of a continuing education module about evidence-based practice and a presentation about implementation of the recovery model in mental health care at a regional psychiatric nursing conference. She recently developed a 3-hour continuing education offering on domestic violence for the continuing education department. She also serves as a reviewer of articles for a major peer-reviewed nursing journal. She keeps current in her knowledge about mental health nursing and nursing education by reading and evaluating current nursing research and literature and attending relevant nursing workshops and conferences, and she also maintains her accreditation as an APRN. The DNP degree emphasis on leadership has also enabled Dr. P. to serve successfully in significant positions in the local American Nurses Association and the local Sigma Theta Tau chapter. Notably, Dr. P. attained tenure at her institution, a significant accomplishment that would not have been possible without her DNP education.

SUMMARY

- Education is a part of every nurse's role. A DNP degree provides graduates with enhanced knowledge to improve nursing practice and patient outcomes; advanced competencies for extremely complex clinical, faculty, and leadership roles; enhanced leadership skills; and parity with other professions, but the nurse educator is still a less-recognized role of the DNP graduate.
- Graduates of research-focused and practice-focused doctoral programs may need additional preparation in pedagogy, but both can function effectively as nursing faculty members and bring alternate, complementary approaches and expertise to the role.
- Although the *Essentials of Doctoral Education for Advanced Nursing Practice* (AACN, 2006b) does not speak directly to the educator role, there are competencies in every essential that are important and relevant to nurse educators.
- The shortage of registered nurses in the United States could be as high as 260,000 by 2025. Difficulty in filling nursing faculty positions may be the most crucial factor affecting the future supply of nurses.
- There are multiple factors associated with the nursing faculty shortage: aging of current faculty members, entering academia later in life, discouragement of students from careers in academia, compensation, workload, and work environment.
- Innovative strategies and the ability to think outside the box about those who may be able to fulfill faculty roles are needed. Creatively using diversely prepared faculty members and capitalizing on the strengths of individuals' educational preparation are good options. DNP graduates are uniquely positioned to fill the nursing faculty gap.
- Clinical teaching at both undergraduate and graduate levels necessitates advanced clinical knowledge and enhanced practice skills. The DNP graduate is a master teacher and a role model in the area of advanced clinical nursing practice.

- Scholarship is an important part of the nurse educator role. DNP graduates are well prepared to actively participate in scholarship, including publication and presentation of results.
- Promotion and tenure are primarily institutional decisions, but a DNP faculty member should be able to compete favorably with faculty members who hold other practice doctorates. A possible strategy is the partnering of DNP graduates with research-focused faculty to marry the generation of new knowledge with the translation of that knowledge into clinical practice.

REFLECTION QUESTIONS

1. What education preparation and experience do you think is important for a nurse educator to have to teach at the undergraduate and graduate levels?

2. What education preparation and experience do you think is important for a nurse educator to have to pursue scholarly interests?

3. What kinds of scholarly contributions do you think a DNP-prepared faculty member could make?

4. How important do you think it is for nurse educators to have current clinical expertise, either through practice or research?

5. What are some creative ways that DNP-prepared nursing faculty members can partner with research-prepared nursing faculty members to improve nursing practice and patient health outcomes?

6. What contributions can DNP-prepared nursing faculty members make in schools of nursing within universities that are not research intensive, for example, regional universities that offer associate's, bachelor of science in nursing, or master of science in nursing degrees?

7. What contributions can DNP-prepared nursing faculty members make in schools of nursing that reside in research-intensive universities?

8. Despite the factors that contribute to the nursing faculty shortage, serving as a nurse educator offers opportunities to impact many lives—not only the lives of every student, but also those whose lives and care are ultimately entrusted to students throughout their nursing careers. Can you see additional nursing education in your future? If so, how can you make a unique contribution in an educator role by utilizing the knowledge and skills gained from your DNP education?

AUTHOR'S NOTE

The author would like to thank Drs. Melanie Hardin-Pierce and Leandra Price for their friendship and assistance in writing this chapter.

This work is dedicated to my brother, Charles Kraig McBroom, who has always been my best friend. An immensely talented musician and nationally recognized educator, he works every day to enrich the lives of others through music. His unfailing love and support inspire me daily to try to create the same kind of passion for nursing in my students as he creates for music in everyone he touches. Kraig, I love you best.

REFERENCES

Aiken, L., Clark, S., Sloane, D., Sochalski, J., & Silber, J. (2002). Hospital nurse staffing and patient mortality, nurse burnout, and job dissatisfaction. *Journal of the American Medical Association, 288,* 1987–1993.

Alfes, C. (2011). Evaluating the use of simulation with beginning nursing students. *Journal of Nursing Education, 50*(2), 89–93.

American Association of Colleges of Nursing. (1999). *Faculty shortages intensify nation's nursing deficit* (Issue bulletin). Washington, DC: Author. Retrieved from http://www.aacn.nche.edu /Publications/Issues/IB499WB.htm

American Association of Colleges of Nursing. (2001). Strategies to reverse the new nursing shortage. Retrieved from http://www.aacn.nche.edu/publications/position /tri-council-shortage

American Association of Colleges of Nursing. (2004a). *Position statement on the practice doctorate in nursing.* Washington, DC: Author. Retrieved from http://www.aacn.nche .edu/dnp/position-statement

American Association of Colleges of Nursing. (2004b). Doctor of nursing practice programs: Frequently asked questions. Retrieved from http://www.aacn.nche.edu/dnp/faqs

American Association of Colleges of Nursing. (2005). *Faculty shortages in baccalaureate and graduate nursing programs: Scope of the problem and strategies for expanding the supply.* Washington, DC: Author.

American Association of Colleges of Nursing. (2006a). *Custom data report: Nursing faculty.* Washington, DC: Author.

American Association of Colleges of Nursing. (2006b). *Essentials of doctoral education for advanced nursing practice.* Retrieved from http://www.aacn.nche.edu/publications /position/DNPEssentials.pdf

American Association of Colleges of Nursing. (2013a). *2012–2013 enrollment and graduations in baccalaureate and graduate programs in nursing.* Washington, DC: Author.

American Association of Colleges of Nursing. (2013b). *AACN's report of 2012–2013 salaries of instructional and administrative nursing faculty in baccalaureate and graduate programs in nursing.* Washington, DC: Author.

American Association of Colleges of Nursing. (2013c). Nursing faculty shortage fact sheet. Retrieved from http://www.aacn.nche.edu/media-relations/FacultyShortageFS.pdf

American Association of Colleges of Nursing. (2013d). *Special survey of AACN membership on vacant faculty positions.* Washington, DC: Author.

Anderson, C. A. (2000). Current strengths and limitations of doctoral education in nursing: Are we prepared for the future? *Journal of Professional Nursing, 16*(4), 191–200.

Bellini, S., McCauley, P., & Cusson, R. (2012). The doctor of nursing practice graduate as faculty member. *Nursing Clinics of North America, 47,* 547–556.

Berlin, L., Bednash, G., & Alsheimer, O. (1993). *1992–1993 enrollment and graduations in baccalaureate and graduate programs in nursing.* Washington, DC: American Association of Colleges of Nursing.

Berlin, L. E., & Sechrist, K. R. (2002). The shortage of doctorally prepared nursing faculty: A dire situation. *Nursing Outlook, 50*(2), 50–56.

Berlin, L., Wilsey, S., & Bednash, G. (2005). *2004–2005 salaries of instructional and administrative nursing faculty in baccalaureate and graduate programs in nursing.* Washington, DC: American Association of Colleges of Nursing.

Berliner, H. S. M., & Ginzberg, E. (2002). Why this hospital nursing shortage is different. *Journal of the American Medical Association, 288,* 2742–2744.

Boyden, K. M. (2000). Development of new faculty in higher education. *Journal of Professional Nursing, 16*(2), 104–111.

Boyer, E. L. (1990). *Scholarship reconsidered: Priorities of the professoriate.* San Francisco, CA: Jossey-Bass.

Brendtro, M., & Hegge, M. (2000). Nursing faculty: One generation away from extinction? *Journal of Professional Nursing, 16*(2), 97–103.

Broome, M., Riner, M., & Allam, E. (2013). Scholarly publication practices of doctor of nursing practice-prepared nurses. *Journal of Nursing Education, 52*(8), 429–434.

Buerhaus, P., Auerbach, D., & Staiger, D. (2009). The recent surge in nurse employment: Causes and implications. *Health Affairs, 28*(4), 657–668.

Buerhaus, P., Potter, V., Staiger, D., & Auerbach, D. (2009). *The future of the nursing workforce in the United States: Data, trends, and implications.* Sudbury, MA: Jones and Bartlett.

Buerhaus, P., Staiger, D., & Auerbach, D. (2000). Implications of an aging registered nurse workforce. *Journal of the American Medical Association, 283,* 2948–2954.

Committee for Monitoring the Nation's Changing Needs for Biomedical, Behavioral, and Clinical Personnel, Board on Higher Education and Workforce, National Research Council. (2005). *Advancing the nation's health needs: NIH research training programs.* Washington, DC: National Academies Press.

Danzey, I., Fitzpatrick, J., Garbutt, S., Rafferty, M., & Zychowicz, M. (2011). The doctor of nursing practice and nursing education: Highlights, potential, and promise. *Journal of Professional Nursing, 27,* 311–314.

de Tornyay, R. (1989). Who will teach the future nurses? *Journal of Nursing Education, 28*(2), 52.

Division of Nursing, Bureau of Health Professions, HRSA. (2001). *The registered nurse population: National sample survey of registered nurses.* Unpublished report for the American Association of Colleges of Nursing.

Dunbar-Jacob, J., Nativio, D., & Khalil, H. (2013). Impact of doctor of nursing practice education in shaping health care systems for the future. *Journal of Nursing Education, 52*(8), 423–427.

Fawcett, J. (2005). *Contemporary nursing knowledge: Analysis and evaluation of nursing models and theories* (2nd ed.). Philadelphia, PA: F. A. Davis.

Fawcett, J., Watson, J., Neuman, B., Walker, P. H., & Fitzpatrick, J. J. (2001). On nursing theories and evidence. *Journal of Nursing Scholarship, 33*, 115–119.

Fitzpatrick, J. (2002). The balance in nursing: Clinical and scientific ways of knowing and being. *Nursing Education Perspectives, 23*(2), 57.

Fitzpatrick, M. L., & Heller, B. R. (1980). Teaching the teachers to teach. *Nursing Outlook, 28*(6), 372–373.

Goodin, H. J. (2003). The nursing shortage in the United States of America: An integrative review of the literature. *Journal of Advanced Nursing, 43*, 335–343.

Greiner, A. C., & Knebel, E. (Eds.). (2003). *Health professions education: A bridge to quality.* Washington, DC: National Academies Press.

Hathaway, D., Jacob, S., Stegbauer, C., Thompson, C., & Graff, C. (2006). The practice doctorate: Perspectives of early adopters. *Journal of Nursing Education, 45*, 487–496.

Health Resources and Services Administration. (2004). *The registered nurse population: Findings from the March 2004 National Sample Survey of Registered Nurses.* Retrieved from http://bhpr.hrsa.gov/healthworkforce/rnsurveys/rnsurvey2004.pdf

Heifetz, R. A. (1994). *Leadership without easy answers.* Cambridge, MA: Harvard University Press.

Hinshaw, A. (2001). A continuing challenge: The shortage of educationally prepared nursing faculty. *Online Journal of Issues in Nursing, 6*(1). Retrieved from http://www.nursingworld.org/MainMenuCategories/ANAMarketplace/ANAPeriodicals/OJIN/TableofContents/Volume62001/No1Jan01/ShortageofEducationalFaculty.aspx

Institute of Medicine. (2011). *The future of nursing: Leading change, advancing health.* Washington, DC: National Academies Press.

Marion, L., Viens, D., O'Sullivan, A., Crabtree, K., Fontana, S., & Price, M. (2003). The practice doctorate in nursing: Future or fringe? *Topics in Advanced Nursing e-Journal, 3*(2). Retrieved from http://www.medscape.com/viewarticle/453247_1

Melnyk, B. (2013). Distinguishing the preparation and roles of doctor of philosophy and doctor of nursing practice graduates: National implications for academic curricula and health care systems. *Journal of Nursing Education, 52*(8), 442–448.

Mullinix, C. F. (1990). The next shortage—the nurse educator. *Journal of Professional Nursing, 6*(3), 133.

National League for Nursing. (2002, May 18). *Position statement: The preparation of nurse educators.* Retrieved from http://www.nln.org/aboutnln/PositionStatements/preparation051802

National League for Nursing. (2006). *Nurse educators 2006: A report on the faculty census survey of RN and graduate programs.* New York, NY: Author.

National Research Council. (2005). *Advancing the nation's health needs: NIH research training programs.* Washington, DC: National Academies Press.

Neuman, B., & Fawcett, J. (Eds.). (2001). *The Neuman systems model* (4th ed.). Upper Saddle River, NJ: Prentice Hall.

Nicholes, R., & Dyer, J. (2012). Is eligibility for tenure possible for the doctor of nursing practice prepared faculty? *Journal of Professional Nursing, 28*(1), 13–17.

Peterson's Colleges of Nursing Database [Database]. (2002). Lawrenceville, NJ: Peterson's.

Princeton, J. C. (1992). The teacher crisis in nursing education—revisited. *Nurse Educator, 17*(5), 34–37.

Sebastian, J., & Delaney, C. (2013). Doctor of nursing practice programs: Opportunities for faculty development. *Journal of Nursing Education, 52*(8), 453–461.

Smith, D., & Rosenkoetter, M. (2009). Effectiveness, challenges and perceptions of classroom participation systems. *Nurse Educator, 43*(4), 156–161.

Southern Regional Education Board. (2003). *SREB study indicates serious shortage of nursing faculty.* Atlanta, GA: Author. Retrieved from http://publications.sreb.org/2003/02N03-Nursing_Faculty.pdf

Sperhac, A., & Goodwin, L. (2003). Using multiple data sources for curriculum revision. *Journal of Pediatric Health Care, 17*, 169–175.

Tanner, C. A. (1999). Developing the new professorate. *Journal of Nursing Education, 38*(2), 51–52.

U.S. Bureau of Labor Statistics. (2012). Employment projections 2010–2022. Retrieved from http://www.bls.gov/news.release/ecopro.t06.htm

Zebelman, E., & Olswang, S. (1989). Student career goal changes during doctoral education in nursing. *Journal of Nursing Education, 28*(2), 53–73.

CHAPTER 7

The DNP Graduate as Ethical Consultant

Lisa Astalos Chism

The doctor of nursing practice (DNP) graduate may integrate several roles, such as leader, researcher, clinician, policy advocate, and educator. Within each of these roles the DNP graduate will likely encounter various ethical scenarios. Many DNP curricula are including ethics course work to prepare DNP graduates with the skills necessary to evaluate ethical issues. Peirce and Smith believe that "there is a need for an expanded view of required ethics content in the curriculum of Doctor of Nursing Practice programs nationwide" (2008, p. 270).

Ethics is defined as the principles of conduct governing an individual or group (Ethic, 2014a). An ethicist is one who specializes in or is very concerned with ethics (Ethicist, 2014b). Although it may be presumptuous to describe a DNP graduate as an ethicist, a DNP graduate will likely be regarded as an ethical consultant in his or her setting. The DNP graduate may be consulted regarding research, clinical, leadership, and professional ethical scenarios (Peirce & Smith, 2008). Therefore, it is necessary for DNP graduates to develop an understanding of ethical content, including terms, inquiry, and theories. A review of ethical content will enable DNP graduates to evaluate ethical scenarios they may encounter within their settings and specific roles.

This chapter is not inclusive of the ethical content necessary for every potential ethical scenario a DNP graduate may evaluate. Instead, it is intended to introduce or review certain ethical terms, inquiries, and theories that will give DNP graduates the tools to recognize ethical scenarios and obtain the information necessary to evaluate these scenarios. Highlighted concepts in bioethics are also reviewed. Nursing ethics is described, including a tool kit that DNP graduates should be familiar with to evaluate ethical scenarios in their settings. Important content regarding ethical leadership is reviewed as well. Ethical standards regarding Internet and telehealth, also a concern of DNP graduates, are discussed. Finally, specific scenarios are reviewed to assist DNP graduates with ethical discussions.

First a Story . . .

Ethical dilemmas have been debated for centuries among philosophers and scientists. Over the past century, certain events have triggered bioethical concerns. One such event in 1951 involved a young African American woman named Henrietta Lacks who was a tobacco farmer from southern Virginia.

The granddaughter of slaves, Henrietta was raised by her grandfather on a tobacco farm. When she was 30 years old and had given birth to her fifth child, Henrietta began experiencing abdominal pain and knew something was wrong. Finally she asked her husband to drive her to Johns Hopkins Hospital. At the time, Johns Hopkins was the only hospital in the area that would see African American patients for free.

Henrietta was evaluated, and a biopsy confirmed cancer of her cervix. She began radiation treatment, which required her to stay overnight in the hospital twice a month. During her stay, doctors removed several pieces of tissue from her cervix and began growing and studying the tissue. This was done without Henrietta's or her family's consent.

Attempts to grow cancerous tissue outside the body had been made several times without success. The hope was that these cells would help determine what caused cancer and contribute to the development of a cure. Henrietta's cells astonished doctors and scientists by surviving outside her body and continuing to divide. These cells were later named HeLa cells, after Henrietta Lacks.

Unfortunately the doctors could not save Henrietta, and she succumbed to cervical cancer 6 months after she was diagnosed. Her cells, however, continued to thrive and reproduce and were found to be the first "immortal" cells discovered. Her family was not informed of this discovery until many years later.

HeLa cells led to several landmark developments in science and medicine. They were later used to test a polio vaccine that led to the development of a treatment that saved and protected millions of people. Some of the HeLa cells were found to behave differently than others. Scientists learned how to isolate specific HeLa cells, multiply them, and create a new cell line. This discovery led to developments that became the basic techniques for in vitro fertilization and cloning. HeLa cells were also used to discover that humans have 46 chromosomes in 23 pairs, not 48. Because of this discovery, the basis of genetic testing and diagnosis was developed. Finally, anticancer drugs are currently in clinical trials due to the discovery that HeLa cells use an enzyme to repair their DNA.

It was 25 years after the cells were discovered that a scientist contacted Henrietta's family to obtain cell samples from them for further testing. Henrietta's husband had a third-grade education and did not understand what was being explained to him. This event led to a controversial, confusing journey for the family, who never knew Henrietta's cells had been taken. Her cells were in fact the first cells to be bought and sold for research and eventually led to a multibillion-dollar industry.

This story may stir many emotions and raise multiple ethical questions. The people who took the cells had the best intentions in mind, and many wonderful, life-changing discoveries were made as a result of Henrietta's cells. However, cells come from people who may have certain feelings and thoughts about their tissue being used.

Was the means justified by the end? Were Henrietta or her family harmed by the doctors taking the cells? What about all the people who have benefited from HeLa cells and the discoveries that were developed? This true story may help DNP graduates examine their own positions through self-reflection and review of ethical content.

To learn more about Henrietta Lacks's story, please refer to *The Immortal Life of Henrietta Lacks* by Rebecca Skloot (2010).

Back to the Basics

Developing an understanding of ethics will lead to "anticipating and recognizing health care dilemmas and making good judgments and decisions based on universal values that work in unison with the laws of the land, and our constitution" (Pozgar, 2010, p. 3). Further, ethics guides caregivers to "make right judgments as guided by using wisdom to do good" (Pozgar, 2010, p. 3). This section of the chapter provides DNP graduates with a review of basic ethical content, including selected ethical terms, inquiries, and theories.

Ethical Terms

Ethics has been broadly defined as the principles of conduct governing an individual or group. More specifically, Butts and Rich define ethics as "the study of ideal human behavior and ideal ways of being" (2008, p. 4). Butts and Rich also describe ethics as a process, or "doing ethics," whereby one's beliefs are supported by sound reasoning justified by "logical, theoretically based arguments" (2008, p. 5). Ethics emphasizes "the rightness and wrongness of actions, as well as the goodness and badness of motives and ends" (Pozgar, 2010, p. 2). Ethics is also considered a moral philosophy, or discipline, concerned with what is morally right or wrong (Pozgar, 2010, p. 2).

Morals, on the other hand, are "specific beliefs, behaviors, and ways of being derived from doing ethics" (Butts & Rich, 2008, p. 5). The opposite of morality is immorality, which describes "behavior in opposition to accepted societal, religious, cultural or professional ethical standards and principles" (Butts & Rich, 2008, p. 5). Morals may be rooted in culture or religion. The evaluation of morality requires the DNP graduate to reach a decision of what is right or wrong within an ethical scenario.

A code of ethics describes standards of conduct and states certain principles regarding responsibilities and duties of those professionals to whom they apply (Pozgar, 2010). Professionals frequently subscribe to specific values or moral standards written into formal documents referred to as codes of ethics. The American Nurses Association (ANA, 2001) *Code of Ethics for Nurses* and the International Council of Nurses' (ICN, 2006) *Code of Ethics for Nurses* are examples of nursing codes of ethics and should be used as a resource for DNP graduates when evaluating ethical scenarios. These codes of ethics are discussed more fully later in the chapter.

Values have been defined as "ideals, beliefs, customs, modes of conduct, qualities, or goals that are highly prized or preferred by individuals, groups, or societies" (Burkhardt & Nathaniel, 2008, p. 83). Values may influence judgments one may make and reflect what one believes is good or bad. Values may also influence how one behaves or thinks; they may be learned and incorporated at an early age and continue to develop throughout one's life. This may occur through formal teaching by parents, teachers, or professional leaders. More informal values may be developed through socialization and role-modeling (Burkhardt & Nathaniel, 2008).

Reasoning describes the "use of abstract thought processes to think creatively, to answer questions, solve problems, and to formulate strategies for one's actions and desired ways of being" (Butts & Rich, 2008, p. 9). Moral reasoning relates to reasoning that focuses on moral or ethical issues. Socrates believed that moral reasoning was "inherent to rational beings, waiting to be drawn forth" (Forman & Ladd, 1991, p. 1). Conversely, Forman and Ladd believed "one learns to recognize good reasons by engaging in discussion and debate, considering opposite views, and questioning oneself and others" (1991, p. 1).

Ethical Inquiry

The study of ethics includes various types of ethical inquiry. Normative ethics involves prescribing values, behaviors, and ways of being that are considered right or wrong when deciding what to do in a specific situation (Butts & Rich, 2008). This type of ethical inquiry involves evaluating what is right, what is good, and what is genuine (Pozgar, 2010). When applying normative ethics, one is applying accepted moral standards and codes. One form of accepted moral standard is common morality. "Common morality consists of normative beliefs and behaviors that the members of society generally agree about and are familiar to most human beings" (Butts & Rich, 2008, p. 6).

Applied ethics may attempt to explain moral problems that are common in health care, such as assisted suicide and euthanasia. Metaethics involves applying the understanding of the language of morality through the meaning of related concepts such as virtuous and good (Butts & Rich, 2008). Contrary to normative ethics, metaethics does not apply what ought to be done *because it is right* but instead is concerned with the meaning of what a *good* outcome would be. Descriptive ethics is more concrete and describes what one thinks about morality or moral behavior (Butts & Rich, 2008). Descriptive ethics is also referred to as comparative ethics and describes what one believes is right or wrong (Pozgar, 2010). Descriptive ethics also pertains to professional moral values and behaviors that can be examined through research.

Ethical Theories

Ethical theories serve as guidelines when individuals question what they should do or how they ought to be. Ethical theories also provide justification for why one chooses to do something a certain way, especially when faced with a moral dilemma. The following ethical theories are highlighted from Butts and Rich's (2008) nursing ethics textbook titled *Nursing Ethics: Across the Curriculum and into Practice*. These theories were chosen due to their relevance when discussing nursing ethics and the DNP graduate.

VIRTUE ETHICS

Virtue ethics emphasizes the "excellence of one's character and considerations of a sort of person one wants to be" (Butts & Rich, 2008, p. 18). Virtue ethics focuses on the inherent character of a person rather than on specific actions (Pozgar, 2010). This theory is closely linked to the beliefs of Aristotle, who thought a person of virtue was one who was an excellent friend, critical thinker, and citizen. Plato and Hume also described similar approaches to value ethics. Plato described the four virtues of prudence, fortitude, temperance, and justice (Butts & Rich, 2008). Hume related that virtues stemmed from "the natural human tendency to be sympathetic and benevolent toward other people" (Butts & Rich, 2008, p. 19).

Beauchamp and Childress (2009) describe five focal virtues of the healthcare professional: compassion, discernment, trustworthiness, integrity, and conscientiousness. Compassion as a virtue is focused on other people and involves concern regarding their pain, suffering, disability, and misery. Discernment involves the recognition and insight one exhibits when deciding the appropriate action to take in a given situation (Burkhardt & Nathaniel, 2008). Trustworthiness entails the belief that another will act with the right motives consistent with moral norms (Beauchamp & Childress, 2009). Integrity includes soundness, reliability, wholeness, and integration of moral character (Beauchamp & Childress, 2009). Conscientiousness describes one being motivated to do the right thing because it is right and extends the appropriate effort to do so (Beauchamp & Childress, 2009).

NATURAL LAW THEORY

Natural law theory stems from the philosophy of St. Thomas Aquinas. This theory emphasizes that the "law of reason is implanted in the order of nature (usually thought to be implanted by God)" and provides the rules of human nature (Butts & Rich, 2008, p. 21). Natural law theory is frequently associated with Judeo-Christian ethics.

DEONTOLOGY

Deontology, or the study of duty, is an ethical theory that focuses on duties and rules. Deontology also describes the view that the "rightness or wrongness of an act depends upon the nature of the act, rather than its consequences" (Burkhardt & Nathaniel, 2008, p. 39). The term *deontology* is Greek for *duty*. Deontology is sometimes referred to as Kantianism after Immanuel Kant (1724–1804), who was a German philosopher. He prescribed that individuals' moral worth is determined by their dutiful actions. Moreover, if acting from Kant's philosophy, one is bound to duty over love. Many professional codes of ethics are based on Kant's principles, such as the ethical codes used in nursing. These principles within the ANA *Code of Ethics for Nurses* and the ICN *Code of Ethics for Nurses* are so inherent to nursing that they are often unnoticed (Butts & Rich, 2008). Deontology is a useful ethical theory in that it provides clear guidelines for evaluating the wrongness or rightness of an action.

PRINCIPLISM

Principlism uses principles that serve as rules for conduct dictated by duty. Common principles include beneficence and autonomy. Principlism is reflected in the basis of bioethics and positions related to patients' rights.

UTILITARIANISM

Simply stated, utilitarianism describes actions that are judged by their utility. When employing the theory of utilitarianism, emphasis is placed on promoting the greatest good and inflicting the least amount of harm possible (Butts & Rich, 2008). Utilitarianism is also described as a "moral theory that holds that an action is judged as good or bad in relation to the consequence, outcome, or end result that is derived from it" (Burkhardt & Nathaniel, 2008, p. 33). Further, the greatest good for groups, rather than individuals, is emphasized.

CASUISTRY

Casuistry describes considering specific situations individually when making ethical decisions. Additionally, outcomes or similar cases in the past are considered when making ethical decisions. Casuists emphasize the importance of past cases, history, precedents, and past circumstances (Beauchamp & Childress, 2009). Social consensus is formed around past cases, and this consensus becomes authoritative for new cases (Beauchamp & Childress, 2009). Current healthcare ethics committees utilize this theory when considering individual ethical issues related to patients (Butts & Rich, 2008).

NARRATIVE ETHICS

Similar to casuistry, narrative ethics is a story-based approach to making ethical decisions. Narrative ethics focuses on personal life narratives interacting with others' personal life narratives (Butts & Rich, 2008). When evaluating an ethical scenario using this theory, an individual's personal narrative stories are considered when making ethical decisions.

CRITICAL THEORY

Critical theory broadly describes "theories and worldviews that address the domination perpetrated by specific powerful groups of people and resulting in the oppression of other specific groups of people" (Butts & Rich, 2008, p. 27). For example, feminist ethics is utilized to examine how ethical situations affect women. An ethic of care, frequently utilized by nurses, is based on the ethical experiences of women and feminist ethics. Specifically, an ethic of care emphasizes traits that are considered feminine, such as love, compassion, sympathy, and concern for the well-being of other people (Butts & Rich, 2008). Beauchamp and Childress (2009) also describe an ethic of care as traits valued in intimate, interpersonal relationships, such as fidelity and love. Caring is further defined as "to care for, emotional commitment to and deep willingness to act on behalf of persons with whom one has a significant relationship" (Beauchamp & Childress, 2009, p. 36). This theory is familiar ground for many in the nursing profession and is therefore relevant for DNP graduates as a basis of ethical decision making.

Bioethics: Expanding the Basics

Throughout the 20th century, numerous scientific advances, scarcity of medical resources, and unethical research studies led to the development of a branch of ethics termed *bioethics*. Bioethics is defined as "the philosophical study of ethical controversies brought about by advances in biology, research, and medicine" (Pozgar, 2010, p. 403). The following section reviews bioethical principles that are relevant for DNP graduates.

The Birth of Bioethics

Among the many events that led to the birth of bioethics, the Tuskegee syphilis experiment led to the establishment of the Office for Human Research Protections (OHRP) and the federal regulation requiring institutional review boards for the protection of human subjects enrolled in research studies (U.S. Department of Health and Human Services, n.d.). The Tuskegee syphilis experiment was a clinical study conducted between 1923 and 1972 in Tuskegee, Alabama. It was developed by the U.S. Public Health Service to study the progression of untreated syphilis.

The study subjects included 399 impoverished African American sharecroppers from Mason County, Alabama, who were infected with syphilis. The men were not informed of the purpose of the study, nor that they had syphilis. Instead, they were told they had "bad blood," a local term that described several medical illnesses (National Public Radio, 2002). For their participation in the study, the men were given free medical care, free meals, and free burial services. In the 1940s, penicillin was found to be effective in the treatment of syphilis, but many study participants still did not receive this treatment in order to prolong the study and observe full, long-term progression of the disease. In fact, to ensure that men would continue with the painful spinal taps used in the study, a misleading letter was sent out titled "Last Chance for Special Free Treatment." Their burial expenses were not paid for until an autopsy was done for further investigation (Centers for Disease Control and Prevention [CDC], 2011).

In 1972 the Tuskegee syphilis study was made public by a whistle-blower who leaked information to the press, and the study ended. At that time, 74 of the men were still alive, 28 had died of syphilis, 100 had died from complications related to syphilis, 40 of their wives had become infected with syphilis, and 19 of their children were born with congenital syphilis (CDC, 2011). The public knowledge of this study led to a series of developments related to bioethics.

In 1974 Congress passed the National Research Act to regulate studies involving human participants. In 1997 President Clinton apologized on behalf of the nation for the tragic consequences of the Tuskegee syphilis study. In 2001 the President's Council on Bioethics was formed. The CDC provided $10 million in 2004 for the Tuskegee University National Center for Bioethics in Research and Health Center, and in 2006 the Bioethics Center at Tuskegee University was formally opened (CDC, 2011).

As a result of the National Research Act, a commission was created to define the principles supported for research involving human subjects, and a 4-day conference was held at the Belmont Conference Center at the Smithsonian. In 1976 the commission released its report titled the *Belmont Report*. This report outlined three principles for all human subject research: respect for persons, beneficence, and justice (National Commission for the Protection of Human Subjects of Biomedical and Behavioral Research, 1978). The principle of nonmaleficence, or to do no harm, was described in the *Belmont Report* under the principle of beneficence.

In 1979, soon after the *Belmont Report* was released, Beauchamp and Childress published their book *Principles of Biomedical Ethics*, which is currently in its sixth edition (2009). The authors outline four biomedical principles described as autonomy, beneficence, nonmaleficence, and justice. These principles are used today when ethical principlism is invoked to analyze and resolve many healthcare-related ethical scenarios.

Autonomy

Beauchamp and Childress (2009) refer to the ethical principle of autonomy as respect for autonomy. Personal autonomy has been defined as "self-rule that is free from controlling interference by others and from certain limitations such as inadequate understanding that prevents meaningful choice" (Beauchamp & Childress, 2009, p. 103). Respect for autonomy involves more than simply noninterference from others. It includes "building up or maintaining others' capacities for autonomous choice and other conditions that destroy or disrupt autonomous action" (Beauchamp & Childress, 2009, p. 103). According to Beauchamp and Childress, specific moral rules are supported by respect for autonomy. These moral truths include the following: "1) Tell the truth, 2) Respect the privacy of others, 3) Protect confidential information, 4) Obtain consent for interventions with patients, 5) When asked, help others make important decisions" (Beauchamp & Childress, 2009, p. 104).

Informed consent describes the "process by which patients are informed of possible outcomes, alternatives, and risks of treatment, and are required to give their consent freely" (Burkhardt & Nathaniel, 2008, p. 58). Informed consent involves respecting the person's autonomy to make their decisions based on the appropriate information given to them regarding a specific circumstance or potential outcome. Respect for autonomy clearly emphasizes the importance of informed consent.

From a cultural perspective, Dayer-Berenson relates that "how much or how little autonomy a patient wishes to express is culturally mediated" (2011, p. 113). In an effort to be culturally sensitive to a patient's autonomy, the process of informed consent should involve meaningful discussion regarding healing methods and expected or desired outcomes as opposed to a one-sided explanation of specific risks and benefits of a treatment or procedure (Dayer-Berenson, 2011). This process includes the cultural perspectives of others and allows for informed decision making by patients and their families.

Beneficence

The principle of beneficence refers to "the moral obligation to act for the benefit of others" (Beauchamp & Childress, 2009, p. 197). Beneficence describes the acts that are generally doing good, helping others, and showing compassion (Pozgar, 2010). Beyond simply doing good for others, beneficence requires that one knows the beliefs, cultures, and values of others in order to act in their best interest.

Paternalism is a form of beneficence that involves individuals or institutions believing they know what is best for the patient or person and thus makes decisions for them (Pozgar, 2010). Beauchamp and Childress define paternalism as "the intentional overriding of the person's preferences or actions by another person, where the person who overrides justifies this action by appeal to the goal of benefiting or of preventing or mitigating harm to the person whose preferences are overridden" (2009, p. 208). Paternalistic acts may include deception, manipulation of information, lying, nondisclosure of information, or use of force or coercion (Beauchamp & Childress, 2009).

Nonmaleficence

The principle of nonmaleficence describes the obligation to do no harm. Nonmaleficence is concerned with avoiding the infliction of harm on others. Beauchamp and Childress (2009) make a specific distinction between beneficence and nonmaleficence. Beneficence is a more active principle that requires one to take an active role to help others by preventing harm, removing harm, or promoting good. Nonmaleficence simply requires intentionally refraining from doing harm.

Justice

The principle of justice refers to "fairness, treating people equally and without prejudice, and with the equitable distribution of benefits and burdens" (Butts & Rich, 2008, p. 48). Justice involves treating all persons in comparable circumstances similarly. Social justice describes how all people should have the same rights, benefits, and opportunities (Butts & Rich, 2008).

Nursing Ethics

Nursing ethics has been defined as an extension of bioethics where ethical issues are viewed from a nursing perspective (Butts & Rich, 2008). Nursing ethics draws from traditional bioethics and extends the meaning of these principles to scenarios nurses are often faced with in their profession. Further, the focus of nursing ethics is relationship based and involves issues that are related to relationships between nurses and their patients or nurses and their colleagues (Butts & Rich, 2008).

ANA *Code of Ethics for Nurses*

The ANA *Code of Ethics for Nurses* is considered the standard for nurses to refer to as their code for ethical behavior. The ANA code "makes explicit the primary goals, values, and obligations of the profession" (ANA, 2001, p. 9). The ANA *Code of Ethics for Nurses* serves the following purposes:

1. It is a succinct statement of the ethical obligations and duties of every individual who enters the nursing profession;
2. It is the profession's nonnegotiable nursing standard;
3. It is an expression of nursing's own understanding of its commitment to society. (ANA, 2001, p. 9)

The code reflects several approaches to evaluating ethical scenarios, such as using ethical theories, ethical principles, and cultivating virtues.

The ANA code includes nine provisions accompanied by interpretive statements that give more specific guidelines for practice. It provides a framework for nurses to use in ethical evaluation and decision making. The ANA code is essential for all DNP graduates to use when evaluating ethical scenarios. Certain provisions of the code are highlighted in the following sections because they are considered to have focal importance to the ethical scenarios DNP graduates may encounter. However, DNP graduates should become familiar with every provision of the ANA *Code of Ethics for Nurses*, along with the interpretive statements.

Provision 1

"The nurse, in all professional relationships, practices with compassion and respect for the inherent dignity, worth, and uniqueness of every individual, unrestricted by considerations of social or economic status, personal attributes, or the nature of health problems" (ANA, 2001, p. 11).

Interpretive statements within this provision include respect for human dignity, relationship to patients, nature of health problems, right to self-determination, and relationships with colleagues and others (ANA, 2001). DNP graduates will likely reflect on this provision when evaluating patients' individual needs, rights, and values. This provision may also be used as a guide when DNP graduates are evaluating clinical ethical scenarios within their clinician roles. This provision will be essential to informed consent in the clinical setting. Finally, this provision provides guidance when evaluating scenarios related to interprofessional collaboration among colleagues.

Provision 2

"The nurse's primary commitment is to the patient, whether an individual, family, group, or community" (ANA, 2001, p. 14).

The interpretive statements within this provision include primacy of patients' interests, conflict of interest for nurses, collaboration, and professional boundaries

(ANA, 2001). DNP graduates in leadership roles should reflect on this provision when evaluating ethical scenarios related to community programs or resources. Also, DNP graduates in leadership, clinician, education, or research roles will be concerned with conflicts of interest when allocating resources or spending within an organization. Clinicians will also be concerned with this provision when billing directly for services. Collaboration will concern DNP graduates when evaluating ethical scenarios related to interprofessional collaboration, such as participation in multidisciplinary team meetings or ethics committees.

Provision 3

"The nurse promotes, advocates for, and strives to protect the health, safety, and rights of the patient" (ANA, 2001, p. 16).

Interpretive statements within this provision include privacy, confidentiality, protection of participants in research, standards and review mechanisms, acting on questionable practice, and addressing impaired practice (ANA, 2001). DNP graduates in all roles will be concerned with this provision. Potential ethical scenarios for which DNP graduates may use this provision as a guide include any violation of patients' privacy, confidentiality, and informed consent to participate in research. Additionally, DNP graduates in clinical and leadership roles may encounter ethical scenarios related to addressing impaired or questionable practice and use this provision to guide ethical evaluation.

Provision 5

"The nurse owes the same duties to self as to others, including the responsibility to preserve integrity and safety, to maintain competence, and to continue personal and professional growth" (ANA, 2001, p. 23).

The interpretive statements within this provision include moral self-respect, professional growth and maintenance of competence, wholeness of character, and preservation of integrity (ANA, 2001). DNP graduates may use this provision as a guide when evaluating ethical scenarios related to the maintenance of specialty certification for advanced-practice registered nurses. Personally, DNP graduates may reflect on this provision when evaluating their own contributions to the nursing profession. DNP graduates may also use this provision as a guide when threats to personal integrity are evident, such as verbal abuse from patients or coworkers.

Provision 7

"The nurse participates in the advancement of the profession through contributions to practice, education, administration, and knowledge development" (ANA, 2001, p. 27).

Interpretive statements within this provision include advancing the profession through active involvement in nursing and healthcare policy; advancing the profession by developing, maintaining, and implementing professional standards in clinical, administrative, and educational practice; and advancing the profession through knowledge development, dissemination, and application to practice (ANA, 2001). DNP graduates may use this provision as a guide when evaluating ethical scenarios related to the DNP degree itself. DNP graduates in administrative roles may use this provision when evaluating ethical scenarios related to professional standards when employing nurses. Finally, DNP graduates may use this provision as a guide when evaluating scenarios related to scientific inquiry in nursing and related issues.

Provision 9

"The profession of nursing, as represented by associations and their members, is responsible for articulating nursing values, for maintaining the integrity of the profession and its practice, and for shaping social policy" (ANA, 2001, p. 29).

The interpretive statements within this provision include assertion of values, carrying out nursing's collective responsibility through professional associations, intraprofessional integrity, and social reform (ANA, 2001). The DNP graduate is charged with upholding nursing organizations' values and ethical standards. Further, DNP graduates have a role in shaping policy and social reform. Therefore, DNP graduates may use this provision as a guide when evaluating ethical scenarios related to sociocultural issues, such as homelessness, hunger, violence, and the stigma of illness.

ICN *Code of Ethics for Nurses*

The ICN's *Code of Ethics for Nurses* was initially adopted in 1953. The code has been revised several times, most recently in 2005. It should be used as a guide for DNP graduates when evaluating ethical scenarios. The ICN code is based on the four responsibilities of nurses "to promote health, to prevent illness, to restore health, and alleviate suffering" (ICN, 2006, p. 1). The ICN *Code of Ethics for Nurses* has four principal elements that outline the standard of ethical conduct.

Elements of the Code

1. Nurses and People
   - The nurse's primary professional responsibility is to people requiring nursing care. In providing care, the nurse promotes an environment in which the human rights, values, customs, and spiritual beliefs of the individual, family, and community are respected.

- The nurse ensures that the individual receives sufficient information on which to base consent for care and the related treatment.
- The nurse holds in confidence personal information and uses judgment in sharing this information.
- The nurse shares with society the responsibility for initiating and supporting action to meet the health and social needs of the public, in particular those of vulnerable populations.
- The nurse also shares responsibility to sustain and protect the natural environment from depletion, pollution, degradation, and destruction.

2. Nurses and Practice

- The nurse carries personal responsibility and accountability for nursing practice, and for maintaining competence by continual learning.
- The nurse maintains a standard of personal health such that the ability to provide care is not compromised.
- The nurse uses judgment regarding individual competence when accepting and delegating responsibility.
- The nurse at all times maintains standards of personal conduct that reflect well on the profession and enhance public confidence.
- The nurse, in providing care, ensures that use of technology and scientific advances are compatible with the safety, dignity, and rights of people.

3. Nurses and the Profession

- The nurse assumes the major role in determining and implementing acceptable standards of clinical nursing practice, management, research, and education.
- The nurse is active in developing a core of research-based professional knowledge.
- The nurse, acting through the professional organization, participates in creating and maintaining safe, equitable social and economic working conditions in nursing.

4. Nurses and Coworkers

- The nurse sustains a cooperative relationship with coworkers in nursing and other fields.
- The nurse takes appropriate action to safeguard individuals, families, and communities when their health is endangered by a coworker or any other person.

Source: Reprinted with permission of the ICN.

Nursing's Social Policy Statement

Nursing's Social Policy Statement is a document that nurses can use as a framework for understanding nursing's relationship with society and nursing's obligation to those who receive nursing care (ANA, 2010b). Silva and Ludwick (2006) questioned whether or not the DNP degree itself is ethical in relation to *Nursing's Social Policy Statement*. In their discussion they questioned why *Nursing's Social Policy Statement* was not used when the DNP degree's foundational framework was developed. *Nursing's Social Policy Statement* is indeed another tool DNP graduates should use as a guide when evaluating ethical scenarios, especially when faced with social issues. The values of the nursing profession and social responsibility are described within *Nursing's Social Policy Statement*. Additionally, nursing's scope of practice and regulation of nursing practice are described within this statement, which may be needed when DNP graduates in clinical or leadership roles evaluate ethical scenarios related to practice and regulation of practice.

Nursing Ethics Summary

The ANA *Code of Ethics for Nurses*, the ICN *Code of Ethics for Nurses*, and *Nursing's Social Policy Statement* are all necessary elements of the DNP graduate's nursing ethics tool kit. Although every ethical scenario will be unique, DNP graduates should use these tools as guides to ensure that the ethical standards of the nursing profession are upheld. Ways to access the ANA *Code of Ethics for Nurses*, the ICN *Code of Ethics for Nurses*, and *Nursing's Social Policy Statement* are detailed in **Box 7-1**.

Ethical Leadership Tools for the Ethical Leader

DNP graduates will likely be in leadership roles within their clinical setting or academic environment or in more formal leadership roles within healthcare organizations. Gallagher and Tschudin (2009) describe three levels of leadership that nurses may in engage in that will require a grasp of ethical leadership. These three levels are consistent with the envisioned leadership roles that DNP graduates will likely encounter. Gallagher and Tschudin described these levels as follows:

> The micro-level, where nurses provide leadership as role models in their work with individuals and teams; the meso-level, where nurses contribute to organizational discussions and policy development; and the macro-level, where nurses engage politically, lobbying politicians and ensuring their voice is heard in national and international forums. (2009, p. 225)

BOX 7-1

Resources for the DNP Ethical Consultant

- American Nurses Association. (2001). *Code of ethics for nurses.* Silver Spring, MD: Author. http://www.nursingworld.org/MainMenuCategories/EthicsStandards /CodeofEthicsforNurses.aspx
- American Nurses Association. (2010). *Nursing's social policy statement: The essence of the profession.* Silver Spring, MD: Author. http://www.nursesbooks .org/Main-Menu/Foundation/Nursings-Social-Policy-Statement.aspx
- Beauchamp, T. L., & Childress, J. F. (2009). *Principles of biomedical ethics* (6th ed.). New York, NY: Oxford University Press.
- Butts, J. B., & Rich, K. L. (2008). *Nursing ethics: Across the curriculum and into practice* (2nd ed.). Sudbury, MA: Jones and Bartlett.
- Fowler, M. D. M. (2010). *Guide to the code of ethics for nurses: Interpretation and application.* Silver Spring, MD: American Nurses Association.
- iHealthCoalition.org. (2010). *eHealth Code of Ethics.* http://www.ihealthcoalition .org/ehealth-code/
- International Council of Nurses. (2006). *Code of ethics for nurses.* http://www .icn.ch/images/stories/documents/about/icncode_english.pdf

---

DNP graduates in leadership roles must have a firm understanding of ethics content (reviewed earlier in the chapter), traits of ethical leaders, ethical decision-making models, and methods to prevent ethical conflicts. Piper (2007) relates that healthcare leaders need specific knowledge of ethics. This knowledge should include a "definition of ethics, ethical conflict and ethical dilemmas, along with a methodology to examine ethics within an organization" (Piper, 2007, p. 249).

Traits of Ethical Leaders

Paul B. Hofmann, DrPH, FACHE, president of the Hofmann Healthcare Group, presented at an ethics program titled "Rising to the Ethical Challenges of Healthcare Leadership" in fall 2008. He described six specific behavioral traits that are essential for an ethics leader:

1. Ethically conscious, having an appreciation for the ethical dimensions and implications of one's daily actions and decisions;

2. Ethically committed, being completely committed to doing the right thing;

3. Ethically competent, having the knowledge and understanding necessary to make ethically sound decisions;

4. Ethically courageous, acting upon these competencies even when the action may not be accepted with enthusiasm or endorsement;

5. Ethically consistent, establishing and maintaining a high ethical standard without making or rationalizing inconvenient exceptions. Also, be able to rebuff the pressures to equivocate, to accommodate and to justify an action or decision that is ethically flawed;

6. Ethically candid, being open and forthright about the complexity of reconciling conflicting values, be willing to ask uncomfortable questions and be an active, not a passive, advocate of ethical analysis and ethical conduct. (Hofmann, as cited in Buell, 2009, p. 54)

These six traits are admirable and noteworthy. DNP graduates should strive to embody them when encountering ethical scenarios in leadership positions. DNP graduates in leadership roles should regularly reflect on these traits in an effort to ensure they are practicing ethical leadership.

Ethical Decision-Making Model for Leadership

A model for ethical decision making that may be applicable to various scenarios DNP graduates may encounter is reviewed later in the chapter. However, ethical decision making for leaders is somewhat more unique and requires an approach that considers stakeholders and the organizational effects of the ethical decision. When discussing the ethical leader, Sanford (2006) reviews specific steps to ethical management decisions. The model takes into account the effect on organizational politics that leaders who make ethical decisions will have to consider. The model also notes that many stakeholders are involved in decisions that are made. In summary, Sanford asserts that the stakeholders' viewpoints should be considered to ensure that decisions are ethical and do more good than harm (Sanford, 2006). Sanford also offers this insightful advice to DNP graduates regarding ethical leadership: "Ethical leaders realize that a short term 'win' at the expense of the future is not a 'win' at all but smoke and mirrors used to make the manager look good today" (2006, p. 7).

Ethical Conflict

In addition to evaluating ethical scenarios, DNP graduates in leadership roles have a responsibility to prevent ethical conflict within an organization. Although many ethical conflicts are unavoidable, Piper (2007) proposed recommendations to prevent ethical conflicts. These recommendations ensure that an ethical culture exists within the organization, thereby preventing potential ethical conflicts.

First, Piper suggests that "great people" with "ethics as a key principle of their values" are necessary to ensure that ethical conduct is practiced by everyone in the organization (2007, p. 253). Second, "great leadership" is necessary to set the example of ethical conduct (2007, p. 253). The leader must hold everyone in the organization accountable for ethical behavior and create an organizational culture of ethics.

Third, a "great governing board" is necessary to hold the standards of ethical conduct and support the leadership in creating a culture of ethics (2007, p. 253). Fourth, an "ethics policy" should be developed that "addresses ethical behavior and how to address ethical conflicts" (2007, p. 253). The policy should outline a definition of ethics and the principles and guidelines used to handle ethical conflicts. Fifth, an "ethics consultant" with expertise in this area should perform an ethics evaluation (2007, p. 253). This evaluation of the leadership, policies, and procedures would examine the justice and fairness in various departments within the organization, such as human resources, finance, and healthcare delivery (2007).

Summary of Ethical Leadership

The DNP graduate may engage in leadership roles ranging from role-modeling in a practice environment to serving as chief nursing officer in a large organization. Therefore, tools for ethical leadership are imperative for the DNP graduate to successfully evaluate ethical scenarios in leadership roles. These tools include traits necessary for ethical leadership, an ethical leadership decision-making tool, and recommendations for avoiding ethical conflicts. These tools are not inclusive of those necessary for DNP graduates to evaluate ethical leadership scenarios but rather provide exemplars for the DNP graduate to begin the process of ethical leadership.

Telehealth Ethics: Ethical Concerns in the 21st Century

The 21st century and the development of telehealth presents unique ethical scenarios for the DNP graduate. Telehealth, sometimes referred to as telemedicine, encompasses all healthcare delivery that involves information technology. Telehealth spans the use of information technology, from electronic medical records (EMRs) to patients seeking information on the Internet. Telenursing is more specifically "the provision of nursing care utilizing any form of electronic media" (Burkhardt & Nathaniel, 2008, p. 172). With the advent of telehealth comes unique ethical scenarios DNP graduates will likely encounter.

Electronic Medical Records

An EMR is defined as a computer application that electronically stores individually identifiable health data (Layman, 2008). The development of EMRs has raised certain ethical scenarios, most dealing with privacy. It is therefore prudent to make the distinction between *ethics* and *regulation*. Ethics has been defined as the principles of conduct governing an individual or group (Ethic, 2014a). "Codes of ethics are not legally binding but rather voluntary standards a profession or industry adopts" (Simpson, 2005, p. 179). Regulations "include laws and the official policies the healthcare organizations employ" (Simpson, 2005, p. 179).

However, there are scenarios where ethics and regulations are intertwined, and violating an ethical principle may result in legal consequences. The Health Insurance Portability and Accountability Act (HIPAA) of 1996 is an example of a law born from an ethical principle. HIPAA has also been referred to as the Privacy Rule. "A major goal of the Privacy Rule is to assure that individuals' health information is properly protected while allowing the flow of health information needed to provide and promote high quality health care and to protect the public's health and well being" (U.S. Department of Health and Human Services, 2011). The Privacy Rule attempts to protect patients' medical information, both paper and online.

The development of EMRs has prompted ethical discussions related to certain ethical principles. EMRs have been noted by most to be beneficent and purport to do good for others (Layman, 2008). However, EMRs have raised concerns regarding the principle of autonomy, which "requires that the clinician do all he or she reasonably can to respect the patient's right to make an informed decision pertaining to actions the clinician may or may not take on their behalf and to have personal information protected" (Fleming, Edison, & Pak, 2009, p. 798).

Protecting patients' health information is much more challenging with the development of EMRs. EMR data can be "accessed by almost anyone, simultaneously, at anytime, from anywhere" (Phillips & Fleming, 2009, p. 329). EMRs may contain highly sensitive information, such as social and family history, lifestyle information, medications, medical conditions, and genetic information. HIPAA requirements include restrictions for user IDs and passwords to access this information, but unfortunately these regulations are sometimes violated, and so is patient privacy.

EMRs may also be used to promote or hinder the ethical principle of justice. EMRs may be viewed as a source of health information that can increase patients' compliance and self-management (Layman, 2008). However, where inequity exists, such as families and patients who cannot afford a computer, this information may not be accessible. In this instance, lack of access to EMRs may be viewed as injustice (Layman, 2008).

Internet Information Seeking

Patients frequently seek information from the Internet to manage their own health. Patients can access everything from healthcare plans to healthcare providers, insurers, and healthcare facilities (Butts & Rich, 2008). Unfortunately, many cannot adequately evaluate health information on the Internet, and healthcare professionals are faced with helping patients safely navigate the Internet and the vast amount of health information available. An organization called iHealthCoalition.org published an *eHealth Code of Ethics* in an effort "to ensure that people worldwide can confidently and with full understanding of known risks realize the potential of the Internet in managing their own health and the health of those in their care" (2010, Vision Statement, para. 1). This code of conduct is used by "marketers, health professionals, and creators of Web sites in an attempt to enhance a trustworthy environment for consumers of health information, products, and services" (Butts & Rich, 2008, p. 109). The *eHealth Code of Ethics* consists of eight principles based on autonomy, or respect for persons. These principles are as follows:

- Candor: Disclose only information that is beneficial to the consumer. Sites should clearly indicate who owns or has an interest in the site or service and the purpose of the site or service.
- Honesty: Be truthful and not deceptive. Clearly distinguish content intended to promote or sell a product, service, or organization from educational or scientific content.
- Quality: Provide health information that is accurate, easy to understand, and up to date and allows users to make their own judgments about the health information, products, or services provided by the site.
- Informed consent: Respect users' right to determine when and how their personal data may be collected, used, or shared.
- Privacy: Respect and protect the privacy of others.
- Professionalism: Respect ethical obligations to patients and inform and educate patients about the limitations of healthcare information on the Internet.
- Responsible partnering: Evaluate the trustworthiness of the organizations and websites.
- Accountability: Provide the opportunity for users to give feedback, evaluate the website, and monitor compliance with the *eHealth Code of Ethics*.

DNP graduates should become familiar with and use the *eHealth Code of Ethics* when evaluating ethical scenarios related to consumer information on the Internet.

Twitter, Facebook, and Chat: Ethical Perils of Social Networks

The advent of social networks presents a whole new threat to patient privacy. DNP graduates will likely encounter ethical scenarios related to social networking. Unfortunately, violators of patient privacy may involve patients, consumers, and healthcare providers.

Facebook offers subscribers the ability to connect electronically to friends and colleagues all over the world. Facebook has approximately 500 million users worldwide (Wolfe, 2013). Healthcare professionals who use social networks must be mindful of professional boundaries and patients' rights to privacy. The Privacy

Rule, or HIPAA, "applies to any healthcare provider who electronically transfers information in connection with certain transactions including both institutional and individual providers" (Hader & Brown, 2010, p. 271). The Privacy Rule protects any health-related information in paper, electronic, or oral form. Posting patient information, even when seemingly not identifiable, is still a violation of HIPAA and of a patient's autonomy.

The ANA *Code of Ethics for Nurses*, the ICN *Code of Ethics for Nurses*, and the basic principles of bioethics clearly support the need to protect patients' privacy. Blogging, posting, tweeting, or chatting about patients or patients' personal health information is a clear violation of ethics and the law. Due to the novelty of social networks, it is imperative that DNP graduates remain mindful of this new exchange of information and ensure responsible social network interactions among themselves and their colleagues.

In 2011 the ANA published a document to guide nurses regarding their use of social media. The document, titled "6 Tips for Nurses Using Social Media," includes principles for nurses regarding social network interactions and tips to avoid problems. The principles caution nurses against sharing identifiable patient information online and outline the nurse's responsibility in protecting their patients' information (ANA, 2011).

This document advises nurses to remember that online contact with patients crosses the boundary of nurse–patient relationships. This includes the sharing of photos or videos of patients taken with personal electronic devices. Nurses should also avoid posting negative comments about patients, colleagues, or employers, even if they are not identified by name. Any breach in confidentiality or privacy should be reported immediately (ANA, 2011).

In 2011 the National Council of State Boards of Nursing published a white paper that includes guidelines regarding nurses and social media. These guidelines were developed in collaboration with the ANA (National Council of State Boards of Nursing, 2011).

DNP graduates should be aware of these guidelines, principles, and tips. They should role-model ethical behaviors and educate other healthcare professionals regarding ethical behavior and social media.

Telehealth and Ethics Summary

The 21st century has brought wonderful advances to information technology and health care. With these advances come new challenges and responsibilities for DNP graduates. Specifically, DNP graduates have a responsibility to be aware of new ethical scenarios and develop skills to evaluate these scenarios. DNP graduates need both a grasp of ethical content and an understanding of information technologies and new developments within telehealth. Fleming and colleagues stated that "technology is neither ethical nor unethical . . . rather it is the intent and means by which the technology is implemented that impacts the question of appropriate utilization" (2009, p. 797).

An Ethical Decision-Making Model Useful for DNP Graduates

As previously stated, due to their positions in leadership, research, clinical practice, and academia, DNP graduates will likely be asked to evaluate various ethical scenarios in their roles. After a basic understanding of ethical, bioethical, and nursing ethics content is developed, DNP graduates are equipped to begin the process of critically evaluating ethical scenarios. However, evaluation of ethical scenarios is a *process* that DNP graduates will need to develop throughout their careers. With experience, understanding of ethical content, and a diligent commitment to upholding the ethical standards of the nursing profession, DNP graduates will become more proficient at this process.

Burkhardt and Nathaniel (2008) developed an ethical decision-making model that may be useful for DNP graduates when an ethical scenario is presented. This model is based on the premise that ethical decision making is "a process that overlays other dynamic biological, psychological, and social processes—layer upon layer" (2008, p. 128). Further, the process of ethical decision making requires ongoing evaluation and assimilation of information, making way for an evolving perspective that may change over time. This model allows for evolving perspectives as one moves toward a resolution or decision.

Step 1: Articulate the Problem

The first step of Burkhardt and Nathaniel's (2008) model involves clearly describing the ethical problem that has been identified. This is followed by identifying desired goals, which will allow movement toward step 3 of the model, developing strategies. Burkhardt and Nathaniel (2008) relate that because strategies are often dramatic, identifying goals at this time will reduce conflict later in the process. Further, by clearly identifying the problem, it will be defined as an ethical or practical dilemma.

Step 2: Gather Data and Identify Conflicting Moral Claims

After the ethical problem is clearly identified, one should gather the necessary information or facts to provide clarification of the issues involved. Burkhardt and Nathaniel (2008) relate that throughout this process attention should be paid to the societal, religious, and cultural values and beliefs of those involved. In addition, one should identify the participants' ethical perspectives. This is when an understanding of basic ethical content, theories, principles, and perspectives is imperative.

Step 3: Explore Strategies

Identifying the problem and gathering data is followed by identifying possible strategies. Burkhardt and Nathaniel state that "various options begin to emerge throughout the assessment process" (2008, p. 130). In an effort to eliminate unacceptable alternatives, the proposed alternatives should be evaluated for how they best fit the identified goals, beliefs, lifestyles, and values (Burkhardt & Nathaniel, 2008). This step of the ethical decision-making process may take time to develop acceptable strategies and eliminate unacceptable strategies. Further, when a strategy is adopted, one must be ready and willing to act on it (Burkhardt & Nathaniel, 2008).

Step 4: Implement the Strategy

When a strategy is adopted, it is implemented. However, Burkhardt and Nathaniel (2008) relate that this may be the most difficult step. Those involved in the process must feel empowered to make a difficult decision. The emotions that are surely stirred by implementing the strategy should be acknowledged by those involved, and they should be accepted as part of this difficult process (Burkhardt & Nathaniel, 2008).

Step 5: Evaluate Outcomes

Burkhardt and Nathaniel state that upon acting on the decision, "reflective evaluation sheds light on the effectiveness and validity of the process" (2008, p. 132). The effects of the strategy on those involved in the process should be evaluated. This step of the model may involve ongoing evaluation of additional ethical problems that may arise as the situation changes and new data are gathered (Burkhardt & Nathaniel, 2008).

Putting It All Together: Ethical Scenarios with Discussions

As stated earlier in the chapter, DNP graduates are not ethicists, but rather experts in nursing practice who will encounter ethical scenarios within their settings. It is the DNP graduate's responsibility to become familiar with ethical content and nursing's ethical standards for practice. The following are possible ethical scenarios that DNP graduates may encounter in their various roles.

Case Scenario 1

Dr. A. is a DNP-prepared nurse practitioner within a multidisciplinary breast center. As part of her role, Dr. A. cares for patients with breast health issues, including breast cancer. When a new patient in the breast center is evaluated, Dr. A. orders and discusses diagnostic tests with the patient, and, if need be, orders a breast biopsy. The breast center's philosophy of care is designed to be seamless and potentially takes the patient from assessment and evaluation to diagnostics and biopsy—all in the same day. One would think this is an ideal scenario.

Dr. A. sees her first new patient of the day. She assesses the 39-year-old mother of two who is under a great deal of stress due to lack of child care at home. The patient, Ms. B., relates that she found a lump in her breast about 6 months ago, but due to her schedule and lack of child care, she has been unable to come in to the breast center. She has never had a mammogram and has no family history of breast cancer.

As per the standard of care, Dr. A. examines Ms. B., orders a mammogram and ultrasound, and awaits the results. In the meantime, Ms. B. receives a call that her babysitter is late for an appointment and needs to leave soon. Stressed and worried, Ms. B. undergoes the ordered diagnostic testing. While in the ultrasound room, she is informed by the radiologist that there is a mass in her breast that is worrisome and requires a biopsy. In an effort to provide seamless care, the room is prepped. Ms. B., confused and in a hurry, consents to the procedure. While she waits for the radiologist to perform the biopsy, her mind is racing. She wishes her husband had come, she wishes she had made different child care arrangements, she might have gotten a second opinion regarding the biopsy. But, she thinks, the doctors and nurses know best. They told her she needs the biopsy today, so she should have it. Tears stream down her face and she wishes she wasn't there alone. At the end of a 4-hour appointment, seamless care has been provided and precious time is saved by having the biopsy performed so quickly. Ms. B. is diagnosed a week later with stage I breast cancer, and she begins receiving treatment within 1 week of presenting to the clinic.

DISCUSSION

Upon reviewing this scenario, one may note that from a deontological theory, Dr. A. performed her duty to the patient and did what was right by diagnosing cancer and initiating the necessary treatment as soon as possible. However, with regard to beneficence, or doing what benefits the patient, the answers are not so clear. The patient benefitted from an early diagnosis, but at what cost? One should note that the actions of the multidisciplinary team were paternalistic in that the decision was made for Ms. B. that it would be best if she had her biopsy on the same day as her first visit to the breast center. One may consider that Ms. B. was emotionally harmed by the paternalistic actions and nonmaleficence was not supported.

How could this scenario have been handled differently by Dr. A.? Do you think Dr. A. is aware that her actions could be viewed as paternalistic, or do you think she is acting purely out of duty? What would you do if you encountered this scenario?

Case Scenario 2

Dr. B. is a DNP-prepared clinical nurse specialist working in an urban healthcare center serving a multicultural population. Dr. B.'s role includes counseling patients and their families regarding end-of-life care. One of his patients, Ms. C., who is on the renal transplant floor, is suffering from end-stage renal disease and has been denied a second transplant. Dr. B. knows from previous admissions that Ms. C. does not wish to be resuscitated and has previously signed advance directive paperwork. However, during this new admission, the advance directive must be signed again. Ms. C. is from a Middle Eastern country and speaks little English. Her family has been present and translating for her.

Dr. B. is consulted by the nursing staff to renew the advance directive due to the fact that the family is currently refusing to sign the paperwork. Dr. B. arrives on the unit, is met by the English-speaking son of Ms. C. (Ms. C.'s power of attorney) who states, "She is confused; she doesn't know what she wants." Dr. B. tries to counsel Ms. C.'s son and reassure him that this is what Ms. C. had wanted.

Unfortunately, the next day Ms. C.'s condition worsens and she is placed on a ventilator. Ms. C.'s son continues to refuse to sign the advance directive. Dr. B. consults with the medical team, who continues aggressive medical care. Ms. C.'s health declines and she becomes comatose. Ms. C. remains unresponsive and on a ventilator for several more days. She is eventually determined to have minimal brain activity and is finally removed from the ventilator.

DISCUSSION

This scenario involves many ethical concerns ranging from the provision of culturally sensitive care to respect for the patient's autonomy. First and foremost, whenever there is a language barrier, respect for autonomy and informed consent require a translator be present for all medical decision-making discussions. This ensures that all information is appropriately shared with the patient.

At times, healthcare professionals may feel they need to override a patient's autonomous choice to practice nonmaleficence (or do no harm). This involves the art of ethics and requires careful deliberation and ethical reflection. The healthcare providers made decisions based on a deontological perspective—they felt it was their duty to save Ms. C.'s life. In this situation, however, the patient had made her wishes clear in a previous advance directive. "Nurses have multiple ethical obligations, sometimes competing, sometimes conflicting, including those to the patient, the organization or institution in which they work, or other healthcare professionals, and the nursing profession" (Davis, 2010, p. 15). Importantly, the ANA *Code of Ethics for Nurses* makes it clear that the nurse's primary obligation is to the patient. Nurses may need courage to act when dealing with the consequences of an ethical decision (Davis, 2010).

What should Dr. B. have done when the family members refused to sign the advance directive for Ms. C.? Would an ethics committee have a role in this scenario? What would you do in this scenario? What ethical principles would you feel took precedence in this scenario?

Case Scenario 3

Dr. C. is a vice president of nursing at a large tertiary care hospital. She has been having trouble recruiting and keeping nursing staff; as a result some units are short staffed. She is faced with making a choice regarding allocation of resources. She may spread the nurses around the hospital with few nurses on each unit or close certain units and staff the open units adequately. If she closes units, the patients who were already admitted would be cared for, but this decision would limit how many patients could be admitted in the future (Davis, 2010).

DISCUSSION

Evaluating this ethical scenario requires reflection on the principles of justice, non-maleficence, and beneficence. The principle of justice must be considered when resources are limited or managed (Davis, 2010). Distributive justice refers to "the sharing of burdens and benefits in the allocation of resources, sometimes, but not always, under conditions of scarcity or rationing" (Davis, 2010, p. 17). Dr. C. should consider what solution would promote the most good while inflicting the least harm. Dr. C. is faced with scarce resources, and she must evaluate what option promotes care of the patients in her institution.

Would you close some units and provide better staffing for the patients who are currently admitted? What would you do regarding the lack of open beds for new admissions? What ethical principles would you rely on to evaluate this scenario?

Case Scenario 4

Dr. D. is an associate professor in a large university-based school of nursing. Dr. D. teaches students who are second-degree students, or those with a bachelor's degree in another field and are returning to school for a degree in nursing. The majority of Dr. D.'s students are in midlife and have experienced layoffs related to a declining economy within their area.

Many of Dr. D.'s students are doing well in the program and express love for the nursing profession. However, Dr. D. occasionally has a student who clearly is looking for job security rather than expressing commitment to the profession. These students do mediocre academic work and meet the minimum requirements in their clinical rotations, but they lack passion for patient care.

Dr. D. struggles regularly regarding these students and seeks assistance from the administration. She and her colleagues counsel these students regarding their career choice, but many stay in the program, graduate, and enter the nursing profession. Despite her best efforts in her academic setting, Dr. D. is disillusioned with teaching and wonders if she should stay in this setting and what she can do about this ethical scenario.

DISCUSSION

Although there may be nothing Dr. D. can do regarding students who entered the profession for job security, she may reflect on the ANA *Code of Ethics for Nurses* Provision 5: "The nurse owes the same duties to self as to others, including the responsibility to preserve integrity and safety, to maintain competence, and to continue personal and professional growth" (ANA, 2001, p. 23). This provision will remind her that her responsibility to the profession is to ensure competence in the profession. Her students must meet the academic requirements, but she cannot ensure that they love their chosen profession.

Dr. D. is responsible to vigorously counsel students who don't seem to fit with nursing and offer alternate career choices that may better suit them. She may also decline to give letters of recommendation after graduation (Fowler, 2010). It is Dr. D.'s responsibility to ensure competence, but it is not her responsibility to ensure that these students stay within the profession.

How would you counsel these students? What would you do if your students expressed a lack of passion or actual disdain for the nursing profession?

Case Scenario 5

Mr. E. is a busy certified registered nurse anesthetist practicing in a labor and delivery unit within an academic hospital. He has been considering returning to school for a DNP degree and has been researching DNP degree programs. As part of his decision making, he met with his director to discuss reducing his hours to allow time for returning to graduate school. He was met with resistance and questioned why he needed "yet another degree." Mr. E. explained the DNP degree to his director and the reasons he wanted to expand his knowledge base and improve his overall practice.

After this meeting, Mr. E. was somewhat discouraged, and despite the fact that he was committed to advancing his profession and his own professional development, he is now struggling with his decision.

DISCUSSION

Reflecting on the ANA *Code of Ethics for Nurses* may help Mr. E. with his decision to pursue a DNP degree. Provision 7 states: "The nurse participates in the advancement of the profession through contributions to practice, education, administration, and knowledge development" (ANA, 2001, p. 27). Commitment to this provision does not necessarily mean everyone must return to graduate school; however, this provision supports nursing contributing to the profession through ongoing educational efforts and developing nursing's body of knowledge.

The ANA *Code of Ethics for Nurses* states that "administrators must create an environment that is supportive of the ongoing educational needs of nurses and conducive to rapid implementation and innovation" (Drought & Epstein, 2010, pp. 90–91). The nursing profession can advance only through the commitment of nurses who are willing to learn and incorporate new knowledge (Drought & Epstein, 2010). Provision 7 of the ANA *Code of Ethics for Nurses* and Mr. E.'s commitment to his profession should help him evaluate his decision to return to school for a DNP degree.

How would you respond to your director if you encountered resistance regarding returning to graduate school? What ethical perspectives would drive your decision to return to school despite meeting resistance?

Interviews with Nurse Ethicists: Wisdom from the Field

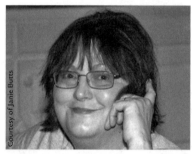

JANIE BUTTS, PHD, RN, AND KAREN RICH, PHD, RN, are nurse ethicists and nursing professors at the University of Southern Mississippi School of Nursing. Their interviews provide valuable insights regarding ethics in nursing and implications for DNP graduates.

THEN . . . 2011

Dr. Butts and Dr. Rich, could you describe your background, including education, nursing, and academic experience, and your current position?

Dr. Butts: My career as a registered nurse involves a 32-year era of my life thus far, occurring in advancing stages. In the first stage of my nursing career I was an associate's-prepared, then a baccalaureate-prepared, clinical practice nurse with a focus in adult health nursing, in labor and delivery, and finally in emergency nursing. In my current and second stage, I have been a nursing educator since 1990—for 21 of my 32 years of nursing—from 1993 to present at the University of Southern Mississippi School of Nursing. My earlier teaching years were from 1990 to 1993 at William Carey University. My love for knowledge and being a nursing educator with a master's of science degree in nursing led me down a path of lifelong learning. A doctor of science degree in nursing (DSN) was earned in 1998 from the University of Alabama at Birmingham School of Nursing with a focus on nursing education and curriculum, clinical intervention research with elders, and behavioral intervention research with at-risk adolescents. In 2002, as I began teaching in the PhD program of nursing, my focus turned sharply to ethics, bioethics, and theory. In response to these areas of interest, I attended several summer seminars and earned certificates in ethics and bioethics at the Kennedy Institute of Ethics at Georgetown and at the University of Washington at Seattle, Departments of Law, Medicine, and Allied Health Care. Then in 2002 I earned a certification in ethics from Rush University in Chicago. A significant amount of my learning came from a self-taught approach of reading, daily reflection and journaling, and studying philosophy, ethics, bioethics, and theory development. The most recent research is a qualitative content analysis on adults who have lost their adult siblings. I have numerous articles in journals and many book chapters in others' books. Dr. Rich and I are coauthors of two books, one nonedited nursing ethics book in its second edition, with a third edition forthcoming, and one new edited book with a variety of book chapters by distinguished nursing and nonnursing authors. In my current position at the university, I teach ethics courses and theory development and analysis courses in the baccalaureate, master's, DNP, and PhD programs at differing levels of complexity.

Dr. Rich: I have been a nurse for 31 years. I began my career as an associate-degree nurse and quickly realized that I wanted to pursue higher education in nursing. I have earned a master's in public health nursing, a postmaster's as a psychiatric–mental health nurse practitioner, and a doctorate in nursing with an emphasis in ethics. Although my plan was to practice as a psychiatric nurse practitioner while I pursued that degree, I became captivated with philosophy and ethics during my doctoral education, and my career took a different direction. Actually, Dr. Butts was one of my teachers and played a big role in my academic development during my doctoral program. We began collaborating on scholarly writing projects, and I became a teacher at the University of Southern Mississippi. Now I teach public health, ethics, professional development, research, and graduate classes in quality improvement. I absolutely love being a teacher.

Dr. Butts and Dr. Rich, could you describe how you define *nurse ethicist*, including how you became a nurse ethicist?

Dr. Butts: The nurse ethicist role can be described in different ways according to the working environment and context. The nurse ethicist is an advanced-practice registered nurse with a degree or advanced certification in ethics education and with ethics expertise. The nurse ethicist in clinical settings manages the ethical issues of professional nursing practice. For instance, one large healthcare system—Clarian Health in collaboration with the Fairbanks Center for Medical Ethics and the Indiana University School of Nursing—created the nurse ethicist role for "creating and sustaining programs in clinical ethics and nursing ethics education with the goal of empowering the ethical lives of nurses in the context of the interdisciplinary environments in which they work" (Wocial, Bledsoe, Helft, & Everett, 2010, p. 287).

In academia we are realizing the need for curricula with more concentrated content in ethics, bioethics, and ethical decision making for the express function of improving and maintaining ethical clinical practice. We are seeing a significant emphasis on students' capacity to show evidence of ethical expertise in their nursing practice integrated throughout the American Association of Colleges of Nursing (AACN) baccalaureate essentials (2008), master's level essentials (2011), and doctoral essentials for advanced nursing practice (2006) documents and the current NCLEX plan (2013). The Institute of Medicine (2010) published recommendations for the future of nursing, emphasizing a higher level of education and expertise in collaboration, which includes ethical collaboration with other healthcare disciplines. I have discovered that students and many faculty are intensely interested in the topics of moral integrity in their personal lives and ethical decision making in nursing practice, one reason being that they are experiencing and observing increased moral distress, indicating ethical conflicts in practice.

I have already described my personal progression of ethics education in the first interview question. My curiosity in and pursuance of ethics and bioethics grew from my interest in ethical issues with at-risk adolescents, such as confidentiality issues and the right to choose or refuse treatment. Studying, teaching, and writing about ethical analysis and decision making have helped me develop the skills of making an argument, that is, providing justification for my stance, both theoretically and pragmatically.

Dr. Rich: I define a nurse ethicist as a nurse with a master's or doctoral degree who has had advanced educational preparation in bioethics and nursing ethics in the form of a specific degree or certificate. A nurse ethicist should have a clear research, scholarship, and practice track focused on nursing ethics. Before I became a nurse educator, one of my favorite practice roles was being a discharge planner at a teaching hospital in the heart of New Orleans. I worked as a team member within the hospital's social services department and took on the role of interacting with, teaching, counseling, and advocating for patients and families during a wide range of physical, social, and psychological stages and conditions related to health and illness. Many of the patients and families with whom I worked were coping with end-of-life care and decisions, which were very ethical in nature.

Other ethics-related issues in my work involved accessing care and resources, addressing issues of social justice, being an intermediary among patients and families and the nursing and medical staff at the hospital, and trying to appropriately confront problems related to autonomy and paternalism. When I began working in home care, I found that many of the same basic ethical issues existed, only in a different type setting. When I entered my PhD in nursing program with an emphasis in ethics, the content felt natural to me. I was thrilled to be able to link theories and concepts to the issues that I had experienced in my practice. One of the things that I always have pondered in my career is why some nurses go the extra mile to help patients and families while other nurses want to do the bare minimum. Why do some nurses seem to tune out, rather than tune in, on being caring, present, and compassionate? Studying ethics helped me find a scholarly way to consider my unanswered questions.

Dr. Butts and Dr. Rich, do you believe that ethics education is important in education for nurses and advanced-practice registered nurses, and if so, why?

Dr. Butts: Yes, I believe that ethics is not just important but also mandatory and should include deliberately placed content at all levels of nursing education, whether as a separate course or integrated into all courses across each and every levels. The American Nurses Association's Code of Ethics for Nurses with Interpretive Statements *(2001) and* Nursing: Scope and Standards of Practice *(2010a) denote that nurses are morally obligated and committed to manifest evidence of a solid ethical practice with farsighted decision making rooted in knowledge and contemplated judgments. To accomplish this level of ethical practice entails that nurses remain well informed, competent, and engaged in clinical skills, professional ethics, bioethics issues, and research.*

Dr. Rich: I absolutely believe that ethics education is important for all levels of nursing. Nursing, to me, is an inherently moral endeavor. Consequently, to practice nursing well, nurses need to work on positively developing their character and moral intellect as well as nursing praxis.

Dr. Butts and Dr. Rich, do you think that nursing curricula prepare nurses and advanced-practice registered nurses in education sufficiently for professional ethical practice? Specifically, is there any fundamental ethical content missing from ethics education in nursing?

Dr. Butts: I believe that nurses and advanced-practice registered nurses are not educationally adept in ethics for professional ethical practice for two reasons. One rationale is that the implementation of ethics education has been sluggish because of not being recognized as a prominent foundation for nursing education. Nursing faculty traditionally prefer to stick with what has been a blueprint for student and faculty success, which has translated to a slow implementation of ethics education. Ethics typically has been considered as only a small portion of the essential content within the typical specialties of graduate nursing education and the subspecialties of undergraduate nursing education (that is, adult health, childbearing mothers, newborns, child family health, psychiatric–mental health, and public health care). I believe this approach is quickly changing as new and different nursing, medical, and organizational demands and societal expectations for ethical practice are brought to the forefront of health care.

The second rationale has to do with the complexity and density of ethical practice. Novice nurses do not yet have the capacity for the full range of complex considerations required for ethical practice, analysis, and decision making—either because of the very nature of graduates being novice nurses without depth in clinical experience, or because in nursing school they often receive only limited ethics education from which to draw. However, with a strong education in ethics, novice nurses will draw from that foundation to build and develop competency for professional ethical practice.

There are several essential parts missing from ethics education at all levels, such as the actual bioethical issues, but in my opinion the biggest part that is glaringly absent at all levels is the theoretical and principled justification for ethical decisions and the associated nursing dialogue. I believe it was Leonardo da Vinci who once said about the theoretical knowledge for drawing and art:

> *Those who are in love with practice without knowledge are like the sailor who gets into a ship without a rudder or compass and who never can be certain whether he is going. Practice must always be founded on sound theory, and to this perspective is the guide and the gateway. And without this nothing can be done well in the matter of drawing. (da Vinci, 2005, p. 299)*

Leonardo's same thoughts about theory and practice can be applied to nursing ethical theory and practice. Practice without theory is futile. Nursing educators need to integrate ethics-based theoretical and principled justification for ethical decisions.

Dr. Rich: Generally I do not believe that nursing curricula adequately prepare nurses in theoretical and applied ethics. The fundamental ethical content that I believe is frequently missing from ethics education in nursing is helping nurses be aware of how often they will confront ethical issues in a place similar to what Schön called the "swampy lowland" (1987, p. 3). The ethical issues that nurses confront most often are not the big, recognizable issues that people hear about in the media. Instead they are the day-to-day decisions that nurses must make in their work. One of my favorite ethics quotes says it all for me: "The great ethical danger, I think, is not that when faced with an important decision one makes the wrong choice, but rather that one never realizes that one is facing a decision at all" (Chambliss, 1996, p. 59). Nurses sometimes become so routinized in their everyday relationships with patients that they forget their work is inherently moral. Opportunities to make ethical decisions are all around them.

Dr. Butts and Dr. Rich, how do you think the domain of ethics should influence the development of the DNP degree?

Dr. Butts: Nurses are taught to treat patients with dignity and human respect in an unbiased, nonjudgmental approach. Educators need to place more detailed ethics content in strategic places and levels within the DNP curriculum so that DNP students can develop complexity in their critical reflection of ethical analysis and decision making. I like what Peirce and Smith (2008) implemented at Columbia University School of Nursing. They have some interesting suggestions regarding integration of ethics in the DNP education. They developed DNP ethical competencies in three of the nine competency domains at that university based on four professional organizations' standards and recommendations: (1) the ANA Code of Ethics for Nurses with Interpretive Statements *(2001); (2) the International Council of Nurses* Code of Ethics for Nurses *(2006); (3) the AACN* Essentials of Doctoral Education for Advanced Nursing Practice *(2006); and (4) the National Organization of Nurse Practitioner Faculties* Practice Doctorate Nurse Practitioner Entry-Level Competencies *(2006). The ethical competencies within the three domains include ethical care based on scientific evidence for patient health and illness, and ethical analysis and decision making in the professional role, which is part of professional accountability.*

Dr. Rich: Nursing ethics is grounded in the moral nature of nurse–patient and/or nurse–caregiver relationships. Nurses with a DNP degree should be mentors and role models for other nurses, especially in their relationships with patients and families. These relationships are at the center of nursing practice for DNP graduates who should provide the highest quality of direct nursing care.

Dr. Butts and Dr. Rich, do you agree that an ethics curriculum should be included in DNP programs? If so, how should this content be integrated in DNP curricula?

Dr. Rich: Of course, I must admit my bias, but I believe that ethics should be taught as a separate course in DNP programs and be threaded throughout other courses in the curriculum.

Dr. Butts: Yes I do, but I do not think enough emphasis has been placed on ethics content for DNP programs. A separate ethics core course and a threading of ethical content throughout the DNP curriculum is my suggestion and Dr. Rich's recommendation. Additionally, I gave an example of one university's development of ethical competencies for its DNP curriculum. I believe that competencies for ethical practice by DNPs need to be created in terms of universal competencies for all DNP programs with specific objectives and strategies for teaching and learning.

Dr. Butts and Dr. Rich, how do you think ethics will affect the future roles that DNP graduates will assume? Is any specific ethics content more essential for future DNP graduates, such as information technology, research, or leadership?

Dr. Rich: I believe that having formal ethics knowledge will be integral to the success of DNP graduates in the future. DNP-educated nurses will be more comfortable in their roles if their feet are on semisolid ground rather than totally in the swampy low ground in terms of ethics. DNP nurses must know an ethics-laden situation when they confront it. They must feel confident in knowing how to make decisions that enhance human flourishing and diminish suffering while practicing according to the nonnegotiable provisions of the American Nurses Association's current Code of Ethics for Nurses with Interpretive Statements, *which was most recently published in 2001. The specific ethics content that I believe will be more essential for DNP graduates in the future is content related to social justice and population health, nurse entrepreneurship, leadership, and technology.*

Dr. Butts: I agree totally with Dr. Rich's summation of the significance of ethics education in DNP programs of study. To Dr. Rich's future essential content list, I also add the ethical theoretical justification component and the translation of ethics research findings to DNP ethical practice.

NOW . . . 2014

Dr. Butts and Dr. Rich, could you briefly provide an update regarding your current positions?

Dr. Butts: Currently I am professor of nursing at the University of Southern Mississippi, Hattiesburg. My experience includes 21 years of teaching nursing in theory, ethics, and professional concepts and issues in the PhD, DNP, MSN, RN to BSN, and BSN programs.

Dr. Rich: Currently I am an associate professor of nursing in my same position at the University of Southern Mississippi. I teach public health, ethics, professional development, research, and graduate classes in quality improvement.

Dr. Butts and Dr. Rich, the last time we spoke you wonderfully articulated your thoughts regarding ethics education in nursing curricula. Do you think the inclusion of ethics content in nursing programs has changed in any way?

Dr. Rich: I believe bioethics continues to be more prevalent in the news media, and the public is increasingly aware of ethical issues related to their health care. I'm currently reading the book Five Days at Memorial *by Sheri Fink, which details the experiences of nurses and physicians who were on duty at Memorial Hospital in New Orleans during and shortly after Hurricane Katrina. The book illustrates the need for nurses to prepare for unexpected ethical situations. I believe nurse educators need to continually strive to do a better job of helping students anticipate ethics-laden work situations and prepare them-selves beforehand about how to act when faced with such situations. Of course, the impor-tance of everyday professional ethics should not be overlooked. Nurses are being asked to do more with fewer resources, and related stresses can lead to cutting corners ethically.*

Dr. Butts: I agree with Dr. Rich about the media emphasis on ethical issues of life and death. Though Hurricane Katrina occurred more than 8 years ago in the southeastern Unites States, many nurses, physicians, and other people affected by the storm experience a raw visceral reaction at the very mention of it. I have not read the Sheri Fink book that Dr. Rich mentioned, but I did watch a new realistic movie, Hours, *which is a fictional account of a pregnant woman who gave birth to a premature infant in a New Orleans hospital just as the storm was approaching. The mother died, but the infant remained alive in critical condition on a ventilator. The electricity was out, and the backup generator failed as water surged into the hospital. Officials ordered hospital personnel to evacuate the building, leaving the father alone trying to keep the infant alive. Days passed while the father used a hand-cranked portable generator to support the ventilator, but he had to recharge the battery every few minutes to sustain the electrical current. The story highlighted one nurse who hesitated to leave the father and infant alone in the dark. She faced an ethical situation—to leave or not to leave. Many hours later, she returned to help, only to die by a looter's hand. The loss of electricity and a failing generator brought about a situation that no one could foresee. Nurse educators would find extreme difficulty in teaching students how to manage this particular situation, but they need to teach students the foundations and practical aspects of ethics that will help guide them in the future on how to think on their feet when they are faced with unexpected situations.*

Dr. Butts and Dr. Rich, specific to DNP programs, do you think the inclusion of additional, separate course work in ethics is being taken more seriously by DNP faculty?

Dr. Rich: I'm concerned that as universities are forced to operate more like corporations rather than student-focused centers of learning, program content is being cut for schools and colleges of nursing to be competitive with other programs. I find that nurse educators sometimes are quick to say that ethics is something that can be threaded throughout courses. This practice seems shortsighted to me.

Dr. Butts: I generally agree with Dr. Rich's concern about universities cutting content to remain competitive in the marketplace, but faculty of some DNP programs are adding an ethics component somewhere in the core courses. For instance, in our DNP program we recently revised the DNP theory course title and content to include professional and practical ethics. Some programs may thread it, but the new ethics content for our program was incorporated only into one course and was not threaded throughout the courses, over and above ethics content that already existed in the program.

Dr. Butts and Dr. Rich, what advice do you have for DNP students or graduates seeking additional information in ethics?

Dr. Rich: There are postgraduate certificate programs in ethics available for graduates. Nurses also can attend intensive ethics programs at major bioethics centers, such as the Kennedy Institute of Ethics at Georgetown University and at the University of Washington. My Five R's approach to ethical nursing practice helps students and graduates increase their knowledge and self-efficacy in ethics: read, reflect, recognize, resolve, and respond. Nurses should not assume that ethics is a matter of subjective opinion. I will give you my Five R's in a nutshell. To cultivate ethical practice, nurses need to do the following: (1) read about ethical philosophy and the ANA's Code of Ethics for Nurses; (2) reflect on their own values, motivations, and attitudes in light of what they read; (3) recognize the bifurcation point when ethical decisions are required, that is, recognize that a situation is ethics laden; (4) resolve to practice intellectual and moral virtues—Aristotle provided basic guidance here; and (5) respond to situations deliberately and habitually as a person with a virtuous character would respond.

Dr. Butts: A certification program in ethics could be advantageous to postgraduates. Faculty and some ethics clinicians have initiated online and hybrid postgraduate ethics certification programs. I encourage more ethics education, but some certification programs are better than others. My advice to postgraduates is to scrutinize the pros and cons of several certification programs before making a decision about which one to begin. I completed an online postmaster's certification ethics program several years ago. It was beneficial for me and facilitated my ethics education.

Dr. Butts and Dr. Rich, as more nurses earn their DNP degrees (more than 200 DNP programs and more than 11,000 students enrolled in DNP programs), do you feel that roles in ethics for DNP graduates are increasing? Have you witnessed any DNP graduates pursuing roles in ethics?

Dr. Rich: I am not seeing our DNP students and graduates pursue a career specifically focused on ethics. Of course, DNP-educated nurses are well suited to be members of ethics committees in healthcare organizations.

Dr. Butts: I agree with Dr. Rich. I have one concern. My wish is for the integration of more ethics in DNP education, thus the eventual initiation of more ethics-specific roles for advanced-practice nurses. We certainly need more opportunities for DNPs to take a lead role in professional and practical ethics.

Dr. Butts and Dr. Rich, do you have any advice a DNP graduate may use to become more involved in roles related to ethics?

Dr. Rich: As I mentioned earlier, I believe DNP graduates should vigorously pursue being included on ethics committees. Also, DNP graduates can take their personal practice experiences related to ethics and develop publications and presentations to disseminate information for discussion and learning in nursing.

    Dr. Butts: To add to Dr. Rich's comments, I believe that dissemination by DNP graduates in the form of discussing and learning ethics should include scenarios that require a much deeper knowledge of ethical foundations and theory with more complex ethical reasoning strategies.

SUMMARY

- Ethics has been broadly defined as the principles of conduct governing an individual or group. More specifically, Butts and Rich define ethics as "the study of ideal human behavior and ideal ways of being" (2008, p. 4).
- Morals, on the other hand, are "specific beliefs, behaviors, and ways of being derived from doing ethics" (Butts & Rich, 2008, p. 5).
- A code of ethics describes standards of conduct and states certain principles regarding responsibilities and duties of those professionals to whom they apply (Pozgar, 2010).
- Values have been defined as "ideals, beliefs, customs, modes of conduct, qualities, or goals that are highly prized or preferred by individuals, groups, or societies" (Burkhardt & Nathaniel, 2008, p. 83).
- Reasoning describes the "use of abstract thought processes to think creatively, to answer questions, solve problems, and to formulate strategies for one's actions and desired ways of being" (Butts & Rich, 2008, p. 9).
- Normative ethics involves prescribing values, behaviors, and ways of being that are considered right or wrong when deciding what to do in a specific situation (Butts & Rich, 2008).
- Applied ethics refers to the application of normative ethics to moral problems (Pozgar, 2010).
- Descriptive ethics is more concrete and describes what one thinks about morality or moral behavior (Butts & Rich, 2008).
- Virtue ethics focuses on the inherent character of a person rather than on specific actions (Pozgar, 2010).
- Natural law theory stems from the philosophy of St. Thomas Aquinas. This theory emphasizes that the "law of reason is implanted in the order of nature (usually thought to be implanted by God)" and provides the rules of human nature (Butts & Rich, 2008, p. 21).

- Deontology, or the study of duty, is an ethical theory that focuses on duties and rules.
- Principlism uses principles that serve as rules for conduct that are dictated by duty.
- Utilitarianism describes actions that are judged by their utility.
- Casuistry describes considering specific situations individually when making ethical decisions.
- Narrative ethics is a story-based approach to making ethical decisions and is similar to casuistry.
- Critical theory broadly describes "theories and worldviews that address the domination perpetrated by specific powerful groups of people and resulting in the oppression of other specific groups of people" (Butts & Rich, 2008, p. 27).
- Bioethics is defined as "the philosophical study of ethical controversies brought about by advances in biology, research, and medicine" (Pozgar, 2010, p. 403).
- In 1974 Congress passed the National Research Act to regulate studies involving human participants.
- As a result of the National Research Act, a commission was created to define the principles supported for research involving human subjects, and a 4-day conference was held at the Belmont Conference Center at the Smithsonian. In 1976 the commission released its report titled the *Belmont Report*. This report outlined three principles for all human subject research: respect for persons, beneficence, and justice (National Commission for the Protection of Human Subjects of Biomedical and Behavioral Research, 1978).
- Personal autonomy has been defined as "self-rule that is free from controlling interference by others and from certain limitations such as inadequate understanding that prevents meaningful choice" (Beauchamp & Childress, 2009, p. 99).
- Informed consent describes the "process by which patients are informed of possible outcomes, alternatives, and risks of treatment, and are required to give their consent freely" (Burkhardt & Nathaniel, 2008, p. 58).
- The principle of beneficence refers to "the moral obligation to act for the benefit of others" (Beauchamp & Childress, 2009, p. 197).
- Paternalism is a form of beneficence and involves individuals or institutions believing they know what is best for the patient or person and thus making decisions for him or her (Pozgar, 2010).
- The principle of nonmaleficence describes the obligation to do no harm.
- The principle of justice refers to "fairness, treating people equally and without prejudice, and with the equitable distribution of benefits and burdens" (Butts & Rich, 2008, p. 48).
- Nursing ethics has been defined as an extension of bioethics where ethical issues are viewed from a nursing perspective (Butts & Rich, 2008).

- The ANA *Code of Ethics for Nurses with Interpretive Statements* is considered the standard for ethical behavior in nursing.
- The ICN *Code of Ethics for Nurses* was initially adopted in 1953. The code is based on the four responsibilities of nurses "to promote health, to prevent illness, to restore health, and alleviate suffering" (ICN, 2006, p. 1).
- Tools for ethical leadership are imperative for the DNP graduate to successfully evaluate ethical scenarios in leadership roles. These tools include traits necessary for ethical leadership, an ethical leadership decision-making tool, and recommendations for avoiding ethical conflicts.
- Ethical scenarios in telehealth may involve many aspects of information technology, such as EMRs, patients seeking information on the Internet, and social networking issues.
- DNP graduates need not only a grasp of ethical content, but also an understanding of information technologies and new developments within telehealth.
- The evaluation of ethical scenarios is a *process* that DNP graduates will need to develop throughout their careers. With experience, understanding of ethical content, and a diligent commitment to upholding the ethical standards of the nursing profession, DNP graduates will become more proficient at this process over time.

REFLECTION QUESTIONS

1. What ethical content do you think is necessary for DNP graduates to understand to effectively evaluate ethical scenarios?

2. Of the four principles of bioethics, which do you think influences your decisions when evaluating ethical scenarios?

3. What character traits do you think are necessary for ethical leadership?

4. Describe some ethical scenarios you are concerned with regarding telehealth. What ethical content would help you evaluate ethical scenarios related to telehealth?

5. Do you agree that evaluating ethical scenarios is a *process*? Why or why not?

6. What types of ethical scenarios do you think you will encounter as a DNP graduate in your setting?

REFERENCES

American Association of Colleges of Nursing. (2006). *Essentials of doctoral education for advanced nursing practice.* Washington, DC: Author. Retrieved from http://www.aacn.nche.edu/publications/position/DNPEssentials.pdf

American Association of Colleges of Nursing. (2008). *Essentials of baccalaureate education for professional nursing practice.* Washington, DC: Author. Retrieved from http://www.aacn.nche.edu/education-resources/BaccEssentials08.pdf

American Association of Colleges of Nursing. (2011). *Essentials of master's education in nursing.* Washington, DC: Author. Retrieved from http://www.aacn.nche.edu/education-resources/MastersEssentials11.pdf

American Nurses Association. (2001). *Code of ethics for nurses.* Silver Spring, MD: Author. Retrieved from http://www.nursingworld.org/MainMenuCategories/EthicsStandards/CodeofEthicsforNurses.aspx

American Nurses Association. (2010a). *Nursing: Scope and standards of practice* (2nd ed.). Silver Spring, MD: Author.

American Nurses Association. (2010b). *Nursing's social policy statement: The essence of the profession.* Silver Spring, MD: Author. Retrieved from http://www.nursesbooks.org/Main-Menu/Foundation/Nursings-Social-Policy-Statement.aspx

American Nurses Association. (2011). 6 tips for nurses using social media. Retrieved from http://www.nursingworld.org/FunctionalMenuCategories/AboutANA/Social-Media/Social-Networking-Principles-Toolkit/6-Tips-for-Nurses-Using-Social-Media-Poster.pdf

Beauchamp, T. L., & Childress, J. F. (2009). *Principles of biomedical ethics* (6th ed.). New York, NY: Oxford University Press.

Buell, J. M. (2009, May/June). Ethics and leadership: Setting the right tone and structure can help others in their decision making. *Healthcare Management Ethics,* 54–57.

Burkhardt, M. A., & Nathaniel, A. K. (2008). *Ethics and issues in contemporary nursing* (3rd ed.). Clifton Park, NY: Delmar Cengage Learning.

Butts, J. B., & Rich, K. L. (2008). *Nursing ethics: Across the curriculum and into practice* (2nd ed.). Sudbury, MA: Jones and Bartlett.

Centers for Disease Control and Prevention. (2011). *The Tuskegee timeline.* Retrieved from http://www.cdc.gov/tuskegee/timeline.htm

Chambliss, D. F. (1996). *Beyond caring: Hospitals, nurses, and the social organization of ethics.* Chicago, IL: University of Chicago Press.

da Vinci, L. (2005). *Leonardo's notebooks* (H. A. Suh, Trans.). New York, NY: Black Dog & Leventhal.

Davis, A. J. (2010). Provision two. In M. D. M. Fowler (Ed.), *Guide to the code of ethics for nurses: Interpretation and application* (pp. 12–21). Silver Spring, MD: American Nurses Association.

Dayer-Berenson, L. (2011). *Cultural competencies for nurses: Impact on health and illness.* Sudbury, MA: Jones & Bartlett Learning.

Drought, T. S., & Epstein, E. G. (2010). Provision seven. In M. D. M. Fowler (Ed.), *Guide to the code of ethics for nurses: Interpretation and application* (pp. 90–102). Silver Spring, MD: American Nurses Association.

Ethic. (2014a). In Merriam-Webster.com. Retrieved from http://www.merriam-webster.com/dictionary/ethics

Ethicist. (2014b). In Merriam-Webster.com. Retrieved from http://www.merriam-webster.com/dictionary/ethicist

Fleming, D. A., Edison, K. E., & Pak, H. (2009). Telehealth ethics. *Telemedicine and eHealth, 15*(8), 797–803.

Forman, E. N., & Ladd, R. E. (1991). *Ethical dilemmas in pediatrics: A case study approach.* New York, NY: Springer-Verlag.

Fowler, M. D. M. (2010). *Guide to the code of ethics for nurses: Interpretation and application.* Silver Spring, MD: American Nurses Association.

Gallagher, A., & Tschudin, V. (2009). Educating for ethical leadership. *Nurse Education Today, 30*(3), 224–227.

Hader, A. L., & Brown, E. D. (2010). Patient privacy and social media. *AANA Journal, 78*(4), 270–273.

iHealthCoalition.org. (2010). *eHealth code of ethics.* Retrieved from http://www.ihealthcoalition.org/ehealth-code/

Institute of Medicine. (2010). *The future of nursing: Focus on scope of practice.* Retrieved from http://www.iom.edu/~/media/Files/Report%20Files/2010/The-Future-of-Nursing/Nursing%20Scope%20of%20Practice%202010%20Brief.pdf

International Council of Nurses. (2006). *Code of ethics for nurses.* Retrieved from http://www.icn.ch/images/stories/documents/about/icncode_english.pdf

Layman, E. J. (2008). Ethical issues and the electronic health record. *The Health Care Manager, 27*(2), 165–176.

National Commission for the Protection of Human Subjects of Biomedical and Behavioral Research. (1978). *The Belmont report.* Washington, DC: U.S. Department of Health, Education, and Welfare. Retrieved from http://videocast.nih.gov/pdf/ohrp_belmont_report.pdf

National Council of State Boards of Nursing. (2011). *A nurse's guide to the use of social media.* Retrieved from https://www.ncsbn.org/NCSBN_SocialMedia.pdf

National Council of State Boards of Nursing. (2013). NCLEX Test Plans. Retrieved from https://www.ncsbn.org/4743.htm

National Organization of Nurse Practitioner Faculties. (2006). *Practice doctorate nurse practitioner entry-level competencies 2006.* Washington, DC: Author. Retrieved from http://c.ymcdn.com/sites/www.nonpf.org/resource/resmgr/competencies/dnp%20np%20competenciesapril2006.pdf

National Public Radio. (2002). Remembering Tuskegee. Retrieved from http://www.npr.org/templates/story/story.php?storyId=1147234

Peirce, A. G., & Smith, J. A. (2008). The ethics curriculum for doctor of nursing practice programs. *Journal of Professional Nursing, 24*(5), 270–274.

Phillips, W., & Fleming, D. (2009). Ethical concerns in the use of electronic medical records. *Missouri Medicine, 106*(5), 328–333.

Piper, L. E. (2007). Ethics: The evidence of leadership. *The Health Care Manager, 26*(3), 249–254.

Pozgar, G. D. (2010). *Legal and ethical issues for health professionals* (2nd ed.). Sudbury, MA: Jones & Bartlett Learning.

Sanford, K. (2006). The ethical leader. *Nursing Administration Quarterly, 30*(1), 5–10.

Schön, D. A. (1987). *Educating the reflective practitioner.* San Francisco, CA: Jossey-Bass.

Silva, M. C., & Ludwick, R. (2006). Ethics: Is the doctor of nursing practice ethical? *The Online Journal of Issues in Nursing, 11*(2). Retrieved from http://www.nursingworld.org/MainMenuCategories/ANAMarketplace/ANAPeriodicals/OJIN/Columns/Ethics/DNPEthical.aspx

Simpson, R. L. (2005). E-ethics: New dilemmas emerge alongside new technologies. *Nursing Administration Quarterly, 29*(2), 179–182.

Skloot, R. (2010). *The immortal life of Henrietta Lacks.* New York, NY: Random House.

U.S. Department of Health and Human Services. (2011). *Summary of the HIPAA privacy rule.* Retrieved from http://www.hhs.gov/ocr/privacy/hipaa/understanding/summary/privacysummary.pdf

U.S. Department of Health and Human Services. (n.d.). Office for Human Research Protections (OHRP). Retrieved from http://www.hhs.gov/ohrp

Wocial, L. D., Bledsoe, P., Helft, P. R., & Everett, L. Q. (2010). Nurse ethicist: Innovative resource for nurses. *Journal of Professional Nursing, 26*(5), 287–292.

Wolfe, L. (2013). How many people use Facebook? Retrieved from http://womeninbusiness.about.com/od/facebook/a/How-Many-People-Use-Facebook.htm

CHAPTER 8

The DNP Graduate as Information Specialist

Catherine Nichols

As we face new challenges regarding healthcare insurance, the delivery of care, a complex healthcare system, and an aging population, the majority of Americans agree that the United States needs major healthcare restructuring. Research by the Commonwealth Foundation, used to inform and guide the development of the Patient Protection and Affordable Care Act (PPACA), showed that 8 out of 10 respondents "agreed that the [U.S.] health system needs either fundamental change or complete rebuilding" (Schoen, Lau, Shih, & How, 2008, p. 1). In addition, in its report *To Err Is Human, Building a Safer Health System*, the Institute of Medicine (IOM) uncovered the magnitude of lives, income, time, and resources lost in the current healthcare system (IOM, 1999).

In 2004 the White House addressed the IOM's report:

> The Institute of Medicine estimates that between 44,000 and 98,000 Americans die each year from medical errors. Many more die or have permanent disability because of inappropriate treatments, mistreatments, or missed treatments in ambulatory settings. Studies have found that as much as $300 billion is spent each year on health care that does not improve patient outcomes—treatment that is unnecessary, inappropriate, inefficient, or ineffective. (White House, 2004, p. 1)

President Bush responded to this shocking report with plans to transform health care through the use of informatics. In his State of the Union Address in 2004, President Bush called for the use of electronic health records (EHR) for every American in every setting to "avoid medical mistakes, reduce health care costs, and improve care" (White House, 2004, p. 1). These three levels of improvements are called the triple aim of health care (Bipartisan Policy Center, 2012). President Bush outlined a 10-year plan for the institution of EHRs and health information exchange technology systems. This plan is known as the Health Information Technology for Economic and Clinical Health Act and became part of the American Recovery and Reinvestment Act of 2009. This was a precursor to the PPACA of 2010

245

(American College of Emergency Physicians, 2013). In an effort to carry out these initiatives, the IOM developed a subsequent report titled *The Future of Nursing: Leading Change, Advancing Health* (2010). The report focused on four key messages to transform both the discipline of nursing and the nation's current healthcare system:

- Nurses should practice to the full extent of their education and training.
- Nurses should achieve higher levels of education and training through an improved education system that promotes seamless academic progression.
- Nurses should be full partners, with physicians and other healthcare professionals, in redesigning health care in the United States.
- Effective workforce planning and policy making require better data collection and information infrastructure. (IOM, 2010)

The IOM's recommendations call for nurses to advance their education, training, and scope of practice and thereby act as change agents in leading the change to ensure safe, quality health care for the nation. Although the fourth recommendation specifically addresses nursing and informatics, the implementation of nursing informatics (NI) will provide a vehicle through which all recommendations can be realized.

Why Information Technology in Nursing

Nurses have been active participants in informatics technology for 25 years (Guenther, 2006). As NI roles evolve, definitions and understanding of NI have changed over the years. In 1984 the phrase *nursing informatics* was first seen in the literature (Guenther, 2006). Understandings of NI began with a narrow definition and a focus solely on the bedside nurse. In 1984 Ball and Hanna developed one of the first definitions of NI as "the use of information technologies in relation to those functions within the purview of nursing, and that are carried out by nurses when performing their duties" (Staggers & Thompson, 2002, p. 256).

Definitions have evolved to include conceptual nursing models and the technical aspect of NI. In 1989 Graves and Corcoran broadened the definition of NI to reflect its value as a force supporting nursing practice and defined NI as "a combination of computer science, information science, and nursing science designed to assist in the management and processing of nursing data, information, and knowledge to support the practice of nursing and the delivery of nursing care" (Staggers & Thompson, 2002, p. 257). Graves and Corcoran's work was among the first to combine nursing information and knowledge, and it was a cornerstone in the development of the Sigma Theta Tau library (Staggers & Thompson, 2002).

NI roles and the nursing discipline continue to evolve and grow and are currently viewed within the larger context of healthcare systems. NI is not merely technology to assist in performing nursing duties or acquiring information, but it is a specialty in its own right that facilitates the interaction and collaboration of the nursing profession within health care and informatics systems.

In 2001 the American Nurses Association (ANA) created a formal definition of nursing information technology (IT) to reflect the change and growth of the nursing discipline. In 2008 the ANA revised the definition to include the concepts of knowledge and wisdom:

> Nursing informatics is a specialty that integrates nursing science, computer science, and information science to manage and communicate data, information, knowledge, and wisdom in nursing practice. Nursing informatics facilitates the integration of data, information, and knowledge to support patients, nurses, and other providers in their decision making in all roles and settings. This support is accomplished through the use of information structures, information processes, and information technology. (ANA, 2008, p. 1)

Developing the ability to access information and acquire knowledge through the use of IT is crucial to nursing and medical practice. However, the mere ability to gain knowledge doesn't guide clinical practice. That's where nursing wisdom plays a role. Wisdom is the nursing attribute that guides the appropriate and ethical application of nursing knowledge within the complexity of healthcare problems or needs (ANA, 2008).

Nursing in Healthcare Informatics

To clarify and fully understand how NI differs from other domains of informatics, it's useful to understand the conceptual model of healthcare informatics. The term *healthcare informatics* is the general, overarching term used to include all disciplines of informatics in health care. In **Figure 8-1** the large oval represents the broad area of healthcare IT and deals with the general "study and management of healthcare informatics" in health care (Saba & McCormick, 2006, p. 267). Under the umbrella term *healthcare informatics* there are four specific disciplines: nursing, medicine, pharmacy, and dentistry. As Figure 8-1 shows, the disciplines are separate, signifying a

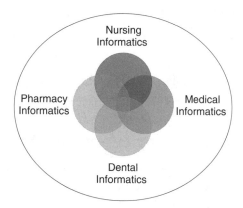

FIGURE 8-1   Healthcare informatics

unique body of IT knowledge for each individual discipline. However, the bodies of knowledge overlap to indicate the areas of IT that are common to each discipline.

The ANA describes NI as a unique discipline that is separate in its foundational theories, knowledge, and practice. The ANA further details the essence of the discipline and its unique attributes:

- Provides a nursing perspective
- Illuminates nursing values and beliefs
- Produces unique knowledge
- Distinguishes groups of practitioners
- Focuses on the phenomena of interest for nursing
- Provides needed nursing language and word context to health informatics (ANA, 2008, pp. 1–2)

Nursing's Response: The Doctor of Nursing Practice

Nursing has responded to the current challenges set forth by the IOM as opportunities to improve healthcare delivery and unite the nursing profession through one terminal nursing degree, the doctor of nursing practice (DNP). The *Essentials of Doctoral Education for Advanced Nursing Practice* (American Association of Colleges of Nursing [AACN], 2006) specifies eight essential elements of education. Although Essential IV specifically addresses IT, Essentials II, III, and V also address various aspects of IT knowledge (AACN, 2006):

- Essential II: Organizational and Systems Leadership for Quality Improvement and Systems Thinking: This essential emphasizes leadership, quality, and safety in the use of IT.
- Essential III: Clinical Scholarship and Analytical Methods for Evidence-Based Practice: This essential emphasizes the use of data analysis for use in clinical practice and, ultimately, care outcomes.
- Essential IV: Information Systems–Technology and Patient Care Technology for the Improvement and Transformation of Health Care: This essential encompasses NI.
- Essential V: Healthcare Policy for Advocacy in Health Care: This essential addresses healthcare policy evaluation for change and development. IT is emphasized as the mode of policy analysis, evaluation, and change.

The DNP-Prepared Nursing Information Specialist

Technology is part of our American culture. It permeates every aspect of our lives: smartphones and apps; texting and tweeting; PCs, iPads, and Kindles; interactive television and entertainment; Skype and video conferences. The current U.S.

healthcare system is no exception to this technology explosion. Within health care there is no lack of data, but there is a lack of utilizing that data to supply quality, efficient patient care. The current U.S. healthcare system is ranked one of the lowest in the world in care quality and efficiency. Among the world's advanced economies, the United States ranks 46 out of 49 in healthcare system efficiency, barely ranking better than Serbia and Brazil. The United States spends the most healthcare dollars with the poorest healthcare outcomes (Bloomberg, 2014).

With advanced education and healthcare systems knowledge, the DNP-prepared nurse is clearly poised at the front line of healthcare leadership and can become a leading force in IT development and delivery. The DNP nursing information specialist can help rescue the current U.S. healthcare system on various levels. First, on the front line of daily clinical practice, DNP NI specialists can use IT to guide their personal practice by utilizing EHRs and accessing personal clinical apps from the Internet. Second, they can serve as data and information managers and IT collaborators for system development and improvement. Third, they can function as informatics innovators, researchers, systems designers, and population health managers (Curran, 2003). DNP information specialists have the advanced education and knowledge to facilitate access to care, care delivery, and quality improvements, and to be accountable for efficiency and spending in the nation's healthcare delivery system.

DNP-Prepared Nursing Information Specialist Roles

Opportunities for nursing information specialists are evolving and growing, and formal roles for IT nurses are in their infancy. Several nursing information specialists roles are as follows:

- Project manager: The project manager analyzes, reviews, revises, and designs current health policy and delivery of care within the existing healthcare system. The NI specialist designs policy and processes according to the nursing scope of practice and healthcare and institutional guidelines. Team building, collaboration, and delegation are key aspects of the project manager's role. The goal of the project manager is to provide evaluation of current processes and systems and their effectiveness, and develop improvements in care quality, efficiency, and patient care outcomes (ANA, 2008).
- Consultant: The NI consultant acts as a resource, supplying specialized knowledge and experience to both internal and external clients. The NI consultant can act as a project manager in designing and developing an informatics system or project, or the consultant may be an assistant to the project manager. Other consulting functions might include designing, implementing, and reviewing NI initiatives. The NI consultant has the

knowledge to review and relay marketing strategies and has the written, oral, and interpersonal skills to provide NI consultative presentations and written reports. Employment opportunities range from hospitals to private practice, academia, corporations, and freelance work (ANA, 2008).

- Educator: NI education is crucial to the success of the information specialist. In this new and developing role, the NI educator is an informatics expert who teaches staff nurses, patients, healthcare leaders, and employees how to use current systems. The educator also instructs nursing students and designs and develops NI courses and curricula in this evolving role. As with the rest of nursing, NI educators are in great need because of the phenomenal expansion of informatics in health care. DNP-prepared nursing information specialists are innovators who are poised to create and promote informatics as part of the nursing discipline (ANA, 2008).

- Researcher: The NI researcher probes every aspect of healthcare informatics. The NI researcher may conduct research on the level of nursing's IT knowledge and effectiveness regarding NI. The NI researcher may also evaluate healthcare outcomes related to patient use of IT (ANA, 2008).

- Product developer: Healthcare systems are quickly learning that information systems, hardware, and software need to be designed and tailored specifically for the healthcare industry to provide efficient, quality, and cost-saving care. The NI product developer designs, develops, and markets these systems for healthcare use. The NI product developer may be employed by a healthcare institution, private practice, or a system and software manufacturer. The DNP-prepared nursing information specialist will have expertise and knowledge of nursing, clinical services, and patient care, as well as advanced understanding of healthcare business and the marketplace (ANA, 2008).

- Decision support and outcomes manager: One way nursing can help shape the future of the U.S. healthcare system is through improving healthcare outcomes. The IOM relays confidence in nursing to do so: "Working together . . . [nurses] can help ensure that the health care system . . . leads to improved health outcomes" (IOM, 2010). The NI specialist can analyze current aggregate data to develop correlations between practices and outcomes measures. These data may then guide theory, policy, practice, and role development (ANA, 2008).

- Advocate and policy developer: Historically, nursing prides itself as the patient advocate at the bedside. Current practice standards set by the ANA in the *Code of Ethics for Nurses* may guide nurses to promote patient advocacy. Provision 3 of the code specifically calls nurses to advocate for the health and rights of the patient (ANA, 2010). The NI advocate and policy developer functions on the international, national, state, local, and organizational levels to design and develop policy regarding the use of healthcare data. Areas of interest include data security, patient safety and anonymity, systems development, and economic aspects. Policy and advocacy are areas of nursing ethics, and the NI specialist has the knowledge and ethical guidance to promote the use of informatics ethically and justly (ANA, 2008).

- Nurse informatics executive: The IOM report on the future of nursing goes far beyond transforming the nursing discipline itself. Nursing is called upon to be a key player in the reformation of the U.S. healthcare system. "As a result, a new type of nurse leader role is emerging: the 'Nurse Informatics Executive'" (Healthcare Information and Management Systems Society [HIMSS], 2014, p. 7). The DNP NI executive embodies the vision to guide the current use of EHRs from a healthcare record to a healthcare documentation system, providing a repository of clinical data. The NI executive can then use the data repository to facilitate improvements in current clinical practice and improve health outcomes (American Organization of Nurse Executives, 2012).

Nursing Informatics as a Specialty

To be fully prepared for one of the NI roles, certification in NI is recommended. In 1995 the American Nurses Credentialing Center (ANCC) established a formal process for NI certification and competencies. The competencies include areas of decision making in client care, research, education, and administration, as well as information and data organizing, processing, analyzing, and communicating (Saba and McCormick, 2006).

Competencies continue to expand and evolve as IT in health care grows exponentially. The ANCC is the official certifying body for nursing informatics. The current prerequisites for certification are as follows:

- Hold a bachelor's or higher degree in nursing or a bachelor's degree in a relevant field.
- Have practiced the equivalent of 2 years full-time as a registered nurse.
- Have completed 30 hours of continuing education in informatics nursing within the last 3 years.
- Meet one of the following practice hour requirements:
  - Have practiced a minimum of 2,000 hours in informatics nursing within the last 3 years.
  - Have practiced a minimum of 1,000 hours in informatics nursing in the last 3 years and completed a minimum of 12 semester hours of academic credit in informatics courses that are part of a graduate-level informatics nursing program.

- Have completed a graduate program in informatics nursing containing a minimum of 200 hours of faculty-supervised practicum in informatics nursing. (ANCC, 2014)

The certification requires nurses to have a solid background and knowledge of IT. Several programs have developed competencies for IT education over the years to facilitate the credentialing of nurses. National NI programs are easily accessible online. A few national organizations worth considering are the Alliance for Nursing Informatics and the International and American Medical Informatics Association (IMIA/AMIA). The AMIA has a working group called Nursing Informatics. The National League for Nursing is an excellent resource for NI programs and educators. Additionally, the HIMSS has developed an informatics certification for healthcare professionals that is not related to nursing, and the eligibility criteria are based on business and management experience, not on health care or nursing experience. Most accredited universities now have nursing informatics courses and programs that can be completed online.

The HIMSS has conducted research regarding NI specialists and role development. They have surveyed NI specialists every 3 years since 2004 in an effort to determine advantages and trends in NI and certification. In 2014 the HIMSS published a report titled *2014 Nursing Informatics Workforce Survey*. The results of this report are encouraging for nursing. A key finding was the reported increase in salary of nearly 20% since 2007, and more than 44% since 2004 (HIMSS, 2014). The average salary of an NI specialist in 2014 was $107,170. It was approximately $15,000 more for nurses who are certified in IT (HIMSS, 2014). The highest-paying positions were found in consulting firms, preferred provider organizations (PPOs) and health maintenance organizations (HMOs), and vendor companies, in that order. In 2013 *U.S. News and World Report* identified NI as one of the "top new college majors for the future" (AllHealthcareDegrees, 2013). AllHealthcareDegrees also reported on the top emerging career opportunities in NI (**Table 8-1**).

TABLE 8-1   Nursing Informatics Career Opportunities

Chief Information Officer	Chief Clinical Information Officer
Director of Nursing Informatics	Nursing Informatics Specialist
Nursing Informatics Analyst	Informatics Nurse Educator
Clinical Decision Support Specialist	Nursing/Health Informatics Consultant
Chief Nursing Information Officer	Implementation Consultant

Source: Data from AllHealthcareDegrees (http://www.allhealthcaredegrees.com/informatics_nursing.htm)

Interview with an NI Leader

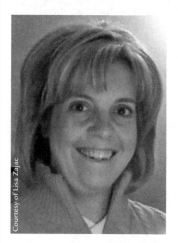

Courtesy of Lisa Zajac

LISA ZAJAC, RN, MSN, ANP-BC, OCN, DNP STUDENT, AND NI SPECIALIST, is an NI pioneer at one of the nation's 41 Designated Comprehensive Cancer Centers accredited by the National Cancer Institute. She currently practices at Karmanos Cancer Institute in Detroit. In this interview she discusses her role as an NI specialist within an oncology healthcare setting.

Ms. Zajac, will you describe your current position and role?

In my current position as the quality, education, and informatics specialist, I oversee nursing education, acute and critical care nursing informatics, and nursing quality at the Karmanos Cancer Center in Detroit, Michigan. Although I have been in this combined role for just over 1 year, I have been involved in informatics since 2010. In my informatics role I was instrumental in the initial design and implementation of, and in the ongoing conversion to, electronic medical records (EMRs) in inpatient areas. In 2013 I was presented with an opportunity to manage the nursing education department and nursing quality initiatives. This innovative approach to blending these areas of responsibility has contributed greatly to the delivery of high-quality patient care at our cancer center.

Ms. Zajac, what was your motivation for pursing your current position?

Although it was difficult to leave direct patient care in 2010, I knew I would be able to indirectly impact all healthcare delivery at my organization. This, combined with the excitement of being able to design and implement an EMR, were the motivating factors. With an EMR, there is always something that can be done to enhance the system to ease the work flow of the end users. Although instant gratification does not occur when implementing anything in the EMR, nothing replaces the feeling I get with successful execution of a new process or function. The motivation for the blended role with nursing education and quality came from my desire to have a larger impact on the quality data from the EMR. I believe that with effective education and correct documentation, the quality of care provided by the patient care staff should be visible throughout the medical record.

Ms. Zajac, how do you see advanced-practice registered nurses (APRNs) affecting the delivery of care using health information technology (HIT) in our nation's healthcare system?

APRNs are in a unique role because, while they don't always possess formal informatics training, they have an extensive background in the patient care delivery system. APRNs play a significant role in HIT by bridging care delivery and documentation in the EMR. For example, I had not had any formal informatics education when I began my role in informatics. I was selected for the role of informatics nursing specialist because of my background in nursing at my place of employment. I came into the role with a history of being a student nurse, registered nurse, and nurse practitioner all at my institutions. I was able to understand the work flow process of the unlicensed assistive personnel, nursing staff, and provider. The informal informatics education was learned on the job. I have learned that when you understand the foundation of the functionality of the EMR, the systems can be designed and implemented with ease.

Ms. Zajac, what motivated you to pursue the DNP degree?

The motivation to pursue the DNP degree came from a combination of my thirst for knowledge and the advice of a mentor. I began my career as an associate's-degree nurse and then earned a bachelor of science degree in nursing, a master of science degree in nursing (MSN) as a primary care nurse practitioner, and a post-MSN certificate as a health educator. It seemed natural that I would go back to school for a terminal degree. When looking into the plans of study, I was intrigued by the DNP, the terminal practice degree. I have always worked in a hospital setting and know that is where I would like to remain throughout my career. Additionally, since my ultimate career goal is to be a nurse executive, when a mentor told me that nurse executives of the future will require a terminal degree, I began my DNP journey.

Ms. Zajac, how will the DNP degree better prepare you for your role in HIT?

At this time, many quality measures and regulatory guidelines depend on the documentation of an assessment, task, or process. By incorporating the Essentials of Doctoral Education for Advanced Nursing Practice *into my practice, HIT will be enhanced in my organization. The blending of information technology with organizational and systems leadership, clinical prevention, interprofessional collaboration for improving patient outcomes, and healthcare policy is required as we move forward with technology in the healthcare setting. Regulatory agencies continue to increase care delivery and documentation requirements. With a DNP degree I will be able to quickly devise and execute the needed EMR enhancements to meet these regulations in any organization.*

Ms. Zajac, where do you see yourself in 5 years, and how is HIT a part of that vision?

In 5 years I hope to have continued my career advancement, moving toward my goal of being a nurse executive. HIT will always be part of my vision because I can see health-care systems becoming more technologically advanced as we head into the future. With my background in nursing informatics, I know I will be an asset to any healthcare organization.

Ms. Zajac clearly brings a nursing perspective of IT to her healthcare institution. She is an example of a nursing pioneer in the developing NI role. She has the vision and systems thinking to adapt and progress as an IT leader. As she continues her lifelong commitment to nursing and Karmanos, Ms. Zajac will guide and educate other NI APRNs, and she can be an inspiration and resource for the future of nursing.

Conclusion

Nursing has historically been called upon to aid an ailing healthcare system. Florence Nightingale had a historical impact on saving lives through evidence-based practice and her groundbreaking work with infection control. Clara Barton used her nursing vision and risked her life to aid a population—the Civil War soldiers on the battleground. Her development of the American Red Cross stands as a beacon to the world for emergency and disaster relief and healthcare needs. Mary Breckenridge developed a rural healthcare delivery system, helping the frontier population to gain access to care. The instances of nurses affecting health and healthcare delivery, both internationally and nationally, are boundless, proving time and again that nursing is a major driving force for healthcare reform.

The 21st century finds itself calling on nursing to affect change. The IOM, the PPACA, and the U.S. Department of Health and Human Services have charged nursing to transform the current broken healthcare system. As leaders, nurses are progressively leading the healthcare industry as nurse executives of major healthcare systems, deans of nursing universities, and members of governmental cabinet and committees. And they are always on the front lines of healthcare provision. The *Essentials of Doctoral Education for Advanced Nursing Practice* are the underpinnings for the future of DNPs to be leaders and pioneers in this frontier of new healthcare delivery. The future of nursing is the future of the American healthcare system. DNP APRNs will lead the way, and they will not let the American people down.

SUMMARY

- The U.S. healthcare system is faced with unprecedented changes and challenges and is in desperate need of restructuring. The IOM published *The Future of Nursing: Leading Change, Advancing Health* in 2010, which outlines nursing's role in restructuring the current healthcare system. The report focuses on four key messages to transform both the discipline of nursing and the nation's current healthcare system.

- The IOM's recommendations call on nurses to advance their education, training, and scope of practice and thereby act as change agents to lead and ensure safe, quality health care for the nation. The implementation of nursing informatics will provide a vehicle through which all recommendations can be realized.

- IT education recommendations are expressed throughout the *Essentials of Doctoral Education for Advanced Nursing Practice*.

- The practice focus of DNP NI specialists ranges from individuals at the bedside to data managers and informatics innovators who design systems and manage population health systems.

- Opportunities for NI specialists are evolving and growing, and formal roles for IT nurses are in their infancy. The ANA has outlined seven NI roles: project manager, consultant, educator, researcher, product developer, decision support and outcomes manager, and advocate and policy developer.

- To be fully prepared for an NI role, certification in NI is prudent. The ANCC established a formal process for NI certification and competencies. Several programs have developed competencies for IT education over the years to facilitate nurse credentialing. Professional organizations and most accredited universities offer IT education, and most programs can be completed online.

- IT certification was shown to increase annual salaries by at least $15,000. The highest-paying IT positions were found in consulting firms, PPO and HMO organizations, and vendor companies, in that order.

- The 21st century finds itself calling on nursing to affect change. The IOM, the PPACA, and the U.S. Department of Health and Human Services have charged nursing to transform the current broken healthcare system. *The Future of Nursing* (IOM, 2010) outlines the future of the American healthcare system. DNP APRNs are clearly poised at the front line of healthcare leadership and will lead changes in the nation's much-needed healthcare reform efforts.

REFLECTION QUESTIONS

1. How do you see using IT in your personal practice to advance health care in your current setting?

2. How do you see the DNP NI specialist changing healthcare delivery systems in the United States?

3. Would you consider involvement in health care as a DNP NI specialist? Why or why not?

4. If so, would you seek IT certification? Why or why not?

5. How can nursing ensure patient confidentiality and enforce Health Insurance Portability and Accountability Act standards in an NI role?

REFERENCES

AllHealthcareDegrees. (2013). *Nursing informatics career overview and degrees.* Retrieved from http://www.allhealthcaredegrees.com/informatics_nursing.htm

American Association of Colleges of Nursing. (2006). *The essentials of doctoral education for advanced nursing practice.* Retrieved from http://www.aacn.nche.edu/dnp/Essentials.pdf

American College of Emergency Physicians. (2013). *Health information technology.* Retrieved from www.acep.org/Advocacy/Health-Information-Technology/

American Nurses Association. (2008). *Nursing informatics: Scopes and standards of practice.* Silver Spring, MD: American Nurses Association.

American Nurses Association. (2010). *Code of ethics for nurses.* Retrieved from http://www.nursingworld.org/MainMenuCategories/EthicsStandards/CodeofEthicsforNurses/Code-of-Ethics.pdf

American Nurses Credentialing Center. (2014). Informatics nursing certification eligibility criteria. Retrieved from http://www.nursecredentialing.org/Informatics-Eligibility.aspx

American Organization of Nurse Executives. (2012). *Position paper: Nursing informatics executive leader.* Retrieved from AONE_Technology_Committee_CNIO_Position_Paper.pdf

Bipartisan Policy Center. (2012). *Transforming health care: The role of health IT.* Retrieved from http://bipartisanpolicy.org/sites/default/files/Transforming%20Health%20Care.pdf

Bloomberg. (2014). Most efficient health care 2014: Countries. Retrieved from http://www.bloomberg.com/visual-data/best-and-worst/most-efficient-health-care-2014-countries

Curran, C. R. (2003). Informatics competencies for nurse practitioners. *Advanced Critical Care, 14*(3). Retrieved from http://journals.lww.com/aacnadvancedcriticalcare/toc/2003/08000

Guenther, J. T. (2006). Mapping the literature of nursing informatics. *Journal of the Medical Library Association.* Retrieved from http://www.ncbi.nlm.nih.gov/pmc/articles/PMC1463042/

Healthcare Information and Management Systems Society. (2014). *2014 nursing informatics workforce survey*. Retrieved from http://www.himss.org/ni-workforce-survey

Institute of Medicine. (1999). *To err is human: Building a safer health system*. Retrieved from https://www.iom.edu/~/media/Files/Report%20Files/1999/To-Err-is-Human/To%20Err%20is%20Human%201999%20%20report%20brief.pdf

Institute of Medicine. (2010). *The future of nursing: Leading change, advancing health*. Retrieved from http://www.iom.edu/Reports/2010/The-future-of-nursing-leading-change-advancing-health.aspx

Saba, V. K., & McCormick, K. A. (2006). *Essentials of nursing informatics* (4th ed.). New York, NY: McGraw-Hill.

Schoen, C., Lau, J., Shih, A., & How, S. K. H. (2008). *Public views on U.S. health system organization: A call for new directions*. Retrieved from http://www.commonwealthfund.org/publications/data-briefs/2008/aug/public-views-on-u-s-health-system-organization-a-call-for-new-directions

Staggers, N., & Thompson, C. B. (2002). The evolution of definitions for nursing informatics: A critical analysis and revised definition. *Journal of the American Medical Informatics Association*, *9*(3), 255–261. Retrieved from http://www.ncbi.nlm.nih.gov/pmc/articles/PMC344585/

White House. (2004). Promoting innovation and competitiveness: Transforming health care: The president's health information technology plan. Retrieved from http://georgewbush-whitehouse.archives.gov/infocus/technology/economic_policy200404/chap3.html

PART II

Professional Issues Related to the Doctor of Nursing Practice Degree

P art I of this text describes the various roles DNP graduates may develop and integrate to meet the demands of today's complex healthcare environment. As these roles are developed, DNP graduates may be faced with unique challenges that result from their distinct educational preparation and goals. These challenges include dealing with issues such as deciding to return to graduate school, the unique challenges and recommendations related to the BSN-DNP pathway to the DNP degree, using the title "doctor," educating others about their educational preparation, marketing themselves as DNP graduates, and discussing the debate and new concerns regarding this innovative degree.

Doctor of Nursing Practice graduates are charged with the responsibility to lead the way. Indeed, the ways in which DNP graduates manage these issues will shape the future of healthcare delivery and nursing education. The following chapters specifically discuss these issues and provide direction regarding the continued transition for DNP graduates.

CHAPTER 9

Do You Want to Go Back to School? Exploring How to Make the Big Decision

Elizabeth Johnston Taylor

Should I incur debt to go back to school? Can I really afford a doctor of nursing practice (DNP) degree? Should I sacrifice time with my family to devote time to school? Can I really spend less time with my family? Should I forfeit my relatively stress-free lifestyle for the more stressful (albeit temporary) life of a DNP student? Can I remain healthfully balanced amidst the stress of school? How much are balance and health important to me? These and myriad other questions are inherent in the decision about whether to return to graduate school for a DNP.

The purpose of this chapter is to support you as you make this big decision. It is a decision that could be life changing. Indeed, by carefully processing this decision—critically examining how and why you make the decision you make—you may find that your self-awareness and perspective on life are enhanced. Life presents tough decisions, such as what career to pursue, whether to discontinue a hurtful relationship, how to spend a large sum of money, and whether to have a child. Studious attention to the decision of whether to go for the DNP will improve your ability to make other big choices in life.

Some readers may have uncertainty about whether to get a DNP degree, and others may have already confirmed their decision. This chapter can help the latter readers by bringing to their awareness the hows and whys of the decision, allowing them to affirm the decision, and increasing their inner motivation. For some the process of decision making will end in a choice to pursue the DNP degree, and for others it may lead to a rejection of further advanced-practice training (even, perhaps, for some who initially think they want it). This author posits that purposeful deliberation, regardless of outcome, is beneficial; nothing in life is wasted.

After a cursory review of some pertinent points for making a DNP decision, this chapter reviews some of the decision-making theory and research and presents selected practical decision-making strategies. Because much of this literature is devoid of the spiritual dimension regarding discernment, advice from spiritual giants about how to make a decision is reviewed. The chapter ends with a discussion of how to live with the decision after it is made.

To Be a DNP or Not to Be: Relevant Facts

You may be an undergraduate or graduate nursing student considering what preparation you need for the nursing career you want. Or you may already be an advanced-practice registered nurse (APRN) and are wondering whether to obtain further education. Your question may be whether to become a master's- or doctorate-prepared APRN. If you want a doctorate, you may be wondering whether to obtain the DNP or the PhD degree (or another more research-oriented doctorate). If you are a bachelor of science in nursing (BSN) graduate, you may be concerned about the time commitment involved with a BSN-to-DNP path.

Most nurses who choose the DNP over the PhD do so because their primary interest is in promoting excellence in clinical practice rather than scholarship (Loomis, Willard, & Cohen, 2007). Others choose the DNP degree because it requires less time; it is impractical for an APRN who is in the last several years of his or her career to invest in a DNP. Some find confirmation of their preference for an advanced-practice career when they perceive that PhD professors are occupants of an ivory tower, and they yearn for instruction that enhances their abilities to improve clinical care (Loomis et al., 2007).

Grandfathering

For those who are choosing between the DNP and remaining as master's-prepared APRNs, there may be worry that after 2015 they will not be able to continue to practice as APRNs. In their review of the issues surrounding the implementation of the DNP degree, Fulton and Lyon (2005) identified the need to reassure master's-prepared APRNs that they will be grandfathered—they will be able to continue to practice without additional education. Subsequently, the American Association of Colleges of Nursing (AACN) mandated a DNP Roadmap Task Force to explore this and other issues in transitioning toward 2015. The task force report (accepted by the AACN in July 2006) says, "State and national regulatory boards are encouraged to review all statutes and regulations governing advanced or specialty nursing practice and clarify language to require a graduate level degree as minimum preparation for practice as an APN" (American Association of Colleges of Nursing [AACN], 2006, p. 21).

However, each state's board of nursing determines the regulations under which APRNs may practice. Portability of state licensure may be a concern. APRNs "must then consider closely their future and decide if mobility is important, as well as how long they wish to practice" (Clinton & Sperhac, 2009). Although licensure may be grandfathered, APRNs must also consider if employers who seek DNP-prepared APRNs will value experience over the DNP degree (Clinton & Sperhac, 2009).

The AACN *Consensus Model for APRN Regulation: Licensure, Accreditation, Certification & Education* (2008) describes the graduate educational requirement for APRN practice as a master's or doctorate degree in nursing. Although future law cannot be guaranteed, it is clearly the intent of the AACN to promote grandfathering. Indeed, grandfathering has historically been a necessary component of transitions such as this.

Decision-Making Research

The study of decision making has advanced substantially over the past few decades. Although it started as a topic for psychologists and economists, decision science now is a very widely encompassing multi- and interdisciplinary field. Researchers are investigating not only the economic, ethical, and sociopsychological aspects of decision making, but also the neurobiological processes involved in decision making.

Here is a smattering of findings from recent research (albeit isolated studies) on decision making:

- When an environment feels normal, trustable, and safe, a decision maker with a trusting state of mind will tend to make the decision using routine decision-making strategies and outperform a distrusting decision maker. Conversely, when a person is in an unusual situation that would benefit from a nonroutine decision-making strategy, a distrustful stance works best (Schul, Mayo, & Burnstein, 2008).
- Whether information is framed positively or negatively influences a decision maker. For example, when adults were asked whether they would choose resuscitation or comfort care for a premature baby, those who were presented with the baby's survival data were apt to decide on resuscitation, whereas those who were presented with the negativity of mortality data were likely to choose comfort care. Except for the participants who were highly religious, the framing significantly influenced their decision making (Haward, Murphy, & Lorenz, 2008).
- Persons who are indecisive have tunnel vision that limits how they gather information during the process of making a decision. They tend to limit their data collection to data that supports what they ultimately choose (Rassin, Muris, Booster, & Kolsloot, 2008).

- A sad mood while making a decision usually prompts people to analyze information very carefully before making a decision, and a happy mood tends to contribute to decisions that are based more on feelings and intuition. When there is a matchup of mood and decision-making strategy, the decision maker values the decision outcome more than when there is a mismatch of mood and strategy (de Vries, Holland, & Witteman, 2008).
- A biologic basis has been established that shows emotion plays an integral role in decision making (van 't Wout, Kahn, Sanfey, & Aleman, 2006).

This bit of psychological research highlights some aspects to consider as you begin your decision making. You may want to think about how you or others are positively framing this decision (and how you frame it for your family). Likewise, this research should stimulate you to consider how you might be using tunnel vision and narrowing your options prematurely or to notice what mood you are in and how it affects your decision making.

Practical Tools for Decision Making

Several practical strategies have been developed to guide an individual or group in making a decision. These strategies can help managers make business decisions, and they can also help individuals make important personal decisions. Many of these strategies are presented in an easy-to-use format on the Mind Tools website (http://www.mindtools.com). Because of their simplicity and fit for the decisions surrounding DNP education, the following strategies will be described and illustrated here: Force Field Analysis, Thinking Hats, and Grid Analysis.

Force Field Analysis

Mark Lee, MSN, APRN, is a 33-year-old who is working full time in a public health clinic. He is happily married to Sue, who stays at home with their twin toddlers. Although he is fairly content with his level of clinical knowledge, he is naturally curious and interested in learning more about healthcare policy, research utilization, and ethics. Plus, to be really honest, he would love to be a doctor. Mark knows that if he could, he would go for the DNP degree. Sue, however, is seriously concerned that his doing so would make their marriage and financial situation suffer. He questions, "Should I get the DNP? Is it appropriate to let my family suffer, even for a few years? Should I ask my wife to go to work and put the kids in day care?"

Force Field Analysis is a decision-making strategy that requires one to specify the desired plan and then identify the forces that support the plan and the forces that are working against it. When this is done, assign a score to each force using a scale of 1 (weak) to 5 (strong). **Figure 9-1** illustrates Force Field Analysis by showing how Mark might weigh the pros and cons of getting a DNP degree.

Forces Supporting Plan	Plan	Forces Against Plan
+1 Wife benefiting from social connectedness at work ⇑	**To get the DNP while minimally stressing himself and his family; wife working part-time while twins are in preschool**	⇓ Less time for wife, marriage stressed −3
+1 Kids supposedly benefit from part-time preschool ⇑		⇓ Less engaged with kids' development during pivotal years of their lives −3
+1 Increased income potential after DNP ⇑		⇓ Financial debt for several years −3
+3 Increased marketability and prestige with DNP ⇑		
+4 Personal benefit of stimulating academic experience ⇑		
+10	*versus*	−9

FIGURE 9-1   Mark Lee's Force Field Analysis

Mark's analysis suggests that, by one point, forces favor him pursuing the DNP degree. Given how close the pros and cons balance each other out, however, Mark will want to explore ways that he can minimize the negative forces, especially the strong ones. In this case, for example, he may want to consider how he and his wife can shore up their marriage before the DNP program starts or receive marriage counseling on how to allow stress to strengthen their marriage. Or Mark may choose a DNP program that allows him more time around his twins (i.e., distance and part-time programs). Likewise, Mark and Sue may decide to downsize their living accommodations to save money. Force Field Analysis leads one to see the changes that could be implemented to minimize negative forces and promote positive forces.

Thinking Hats

Sarah Brown, BSN, RN, is a 24-year-old intensive care nurse with 2 years of nursing experience. She realizes that she does not want to work in an acute care setting much longer and is quite sure she would love to work as an APRN in some sort of outpatient clinic. She knows from visiting the AACN website and talking with the recruiter from a university in her city that getting a DNP degree is definitely the way to go. She is unmarried and lives near her parents. She still owes about $30,000 on the loan she got for her BSN degree. Although there is a DNP program in her city, she is attracted to the curriculum at a DNP program in a city several hours away. Sarah is wondering,

"Should I get the DNP now or later? Should I get it from the local university or from the one several hours away? Is it fiscally wise to get the DNP now?"

Thinking Hats is a decision-making strategy devised by Edward de Bono (http://www.deBonoConsulting.com). It is a strategy that allows one to systematically look at a decision from several different perspectives or with different styles of thinking, not just the habitual way. That is, one puts on each of the following hats during the process of decision making:

- White hat, which encourages intellectual analysis. What do I know from the past that could influence the present situation? What factual information do I need to make a good decision? For example, Sarah would calculate the expenses involved in studying full time versus part time and of moving to be near the preferred program versus commuting to it—and check to see if commuting is even possible. She would carefully compare all the curricula of the competing programs. She would project her financial future given her added debts and potential increased income with a DNP degree. She would examine financial aid packages.

- Red hat, which respects intuition and emotional inclinations. For example, Sarah would more deeply explore her gut response to each of the DNP programs that she is considering. She would also do well to listen to her inner energy, to decide if it is best to save more energy or to spend it now on the DNP program.

- Black hat, which supports a pessimistic stance and thereby allows one to see the fatal flaws or pitfalls and develop contingency plans. For example, Sarah would do well to think about the emotional and financial hardships of doing the DNP program now versus later. (Going to school now might mean feeling the pain of leaving her parents and known community and incurring further debt. Choosing to postpone her education could mean it might be compromised by the distraction of marriage or childbearing.)

- Yellow hat, which encourages positivity, optimism, and a look at what might be the benefits of the options being considered. Sarah might compare the positives of starting a DNP program now versus later (e.g., getting it done while she is unmarried, increased earning potential sooner versus paying off immediate debt, and enjoying a less stressful life now). She can also compare the positives of studying locally instead of away from home (e.g., the comfort of being home in contrast with the benefit of cutting the apron strings).

- Green hat, which symbolizes energy for creativity and thinking outside the box about options. For example, Sarah might consider ways to pursue the DNP program while living at home or in inexpensive living accommodations to minimize her debts. She might also consider how she can live near her parents and loved ones and still attend the DNP program that is more distant. Or she might look elsewhere for long-distance programs or weekend programs that would allow her to continue to work.

- Blue hat, which is the control or process-oriented thinking that decision making requires. For example, if Sarah observes that she is focusing on all the positives, she may realize that putting on the black hat would be helpful; if she senses she is stuck on a problem that she wishes to eliminate, she may put her green hat on.

The Thinking Hats strategy fosters self-awareness about the different perspectives that are all essential to use in a decision-making process. A decision should not be only a rational decision. It must also recognize the value of intuition, thinking outside the box, and even pessimism.

Grid Analysis

Kim Fitzhugh, BSN, RN, is a 40-year-old volunteer parish nurse at a large local congregation. She quit the stressful work of staff nursing on an oncology unit when she began suffering from chronic fatigue and fibromyalgia syndromes 2 years ago. She feels that she is recovering and is eager to do something. The idea of working in an academic setting stirs her passion. Her four children (ages 10–16 years) are all in school, yet she wants to be there for them physically and emotionally when they are home. (To work as an academic would be less physically challenging and would mean flexible work hours and an academic calendar that synchronizes with her children's school year.) Her husband, who is probably eager to see her become "normal" again, is supportive of her returning to school for a DNP degree. The DNP program would pose minimal financial threat to Kim's family. Part-time and full-time DNP programs are available to Kim, but she is ambivalent: "Can I really do this? What if it makes me relapse? And then that prevents me from keeping close to the kids! And can I do the DNP without sacrificing the quality of my relationships with my teenagers? Should I really quit the parish nursing? It's been so fulfilling for me, and I am so close to the people of the congregation. And dare I go full time, or should I try part time and take forever to get through? Or should I be content with a master of science in nursing (MSN) degree, which would make me less marketable to a nursing school?"

Grid Analysis (or Decision Matrix Analysis) is an especially helpful strategy when there are several options to choose from and multiple factors to consider. This strategy requires you to list all the possible options being decided (in rows) and then identify all the factors that are important to consider (in columns). Each factor should then be given a weight between 0 (not at all important) and 5 (extremely important). When this grid is established, you can use the same scoring system to give a score to each option for each of the factors. That is, you can ask how an option

Options	FACTORS (WEIGHTS):					
	Health (5)	Personal fulfillment with further education (2)	Satisfying/ flexible work outside home (3)	Want to please husband (1)	Time with children (4)	Totals (Factor × Option):
DNP full time, quit PN role	1 (5) = 5	5 (2) = 10	5 (3) = 15	3 (1) = 3	3 (4) = 12	45
DNP part time, may need to quit PN role	3 (5) = 15	5 (2) = 10	5 (3) = 15	4 (1) = 4	4 (4) = 16	60
MSN, likely to need to quit PN role	3 (5) = 15	4 (2) = 8	4 (3) = 12	4 (1) = 4	4 (4) = 16	55
Be content with BSN only, keep PN role	5 (5) = 25	0 (2) = 0	2 (3) = 6	2 (1) = 2	5 (4) = 20	53

FIGURE 9-2   Kim Fitzhugh's grid analysis strategy

allows you to meet or satisfy the factor. When each factor has been scored, multiply that score by the weight you have already assigned to that factor. Finally, you add all the scores for each row (i.e., each option). The row or option with the highest score may be the best choice.

The Grid Analysis strategy is illustrated in **Figure 9-2** using Kim's situation. Of course, more factors could be added, and pursuing the MSN degree full time and part time could have been included as options. Using this strategy, however, shows that Kim's best option is to choose part-time DNP study. This strategy brings to full awareness how much health is a pivotal factor for her decision; she weighted it as 5. Thus, Kim may predetermine some contingency plans in case the part-time DNP study is too stressful for her body. This process may also make plain that dropping the parish nurse role is one way Kim can increase her chances of staying healthy and pursuing her professional goals.

Consulting Others

Although these techniques imply that you will get information from others to make your decision, it is indeed pivotal that you consult others in your close circle of family and friends as you make this decision. Your family members who are significantly affected by the outcome of this decision should be integrally involved in the decision making if mutual respect and harmony are to be maintained in the relationship. Although it is perhaps less important, it can be extremely helpful to consult friends who can honestly give you feedback on your decision-making process and on their observations about who you authentically are and how that ought to inform the decision, or they can simply be a sounding board. When discussing your decision with others, try to keep an open or neutral stance toward your decision so you can more fully hear what your friend or loved one is saying.

Spiritual Approaches to Decision Making

Although systematic strategies such as those previously described are invaluable for making a big decision, they can fail to respect the spiritual element of decision making. Given that most Americans (and hence, most nurses) describe themselves as at least moderately spiritual (Gallup & Jones, 2002; Wuthnow, 1998)—and for many this means religious—it is important to consider spiritual approaches to decision making. Spirituality explains the human quest for purposefulness of work, the need for a reason or mission for living, a desire for inner peace and joy, a desire to connect with and serve others, and a yearning for harmony with others, nature, and an ultimate other (Taylor, 2002). (Given the predominance of the term *God* in American society [Gallup & Jones, 2002], that language will be used subsequently in this discussion.) Decision making that fails to recognize these spiritual yearnings is incomplete and may lead to outcomes that are not congruent with what is ultimately important for the individual. Therefore, for those who experience this spiritual aspect of personhood, it is vital that spiritual approaches and strategies be included in decision making.

Steps in a Spiritual Approach to Decision Making

Although the following steps are somewhat linear, they are better envisioned as concurrent aspects of a decision-making process. They might also be better thought of as subgoals. The primary goal of a spiritual approach to decisions is coorientation, communion, and collaboration with God, or a beckoning to listen to the inner light or inner wisdom. Although sometimes decisions are agonizing, they nevertheless manifest a God whose love means the freedom to choose.

A difficult decision can be viewed as an opportunity to intensely encounter God. In contrast, some might find that making a decision from a spiritual perspective is about trying to maintain control (but attributing control to God's will) or about abdicating the decision to God (and the default answer becomes God's will). Regardless, how an individual makes a decision will speak volumes about how that person relates to and perceives God.

STEP 1: ASSUMING HUMILITY

Spiritual giants of centuries ago advise that seeking humility is essential as one faces an important decision. Catherine of Siena, for example, stressed how one should assume a stance of respecting the allness and centrality of God in the universe instead of the prideful position of self-centeredness (Schneiders, 1982). Ignatius of Loyola wrote that such humility "occurs when I do not find myself desiring riches more than poverty, honour more than dishonour, a long life more than a short one, and feel that the service of our Lord God and the salvation of my soul are equally important" (Backhouse, 1989, p. 39). The rationale for such humility is that it is required to be able to take a neutral or indifferent position toward the outcome of the decision-making process.

STEP 2: REACHING NEUTRALITY

Having such a neutral position toward the decision will allow the decision maker to recognize and weigh determining factors objectively. This is not to undermine the value of feelings that should inform a decision but to encourage the decision maker to consider the meaning of the feelings while holding them in check. Ideally, the decision maker will arrive at a perch atop a fulcrum where there is a sense that life will be good regardless of which outcome is chosen (Ignatius, as cited in Backhouse, 1989).

STEP 3: CONSIDERING PERSONAL CONTEXT: PURPOSE OF LIFE

When deciding whether or not to pursue a DNP degree, it is beneficial to stage this question in the context of what is the bigger picture: what do you think is the purpose for your existence? For some the answer may be very specific: to help find a cure for cancer. For others, it may be broad but nevertheless clear: "to praise, reverence, and serve our Lord God," as Ignatius of Loyola believed (Backhouse, 1989, p. 39). Regardless of what your life purpose is, it is essential that your decision for or against the DNP line up with this life purpose.

When thinking about vocation or purpose in life, it is necessary to think about who we are. That is, who we are authentically. McGraw describes it this way:

> The authentic self is the you that can be found at your absolute core. It is the part of you that is not defined by your job, or your function, or your role. It is the composite of all your unique gifts, skills, abilities, interests, talents, insights, and wisdom. It is all your strengths and values that are uniquely yours and need expression, versus what you have been programmed to believe that you are "supposed" to be and do. It is the you that flourished, unself-consciously, in those times in your life when you felt happiest and most fulfilled. It is the you that existed before and remains when life's pain, experiences, and expectancies are stripped away. (2001, p. 30)

As one considers whether or not to become a DNP, knowing whether it fits one's life purpose is vital, and one's life purpose will inherently match up with who one is authentically (McGraw, 2001).

Self-exploration to discover or reaffirm one's authentic self is expedient during the decision-making process. Exercises that can help one to become more aware of the authentic self, and hence one's vocation and purpose, include the following:

- List all the qualities, talents, and personality traits that describe you. Circle the ones that you sense, deep down, are really you.
- List all your roles. Cross off the ones that do not bring joy because they do not allow you to be you. (Remember that roles are distinct from relationships.)
- Write your obituary. Then write down what you need to do so the obituary will be realized.

Getting to know your authentic self will not only help you make a decision regarding your education, but it will also guide you at other times to make choices that are consistent with who you are.

STEP 4: CONSIDERING PROS AND CONS IN LIGHT OF LIFE'S PURPOSE

Given your newfound appreciation for who you are and what your life purpose is, proceed to listing the positives and negatives associated with the choices you face.

Follow a strategy such as the one previously described. Hold your preferences or biases in check. Consider the options in the context of how they conform to who you are created to be and to what you sense your life's purpose to be. If you share Ignatius's life purpose, you would ponder the options in terms of which one would most glorify and praise God.

The 19th-century Protestant cleric Oswald Chambers, in his popular devotional book, suggested further reference points for those who are facing decisions. His writing suggests that the following guidelines be considered (Chambers, 1992):

- The choice that requires a huge amount of faith and courage, forcing you to lean, trust, depend, and rely on God more, may likely be where God is leading. For this will stretch and challenge you, helping you to grow and become more authentic.
- The choice that is new and frightening, perhaps something that you never thought possible, may well be the way God is leading.
- Usually God's leading involves a steady, quiet persistence in the direction God wills. Your heart is at peace when you consider it.

As Chambers indicates, often what is the best choice is also the hardest choice. Indeed, those decisions in life that are agonizing are often so because we are resisting what seems to be the most difficult choice.

BOX 9-1

Questions to Guide a Spiritual Approach to Decision Making

- Which option allows me to live more fully, authentically, more wholly and holy?
- At my deepest level, what do I want? Which option would make me feel most free inside?
- What effect will the choice have on life's meaning?
- What is my body saying?
- What does my wisest elder (an internal or external sage) say?
- How do mind, body, and spirit line up with an answer? What do my head and heart say when considered in concert?
- Which option do I sense would bring consolation (versus desolation)—a sense of inner peace, a lightness?
- Which option energizes me and makes me feel at rest inside?
- Which choice would foster greater humility (versus pride)? Which choice would encourage trust and communion with God?
- If I were on my future death bed, what would I advise myself to do today?
- If I were at the Last Judgment (or at an imagined time when your ultimate worth and goodness are calculated), what would I retrospectively choose for now?

A list of questions that can support your decision making is offered in **Box 9-1**. Using these questions as a starting point for prayerful meditation or journal writing may prove to be very informative.

STEP 5: LISTENING AFTER THE DECISION IS MADE

When possible, it is good to allow time to live with a decision before it is made public and action is taken to implement it. A good decision is one that brings consolation or initiates interior movement toward one's creator and strengthens the soul—versus desolation or an increased slothfulness of heart and inner darkness, as Ignatius described it (Backhouse, 1989). Listen to your heart (inner wisdom or God) to sense how your choice rests inside. Offer your choice up to God for a blessing. An inner peace may come that affirms your choice. No response may be evident within; God may be stretching you to make a leap of faith.

If you experience discomfort or doubt the decision, it may indicate you have made the wrong choice. Recognize the source of those feelings; many decisions inherently mean loss as well as gain. For example, if you have made a decision to move to another city to pursue the DNP degree and sense that your decision is what best praises God, you will undoubtedly also mourn the losses that will occur in moving on. Recognizing the source of your grief will allow you to make the transition without waffling.

You may notice other indicators of good decisions. In addition to consolation, you will notice that you have patience with the ensuing challenges and chaos that the decision may bring. This patience results from the inner peace of living a congruent and faith-filled life. You may also notice within you more reverence toward all things.

Spiritual Tools for Decision Making

A spiritually sensitive person will find several tools that support the decision-making process. Among these tools are prayer and meditation, journal writing, spiritual direction, and dream reflection.

PRAYER AND MEDITATION

One typology of prayer suggests that Americans use petitionary, ritual, conversational, and meditational prayer (Poloma & Gallup, 1991). Although petitionary and ritual prayers are often used during times of crisis, conversational and meditational prayers are more helpful to decision making. Conversational prayer (likely the most common form of prayer in America) is characterized by an individual thinking or verbalizing his or her inner experience for God. Just as human-to-human conversation involves both expression and listening, so does conversation with God. A sense of desolation or getting stuck saying the same things repeatedly are indicators that conversational prayer is one sided.

Meditational prayer, which focuses on listening to God, can ameliorate this condition. Meditational prayer can involve simply spending time in nature or some quiet, sacred space with your heart open toward God. There is no agenda other than to be attentive to whatever may nudge your attention (e.g., a thought, a leaf, the warmth of the sun, a bird's song). Assuming such a receptive and neutral stance allows one to be available to God-sent impressions and insights that are pertinent to the decision.

JOURNAL WRITING

Keeping a journal that is private, unstructured, and unedited can allow you to document not only the various analytical strategies (previously discussed) but to record your feelings, thoughts, and informal observations about your inner life and struggle. The journal can also allow you to record your dreams, conversations, readings, and other sources of insight. For some, it is not until these inner processes get concretized in writing that the best insight occurs. Also, rereading the journal can allow you to see recurrent themes that you otherwise might fail to acknowledge.

SPIRITUAL DIRECTION

Spiritual directors or mentors are soul friends or holy listeners. These lay or professionally trained spiritual directors typically have studied spiritual formation and counseling to some degree. Someone who intentionally desires spiritual development will seek out a spiritual director on a regular basis (e.g., once per month), and an individual amidst the crisis of making a major decision may want biweekly visits with a spiritual director. These sessions (typically 1 hour) will allow the decision maker to explore how to discern God's will, which may lead to discussion about how to encounter God or how God is perceived. A spiritual director can give tips on how to meditate, how to explore one's inner life, and provide support as the seeker draws up courage to make a difficult choice. You can find a spiritual director by consulting the Spiritual Directors International website at www.sdiworld.org.

DREAM REFLECTION

Although a discussion of how to analyze and make sense of your dreams is beyond the scope of this chapter, it is valuable to remember that your dreams will provide you with extremely helpful information during your decision-making process. Your dreams may tell you what you are not able to recognize in waking life. They, in a sense, will help you know your authentic self. A good spiritual director or a trained therapist can assist you, and there are several excellent books on the topic to guide you (e.g., Berne & Savary, 1991; Sanford, 1978).

Living with the Decision

Regardless of the option a decision maker chooses, there are potentially ensuing problems or imperfections. Just because a choice leads to seemingly insurmountable challenges does not mean it is the wrong choice. To address such challenges, it is good to keep centered on what prompted the choice in the first place; that is, to remember how this choice lines up with your overall mission in life and allows fulfillment of who you really are. Victor Frankl (1984) was fond of quoting Nietzsche, who posited, "He who has a why to live for can bear almost any how." Indeed, if your decision supports your overall life purpose, you will find it easier to bear the hardships that result from it.

If your decision-making process leads you to choose the DNP degree, there are ways to cope with the stressors of schooling. Some of them include the following:

- Focusing on what you have yet to do rather than on what you have done to date. According to Koo and Fishbach's (2008) research, this frame of mind is associated with greater goal adherence.
- Simplifying your life. This may require you to think outside the box. Have no more than three foci in your life (e.g., school, family, work). This may require you to resign much-loved roles and forfeit some activities that are wonderful.

You might ask yourself if you would rather do a few things well or several things poorly. If living simply means earning a lower income, find the joy in having less money. (Home cooked beans and rice can taste delicious, and old cars may be less likely to be stolen!)

- Delegating some tasks that are not necessary for you to do. Draw together a supportive network of family and friends who can help you with such tasks and support you emotionally.

- Accepting that you may need to be more disciplined than ever now. You may need to restrict your television viewing, eliminate sweets and high-fat foods that make you sluggish or depressed, and exercise and drink water much more to enhance your energy level.

- Appreciating that the best grade for you in courses may be a B (for balance). Although you always want to do your best, your best while maintaining a balanced life may be not to earn top grades.

Such suggestions for coping with the challenges of DNP study require a proactive (rather than reactive) stance.

Conclusion

This chapter describes some classic strategies for making a decision. It also emphasizes the importance of considering the underlying spirituality inherent in decisions, such as whether to pursue a DNP degree. Although the outcome of a decision will shape who you become, it is just as true that the process of making a decision will reflect who you are. Thus, this decision presents you with an opportunity to reflect on who you have been and who you want to be.

SUMMARY

- Most people who choose the DNP over the PhD do so because their primary interest is in promoting excellence in clinical practice rather than scholarship (Loomis et al., 2007). Others choose the DNP because it requires less time; it is impractical for an APRN to invest in a DNP degree in the last several years of his or her career.

- Although future law cannot be guaranteed, it is clearly the intent of the AACN to promote grandfathering. That is, if you are an APRN now, it is unlikely that you will need a DNP degree to remain an APRN.

- Research about decision making suggests it is important to consider if you are positively or negatively framing the options, your emotions that will influence the decision making, and how you might be using tunnel vision and narrowing your options prematurely.

- Force Field Analysis is a decision-making strategy that requires one to specify the desired plan and then identify the forces that support that plan and the forces that are working against it (i.e., systematically weigh the pros and cons).

- Thinking Hats analysis allows one to look at a decision from several different perspectives or with different styles of thinking (e.g., intellectual, intuitive, optimistic, pessimistic, outside the box).

- Grid Analysis requires you to list all the possible options being decided (in rows) and then identify all the factors that are important to consider (in columns). Each factor should then be given a weight between 0 (not at all important) and 5 (extremely important). When this grid is established, you can then use the same scoring system to give a score to each option for each of the factors.

- Decision making that fails to recognize spiritual yearnings is incomplete and may lead to outcomes that are not congruent with what is ultimately important for the individual.

- A difficult decision can be viewed as an opportunity to intensely encounter God.

- As one considers whether or not to become a DNP, knowing whether it fits one's life purpose is vital.

- Often the best choice (e.g., that which will stretch us, humble us, transform us) is also the hardest choice. The decisions in life that are agonizing are often so because we are resisting what seems to be the most difficult choice.

- Tools that a spiritually sensitive decision maker may find helpful include prayer and meditation, journal writing, spiritual direction, and dream reflection.

- Just because a choice leads to seemingly insurmountable challenges does not mean it is the wrong choice. To address such challenges, it is good to keep centered on what prompted the choice in the first place; that is, to remember how this choice lines up with your overall mission in life and allows fulfillment of who you really are.

REFLECTION QUESTIONS

1. What are the reasons for why I want further education? (Go deep to the most fundamental reasons. For example, you may initially answer with "because I want to know more." Then ask yourself why you want to know more.)

2. What is the principal purpose for my existence? What is my mission in life? How might getting a DNP degree (or not) contribute to my life vocation or mission?

3. Whose input about this decision do I value? What impressions do they have about my returning to school?

4. How am I relating to this decision? Is it bringing dread? Does it excite me? How will the rest of my life be affected by this decision?

5. Please see **Box 9-1** for further reflective questions that are important to the decision-making process.

REFERENCES

American Association of Colleges of Nursing. (2006). *Doctor of nursing practice roadmap task force report.* Retrieved from http://www.aacn.nche.edu/dnp/roadmapreport.pdf

American Association of Colleges of Nursing. (2008). *Consensus model for APRN regulation: Licensure, accreditation, certification & education.* Retrieved from http://www.aacn.nche.edu/education-resources/APRNReport.pdf

Backhouse, H. (Ed.). (1989). *The spiritual exercises of St. Ignatius Loyola.* London, England: Hodder & Stoughton.

Berne, P. H., & Savary, L. M. (1991). *Dream symbol work: Unlocking the energy from dreams and spiritual experiences.* New York, NY: Paulist Press.

Chambers, O. (1992). *My utmost for his highest: An updated edition in today's language: The Golden book of Oswald Chambers.* Grand Rapids, MI: Discovery House.

Clinton, P., & Sperhac, A. M. (2009). The DNP and unintended consequences: An opportunity for dialogue. *Journal of Pediatric Health Care, 23*(5), 348–351.

de Vries, M., Holland, R. W., & Witteman, C. L. M. (2008). Fitting decisions: Mood and intuitive versus deliberative decision strategies. *Cognition & Emotion, 22*(5), 931–943.

Frankl, V. (1984). *Man's search for meaning.* New York, NY: Washington Square Press.

Fulton, J. S., & Lyon, B. L. (2005). The need for some sense making: Doctor of nursing practice. *Online Journal of Issues in Nursing, 10*(3). Retrieved from http://www.nursingworld.org/MainMenuCategories/ANAMarketplace/ANAPeriodicals/OJIN/TableofContents/Volume102005/No3Sept05/tpc28_316027.aspx

Gallup, G., Jr., & Jones, T. (2002). *The next American spirituality: Finding God in the twenty-first century.* New York, NY: NexGen.

Haward, M. F., Murphy, R. O., & Lorenz, J. M. (2008). Message framing and perinatal decisions. *Pediatrics, 122*(1), 109–118.

Koo, M., & Fishbach, A. (2008). Dynamics of self-regulation: How (un)accomplished goal actions affect motivation. *Journal of Personality and Social Psychology, 94*(2), 183–195.

Loomis, J. A., Willard, B., & Cohen, J. (2007). Difficult professional choices: Deciding between the PhD and the DNP in nursing. *Online Journal of Issues in Nursing, 12*(1), 6. Retrieved from http://www.nursingworld.org/MainMenuCategories/ANAMarketplace/ANAPeriodicals/OJIN/TableofContents/Volume122007/No1Jan07/ArticlePreviousTopics/tpc28_816033.aspx

McGraw, P. C. (2001). *Self matters: Creating your life from the inside out.* New York, NY: Simon & Schuster.

Poloma, M. M., & Gallup, G. H., Jr. (1991). *Varieties of prayer: A survey report.* Philadelphia, PA: Trinity Press.

Rassin, E., Muris, P., Booster, E., & Kolsloot, I. (2008). Indecisiveness and informational tunnel vision. *Personality and Individual Differences, 45*(1), 96–102.

Sanford, J. A. (1978). *Dreams and healing: A succinct and lively interpretation of dreams.* New York, NY: Paulist Press.

Schneiders, S. M. (1982). Spiritual discernment in the dialogue of Saint Catherine of Siena. *Horizons, 9*(1), 47–59.

Schul, Y., Mayo, R., & Burnstein, E. (2008). The value of distrust. *Journal of Experimental Social Psychology, 44*(5), 1293–1302.

Taylor, E. J. (2002). *Spiritual care: Nursing theory, research, and practice.* Upper Saddle River, NJ: Prentice Hall.

van 't Wout, M., Kahn, R. S., Sanfey, A. G., & Aleman, A. (2006). Affective state and decision-making in the ultimatum game. *Explorations in Brain Research, 169*(4), 564–568.

Wuthnow, R. (1998). *After heaven: Spirituality in America since the 1950s.* Berkeley: University of California Press.

CHAPTER 10

The BSN-to-DNP Path: Opportunities and Challenges for DNP Students and Graduates

Mary Ellen Roberts and Donna Behler McArthur

This chapter describes the development of postbaccalaureate doctor of nursing practice (DNP) preparation and the opportunities and challenges for students and faculty. Throughout the chapter selected insights will be directed at current or potential bachelor of science in nursing (BSN) to DNP students. Regardless of the pathway, the DNP degree represents the highest level of formal education for advanced nursing practice. The evolution of the degree occurred within the context of burgeoning knowledge, changes in healthcare delivery, escalating demands of chronic illness care, diverse patient populations, and globalization. Likewise, propelling forces from the Institute of Medicine (IOM) and the American Association of Colleges of Nursing (AACN) aligned with early adopters and national initiatives. Criticisms of the timing of DNP programs were related to nurse practitioner (NP) capacity in the face of the Patient Protection and Affordable Care Act. The challenges moving forward continue to surround rigor and program variability—such as BSN-to-DNP and master of science in nursing (MSN) to DNP—as well as the nature of scholarly projects and capstones. The practice doctorate is a program of study that develops specialty practice expertise and core knowledge regarding the integration and application of evidence into practice and leadership strategies for translation of evidence to include quality improvement initiatives (McArthur, 2014).

Background for the BSN-to-DNP Transition

Numerous authors have described the evolution of the DNP degree within the context of major initiatives (Ahmed, Andrist, Davis, & Fuller, 2013; Chism, 2013; Moran, Burson, & Conrad, 2014; Zaccagnini & White, 2011). Consider these initiatives through the lens of a newly graduated nurse with a BSN degree contemplating a DNP degree. More than a decade ago several hallmark reports from the

IOM called for sweeping changes in the way healthcare professionals are educated to meet the challenges of the 21st century: *To Err is Human: Building a Safer Health System* (1999); *Crossing the Quality Chasm: A New Health System for the 21st Century* (2001); and *Health Professions Education: A Bridge to Quality* (2003a). The core competencies for healthcare professionals included the following: (1) provide patient-centered care; (2) work in interdisciplinary teams; (3) employ evidence-based practice; (4) apply quality improvement; and (5) utilize informatics (IOM, 2003a). Given the dynamic nature of the science and evidence base in health care, innovative educational approaches were needed to teach advanced nursing practice students how to manage knowledge, use effective tools to support clinical decision making, and apply methodological rules to evaluate the evidence (McArthur, 2014). These approaches would help shape the *Essentials of Doctoral Education for Advanced Nursing Practice* (AACN, 2006b).

The concept of advanced nursing practice is confusing to students and faculty alike, and the term *advanced nursing practice* is often used in lieu of *advanced-practice nurse*. For clarification, advanced nursing practice is broadly defined by the AACN (2004) to include the administration of nursing and healthcare organizations and the development and implementation of healthcare policy. Often referred to as *indirect care*, this definition broadens the applicability of the DNP degree beyond advanced-practice registered nurses (APRNs)—such as NPs, certified registered nurse anesthetists, clinical nurse specialists, and certified nurse–midwives—to include master's-prepared nurse administrators, informatics nurse specialists, and healthcare policy experts. The IOM (2003b) acknowledges nurse executives and managers and challenges them to have adequate educational preparation to ensure readiness for participation in executive leadership within healthcare organizations. Hence, the BSN-to-DNP trajectory encompasses myriad advanced nursing practice specialties.

Resurgence of Practice Doctorates

The concept of a practice doctorate is not new, but the validation of such a degree has been slow to unfold. Case Western Reserve University is generally credited with beginning the first nursing doctorate (ND) program as an entry-level nursing degree in 1979; graduates were prepared as generalist nurses with expanded skills and knowledge. In 1990 the ND program was changed from an entry-level program to a postmaster's practice doctorate (Case Western Reserve University, 2013).

As of January 2014 there were more than 241 established DNP programs accepting students with another 59 in the planning stages, representing 49 states and the District of Columbia. More than half the established programs offer a BSN-to-DNP option and a postmaster's option. More than 14,700 students attend these programs. From 2012 to 2013 the number of students enrolled in DNP programs increased from 11,575 to 14,699; the number of graduates increased from

1,858 to 2,443 (AACN, 2014a). These numbers are staggering, considering that in 2003 there were four active ND programs (Case Western Reserve University, Rush University, University of Colorado, University of South Carolina), one DNP program (University of Kentucky), and one doctor of nursing science program (University of Tennessee–Memphis). Several other schools were planning programs, most notably Columbia University, which was developing a doctor of nursing practice (DrNP) program (Marion et al., 2003). Although the ND and DrNP degrees share many components of the current DNP degree, the AACN decided to use one degree designation: DNP.

The new BSN-to-DNP student may be confronted with questions from colleagues and perhaps faculty regarding the role of the DNP. We suggest students and DNP graduates prepare their elevator speeches and clarify that the DNP is a doctorate degree, *not* a role. DNP students and graduates may further clarify that the advanced-practice role is integrated within the BSN-to-DNP program of study.

The Transition to the DNP Degree: The BSN-to-DNP Path

Many nursing organizations have played pivotal roles in advancing the practice doctorate. That said, these organizations often are invisible to BSN graduates who are considering DNP study. Potential students should acquaint themselves with the seminal reports from these organizations, which are available in myriad formats, including online. The National Organization of Nurse Practitioner Faculties (NONPF) Practice Doctorate Task Force was established in 2001 to explore issues surrounding the shift in academic preparation for all NPs. Although research supports the notion that APRNs provide safe, high-quality care in all specialties and practice sites (Brooten et al., 2010; Craigin & Kennedy, 2006; Mundinger et al., 2000; Newhouse et al., 2011; Pine, Holt, & Lou, 2003), APRNs are among the few healthcare professionals educated and then licensed as independent practitioners at the master's-degree level rather than the doctoral-degree level (others include pharmacists, medical doctors, dentists, psychologists, and audiologists). A landmark article supporting the development of the practice doctorate and its commitment to provide leadership in this initiative was authored by members of the NONPF task force (Marion et al., 2003). Encouraging nursing to adopt a shared vision to move the practice doctorate forward, these nurse leaders reiterated the challenges for advanced nursing practice in the face of the need for expert clinical teachers, shifts in information technology, demographic changes, disparities in healthcare delivery and access, and stakeholder expectations. The practice doctorate, focused on direct care of patient populations and leadership, would respond to the following: evaluating the evidence base for care, delivering the care, setting healthcare policy, and leading and managing clinical care units and healthcare systems (McArthur, 2014).

The AACN board of directors took the lead in transforming APRN education and created an 11-member task force on the practice doctorate in nursing. Dr. Betty Lenz, then dean of the School of Nursing at Ohio State University, was the chairperson. The charge put to the task force was to clarify the purpose of the professional clinical doctorate, especially core content and core competencies; describe trends over time in clinical doctoral education; assess the need for clinically focused doctoral programs; identify preferred goals, titles, outcomes, and resources; discuss the elements of a unified approach versus a diverse approach; determine the potential implications for advanced-practice nursing; make recommendations regarding related issues and resources; and describe the potential for various tracks or role options (AACN, 2006b). The work of the task force included performing comprehensive reviews of existing practice doctorates across disciplines, collaborating with NONPF, interviewing key informants (e.g., deans, program directors, graduates) at the eight current programs in the United States, and conducting open discussions at the AACN Doctoral Education Conferences and Master's Education Conferences. The task force findings addressed each charge, including the major recommendation—to make the DNP the terminal degree for advanced nursing practice preparation. This recommendation represented a major paradigm shift for advanced-practice nurse education, such as the BSN-to-DNP degree. An additional finding was that practice-focused doctoral programs should be accredited by a nursing accreditation body, with the DNP degree associated with practice-focused doctoral education. At the time, many master's-prepared APRNs were less than supportive of the recommendation; the task force recommended a transition period to provide a mechanism for master's-prepared nurses to pursue the degree if they desired.

This discussion may give readers pause as to why the master's degree could not remain the terminal degree. Indeed, multiple schools of nursing continue to admit students who will graduate with an MSN degree along with specialty training as an advanced-practice nurse. Support for the DNP degree included a better match of program requirements and credits than with the master's degree. Credit creep has occurred since the evolution of NP programs; for example, the number of credits are equal to those of many PhD programs. Likewise, there was recognition that enhanced core knowledge and leadership skills were needed to strengthen practice and healthcare delivery. In addition, justification included the need for faculty, parity with other professions, and an improved image of nursing (McArthur, 2014).

We suggest that BSN-to-DNP students should read the *AACN Position Statement on the Practice Doctorate in Nursing*, created by the task force, which was reviewed by an eight-member external reaction panel and was approved by the AACN membership in October 2004 (AACN, 2004). AACN member institutions that were represented at the meeting voted to move the current level of advanced nursing practice from the master's degree to the doctoral degree by 2015. The two take-home messages for many institutions were that the DNP degree would be the terminal degree (hence the BSN-to-DNP trajectory), and this would be accomplished by 2015. Deans and other administrators within schools and colleges of nursing immediately began to strategize how to implement the recommendations. Further, the AACN Task Force on the Practice Doctorate in Nursing recommended the development of a document addressing educational standards, indicators of quality for practice doctoral programs, and core content and competencies. The DNP Essentials Task Force was created to develop a document titled *Essentials of Doctoral Education for Advanced Nursing Practice* (AACN, 2006b), which provided a framework to guide program development and accreditation; the document was disseminated in 2006. In addition, the DNP Roadmap Task Force was created and charged with developing an implementation plan that provided a roadmap for achieving the goals of the AACN position statement by 2015 (AACN, 2006a). The essentials document is a must read for potential BSN-to-DNP students. The competencies outlined in the eight essentials have shaped the curriculum and program outcomes for most DNP programs.

From 2004 to 2006, the original AACN Task Force on the Practice Doctorate in Nursing and subsequent task forces concerning the essentials and roadmap documents conducted forums and invitational meetings to collect input on the DNP degree from education and practice stakeholders. Internet surveys of schools were conducted, and regional conferences in cooperation with the DNP Essentials Task Force were held in five locations, including a national stakeholder conference in Washington, DC, which hosted 65 leaders from 44 professional organizations. Major resources were developed, which have been updated and remain in use today by faculty, administrators, potential students, DNP students, and healthcare consumers; the most notable are the DNP Tool Kit (AACN, 2014b) and a Frequently Asked Questions document (AACN, 2012).

In response to the national stakeholder conference, the American Academy of Nurse Practitioners (AANP) published a white paper in favor of the DNP degree, but it recommended a smooth transition for APRNs who hold a master's degree: "It is important, however, that the transition to clinical doctoral preparation for NPs continue to be conducted so that master's prepared NPs will not be disenfranchised in any way . . . The development of such programs must be conducted in a manner that allows for smooth transitioning" (AANP, 2010, pp. 140–141).

Several schools described the development of their DNP programs, which were primarily postmaster's entry, to provide exemplars. Magyary, Whitney, and Brown (2006) described the development of practice inquiry and collaborative research endeavors with DNP graduates as science partners at the University of Washington. They described practice inquiry as the "ongoing, systematic, investigation of questions about nursing therapeutics and clinical phenomena with the intent to appraise and translate all forms of best evidence to practice, and to evaluate the translational impact on the quality of health care and health outcomes" (Magyary et al., 2006, p. 143).

This begs two questions: Are students in BSN-to-DNP programs and new graduates from these programs able to integrate the DNP competencies into a practice inquiry derived from practice? Should the focus be on the acquisition of skill sets as an APRN?

Economic Challenges Related to the BSN-to-DNP Path

Economic challenges facing the United States since the AACN published its position paper in 2004 have had a major impact on the ability of some schools to develop new programs and recruit students, perhaps lessening the overall quality of the programs (Cronenwett et al., 2011. Embracing the 2015 target for the DNP degree to be the terminal degree for advanced-practice nurses, many schools of nursing immediately transitioned their program to the DNP degree without the option of a master's degree exit point, which results in additional years of education before certification and practice, coupled with student financial burdens. From a workforce perspective, questions have been raised regarding the capacity of APRNs, particularly NPs, to meet the healthcare needs of the millions of Americans who are expected to gain health insurance through healthcare reform initiatives (Buerhaus, 2010). Dialogue has continued related to workforce concerns and economic challenges. That said, the number of students enrolling in DNP programs and the continued impact within specific work environments speak to the evolving success of many DNP programs, even in these financially vulnerable times.

Program Variability: Special Considerations for BSN-to-DNP Students

With the rapid rollout and proliferation of programs throughout the United States, variability is inevitable (Mancuso & Udlis, 2012; McArthur, 2014). The institutional infrastructure and support that are necessary for new programs present myriad challenges for institutions without doctoral programs. The approval process for programs may be challenging and can include multiple layers of university approving bodies. When the DNP degree is part of a graduate school, instead of within the school or college of nursing, quality standards may be in place across all doctoral degrees. Hence, there are DNP programs in which students must complete comprehensive written and oral exams. Faculty and students alike must be able to discern the difference between a scholarly project and a dissertation, recognizing both types of scholarship.

In response to the AACN recommendations, many BSN entry-level NP programs with a master's degree exit were converted into BSN-to-DNP programs. Udlis and Mancuso (2012) conducted a cross-sectional, descriptive study to develop a database related to DNP program characteristics and admission criteria. These authors acknowledged that DNP programs are moving forward, but an appreciation of characteristics and trends would inform universities in planning and evaluating their programs. For the potential BSN-to-DNP student, numerous variables should be considered, including the program delivery format. Networking with fellow students and faculty in an effort to create a community of scholars may be difficult with an exclusively online program, which is uncommon for BSN-to-DNP programs. Chism (2012) reiterated that BSN-to-DNP students may have concerns regarding their roles as advanced-practice nurses. She recommends that faculty play a role in helping BSN graduates and students discern appropriate programs that recognize each individual's practice expertise, long-term goals, and learning styles (Chism, 2012; Christenbery, 2012). Likewise, the availability of mentoring within a program is crucial for these students. Potential students would benefit from finding a mentor within their desired specialty before matriculation.

The majority of current DNP programs are offered online with mandatory on-campus activities (blocks) each semester, especially during specialty course work. Likewise, plans of study may be full time or part time, and the program length may vary; the average BSN-to-DNP program is 40.6 months (Udlis & Mancuso, 2012). Most of the early DNP programs had only postmaster's options. These DNP students were certified in their respective specialties, often with years of practice experience. In contrast, BSN entry-level DNP students may be new graduates with minimal experience as RNs. Building on a strong nursing background cannot be assumed by faculty and can present challenges for students. The NONPF templates for BSN-to-DNP programs offer guidance for faculty who are developing BSN-to-DNP programs of study and curricula. One approach is the integration of DNP courses throughout the program of study; the second is front-loading specialty course work. Few programs offer a master's degree exit as part of the BSN-to-DNP sequence. This option enables graduates to complete the specialty certification exam and begin practicing as advanced-practice nurses.

The DNP Scholarly Project and Outcomes: Considerations for the BSN-to-DNP Path

Variability in the types of scholarly projects merits discussion. Reiterating the AACN's description of the final DNP project (AACN, 2004), the project should demonstrate the synthesis of the student's work and lay the groundwork for future scholarship, including mastery of specialty content. In contrast to a dissertation as the deliverable in a research-focused doctoral program, the final DNP project has been called a capstone project, clinical dissertation, system change project, portfolio, translational research project, and practice inquiry, among other titles. Examples include the development of a practice portfolio (Committee on DrNP Competencies, 2003), a practice change initiative, a pilot study, program evaluation, a quality improvement project, an evaluation of a new practice model, a consulting project, or an integrated critical literature review. The scope of projects reflects the diversity of advanced nursing practice specialties, population foci, supporting course work, and faculty mentors. The different pathways to the DNP degree (BSN-to-MSN-to-DNP; BSN-to-DNP; MSN-to-DNP; PhD-to-DNP) create opportunities and challenges for the identification, development, and implementation of a project.

Practice partners may be agencies and organizations with an increased number of group projects. The challenge for faculty and students is to assess available resources within individual DNP programs, recognize the need for students and faculty to identify strengths, and provide guidance to students in identifying meaningful projects that can be implemented within a realistic time frame. While further implementation and evaluation of the project may occur postgraduation, the student should have mastered the competencies necessary to identify, plan, implement, and evaluate the project. Titles and abstracts of DNP projects are located on the websites of organizations (Sigma Theta Tau library, Doctors of Nursing Practice LLC, NONPF) and individual programs. At this time there is no central repository of all projects.

Issues have surfaced regarding the scholarly projects of BSN-to-DNP students, who are new to advanced-practice nursing roles, compared to expert practitioners who enter as postmaster's DNP students. The core DNP courses are identical; the requirements for a scholarly project and a designated number of practice hours in which to integrate DNP course work and develop the project are consistent. However, students may represent distinct differences in their levels of practice expertise and their potential to identify a meaningful inquiry from practice. In addition, BSN entry-level DNP students most likely will require additional semesters of clinical supervision and closer oversight of their projects. Potential BSN-to-DNP students should explore programs most suited to their learning styles (e.g., face to face or hybrid). In addition, clinical placements with expert preceptors and the option for additional clinical experiences with mentors should be offered.

Brown and Crabtree (2013) call for a continuous and rapid adjustment of DNP curricula due to the evolutionary nature of DNP programs. Of particular concern is consensus regarding the DNP project. These pioneer NPs and educators posit that the DNP project should be defined as practice improvement partnerships between academia and community agencies (2013, p. 330). They recognize the growing number of BSN-to-DNP students without nursing or advanced-practice nursing expertise, and they encourage partnerships with knowledgeable practitioners. The role of faculty in these partnerships is crucial to help broker the student–agency relationship. In November 2013 the AACN board formed a task force charged with developing a white paper that will clarify the purpose of the DNP final scholarly product and the practice hour requirements as described in the *Essentials of Doctoral Education for Advanced Nursing Practice*.

As a prelude to the next section, measuring outcomes of DNP student projects merits discussion. Murphy and Magdic (2013) provide broad categories of capstone projects from selected schools and publications disseminated by DNP-prepared nurses. They call for additional research on outcomes related to DNP-prepared nurses to include care-related, patient-related, and performance-related outcome measures.

DNP projects generate practice knowledge despite the heterogeneity in focus, rigor, and outcomes. Projects are designed to be context specific, which means they may not be generalized to other settings, and the impact may be difficult to quantify. This does not negate the potential for leadership in improving and sustaining evidence-based practice and practice change through collaboration with agencies and organizations, or research initiatives with PhD-prepared partners. The impact may be measured through dissemination to key stakeholders at local, regional, and national meetings and through publications. Sharing project abstracts with professional organizations via social media and on school of nursing websites are other venues for dissemination.

Evaluation of DNP Programs

Program accreditation by a nursing or nursing-related accreditation organization that is recognized by the U.S. Department of Education or the Council for Higher Education Accreditation is required. Potential students should verify accreditation by reviewing the school's website or querying key personnel or faculty. The two bodies within nursing that accredit DNP programs are the Commission on Collegiate Nursing Education (CCNE) and the Accreditation Commission for Education in Nursing. Although both organizations accredit BSN and MSN programs, CCNE was the first organization to evaluate and accredit DNP programs, beginning with the 2008–2009 academic year; it currently accredits the majority of programs. DNP programs must be developed in accordance with the *Essentials of Doctoral Education for Advanced Nursing Practice* (AACN, 2006b). In BSN-to-DNP programs that prepare NPs, the revised *Criteria for Evaluation of Nurse Practitioner Programs* must be incorporated (National Task Force on Quality Nurse Practitioner Education, 2012).

In addition to accreditation, DNP programs should be evaluated with each cohort to ascertain student and faculty feedback related to program goals and outcomes. These formative evaluations are valuable for students and faculty because the feedback provides a platform for curricular changes and program development. In contrast to formative studies, summative evaluations occur at the completion of the program of study and are related largely to the performance of graduates. Graff, Russell, and Stegbauer (2007) described the formative and summative evaluation data provided by three student cohorts and graduates from the University of Tennessee Health Science Center College of Nursing practice doctorate program.

Questions posed to the groups focused on perceptions of how their roles may change as a result of the program and how the courses they took will contribute to any role change development. Students noted the evolutionary process with changes in functions and relationships. They described how they approached problems differently and noted that their clinical practices changed (Graff et al., 2007, p. 175). Surveys of students on exit ($n = 57$) and 1 year after graduation ($n = 31$) evaluated the program outcomes. The findings indicated that the program was successful in helping them meet the expected outcomes.

Stoeckel and Kruschke (2013) explored the perceptions of the DNP degree among 12 practicing DNP graduates. The findings in this qualitative study supported that the education of these postmaster's DNP graduates provided them with the skills to meet the needs of populations through evidence-based practice. The literature has a dearth of studies that are specific to BSN-to-DNP graduates, their perceptions of the respective programs, and their evolving roles as DNP-prepared APRNs.

Regardless of entry level, challenges frequently identified by DNP students are related to time management and dealing with new technology. Facilitators include having a community of peers, supportive faculty, and program flexibility. The importance of embracing students' perspectives in program evaluations speaks to a student-centric community and can impact future program development, innovation, and marketing.

The BSN-to-DNP Student and the APRN Consensus Model

To reinforce the IOM's (2010) endorsement of graduate education for nursing and the importance of allowing nurses to practice to the full extent of their education, the training, education, accreditation, certification, and licensure of APRNs need to be consistent across jurisdictions. The changes in educational requirements for APRN practice continue to impact certification and regulation for many specialties. Stakeholders continue to recognize that we are in a time of transition and have many venues to communicate shared initiatives, the major one being the *Consensus Model for APRN Regulation: Licensure, Accreditation, Certification & Education* (APRN Consensus Work Group & National Council of State Boards of Nursing APRN Advisory Committee, 2008). All DNP students need to be conversant regarding this model as it relates to their specialties.

The model for APRN regulation was developed by the APRN Joint Dialogue Group and has been endorsed by 48 professional nursing organizations. The document defines APRN practice, the APRN regulatory model, titling, the definitions of specialties, the emergence of new roles and population foci, and strategies for implementation, which is targeted for 2015. For example, the BSN-entry DNP student must have the appropriate education to sit for a certification exam to assess their national-level competencies of the APRN core (pathophysiology, pharmacology, and health and physical assessment), their clinical role (certified nurse practitioner, certified registered nurse anesthetist, certified nurse–midwife, clinical nurse specialist), and at least one population area of practice (family, adult and gerontology, neonatal, pediatrics, women's health or gender related, psychiatric mental health). Education, certification, and licensure must be congruent in terms of the clinical role and the population foci. The acronym *LACE* reflects the communication mechanism of the regulatory organizations representing APRN licensure, accreditation, certification, and education entities.

Many DNP graduates are evolving practice scholars and expert practitioners who may be well positioned to assume a faculty position. This assumes there is a match between the criteria determined by the institution and the qualifications of the applicant. BSN-prepared DNP students who aspire to teach should consider taking electives, over and above the required course work, related to education. Identifying a faculty mentor who can facilitate appropriate teaching experiences is encouraged.

Interview with Heejin Kim

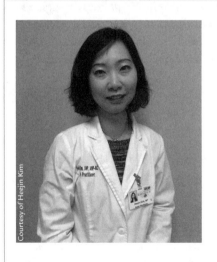

Heejin Kim, DNP, APRN, BC, AOCNP, is a nurse practitioner and BSN-to-DNP graduate.

Dr. Kim, could you please describe your educational and professional background, including your current position?

I earned my BSN degree in 1994, starting my professional journey as an oncology nurse in South Korea. Two years later I enrolled in a master's program, which focused on nursing research and education. In South Korea I earned an MSN degree in 1998 with a master's thesis of "The Effectiveness of Guided Imagery for Chemotherapy Induced Nausea and Vomiting." Since then I kept my professional career as an oncology nurse for more than 15 years in the Bone Marrow Transplant Unit and the Ambulatory Chemotherapy Infusion Center in Canada and the United States.

As a staff nurse working at Karmanos Cancer Center, I earned a DNP degree in 2013 at Wayne State University, Detroit. Currently I am working as an adult nurse practitioner at the Genitourinary Oncology Department at Karmanos Cancer Center, Detroit.

Dr. Kim, could you please explain why you returned to school to earn a DNP degree?

I have been working as a staff oncology nurse for about 20 years since I graduated from a BSN program. I always find strong nursing values and personal rewards through interaction with patients who are in need. Patients who have active cancer diagnoses require tremendous nursing support with clinical oncology nursing knowledge, skills, and compassion. While I was busy with providing nursing care to these cancer patients, I desired to serve them to my best ability. Although I kept up to date on oncology nursing knowledge and meticulous nursing skills, I often found myself struggling with the quality of my nursing care. I realized that my struggles were related to a lack of autonomy and confidence in my nursing practice. Therefore, I decided to enroll in an advanced nurse practitioner program to provide nursing care at an advanced level. Then I entered the master's-prepared advanced nurse practitioner program at Wayne State. In the first year of the program, I learned about a new degree, doctor of nursing practice, which is a terminal degree in clinical nursing practice. I was unsure about what the DNP degree entailed; however, I believed this DNP program would provide all necessary expertise in the clinical setting. With the DNP degree, I valued continual focus on clinical nursing practice, unlike the PhD, where students concentrate on research or academia. Finally, I transferred my MSN program to the BSN-to-DNP program at Wayne State University.

Dr. Kim, would you describe your experience in school while pursuing your DNP degree, including your unique experience as a student in a BSN-to-DNP program?

I did not have a good understanding of the DNP when I entered the program, like other students in my class. Because the DNP degree was very new in the field of nursing at that time, the identity, role, and competency of the DNP were unknown to us. The College of Nursing at Wayne State University started the DNP program a year before I entered the program. During my first year, my class was busy with learning philosophical foundations in the clinical doctorate in nursing practice and discussing the identity and roles of the DNP. We also discussed how the DNP degree has emerged in health care and how the DNP can contribute to nursing practice, the community, and the organization. Improving quality care was mainly centered on our discussion during the DNP core classes. To implement quality care, the DNP program focused on systems thinking, organization theory, leadership, policy change, healthcare disparity, informatics, evidence-based practice, and quality improvement projects. The BSN-to-DNP program also provided advanced nursing practice courses, including pharmacology, pathophysiology, and physical exam, and a clinical practicum in the specialty area.

My unique experience as a student in the BSN-to-DNP program was appreciated in the DNP seminar with case studies, which was the extension of the clinical practicum in the specialty area. While we learned the roles of APRNs at the master's level, we tried to elaborate on unique DNP competences in the clinical setting. Some examples include applying nursing diagnoses and nursing-sensitive outcomes in patient case studies. We also analyzed a particular patient case in view of evidence-based practice and quality improvement by critiquing standard guidelines and current practice. We had an opportunity to perform quality improvement projects during these classes. This experience was extended to our clinical inquiry projects for the DNP program. Retrospectively, I believe these classes assisted students to enrich their knowledge and skills on evidence-based practice and the quality improvement processes.

Dr. Kim, in your opinion, what were the benefits of a BSN-to-DNP program? What were the challenges?

One of the benefits of a BSN-to-DNP program is centered on the shorter course work compared to a MSN-to-DNP program. The traditional MSN program requires core courses and a clinical practicum in the specialty area. If an MSN graduate pursues a DNP program, some of these core courses will be somewhat duplicated. Of course, DNP programs offer core courses at a deeper level with broadened perspectives. However, students in an MSN-to-DNP track may have to revisit the same content that was discussed at the master's level. These core courses may include nursing philosophy and theory, evidence-based practice, and policy change classes. On the contrary, a BSN-to-DNP student will complete these classes in one program instead of two tiered programs.

Another benefit of a BSN-to-DNP program is the professional development that will be offered to an individual who enters the program. Students who enter a BSN-to-DNP program are bachelor's-prepared nurses who have not practiced as an APRN in a specialty area. These individuals have not been engaged in their advanced roles and have not built up their comfort zone. Consequently, these individuals will have an opportunity to develop their professional values, beliefs, and work attitudes at the doctoral level for their new roles. At the entry level of APRN with doctorate, DNP graduates, I believe, will be able to develop a new paradigm of professional values and ethics based on systems thinking, leadership, patient-centered care, and quality of health care. If a DNP degree has emerged to improve current healthcare quality, newly developed professional values and belief are necessary for beneficial change.

The challenges to a student in the BSN-to-DNP program are mainly related to lack of experience in the specialty area. The student has not practiced as an APRN in the specialty area, which would make it difficult for them to identify gaps in the current practice and the standards. Students in the BSN-to-DNP program might be intimidated because of lack of experience in their advanced roles, compared to students in the MSN-to-DNP program. Furthermore, a new BSN-to-DNP graduate who does not have experience in the advanced-practice roles will need to build new knowledge and skills in their specialty area. This may not be easy and comfortable for a DNP who is not confident in the new roles as an APRN. These BSN-to-DNP graduates may feel anxious or uncomfortable before they become an expert in their APRN roles.

Dr. Kim, do you have any recommendations for faculty teaching or developing BSN-to-DNP programs?

There are debates whether BSN-to-DNP students should complete their specialty courses followed by a DNP clinical practicum and the clinical inquiry project (CIP) or capstone project, or if they should complete DNP core courses and a clinical practicum with their project and then take courses in the specialty area. In my opinion, the former is preferable. When BSN-to-DNP students learn their scope of practice in their specialty area, they would have a better idea of how to identify gaps between the current practice and quality health care. This would better assist the student in performing a CIP, which is more relevant to the current clinical setting. An expanded scope of nursing practice as an APRN would better support students in forming ideas and action plans with their CIP. I would like to recommend that faculties take this into consideration when they develop curricula.

I mainly studied in a class with a mixture of BSN-to-DNP students and MSN-to-DNP students. BSN-to-DNP students could be intimidated in class because of their lack of experience and expertise in the specialty area. In addition, MSN-to-DNP students tend to be more experienced than BSN-to-DNP students, not only in the specialty area, but also in the field of nursing. Although lack of experience would intimidate BSN-to-DNP students, a mixture of experience and various backgrounds certainly stimulate abundant discussions in the seminar. I would like faculty members to encourage these BSN-to-DNP students to be actively involved in discussions and provide positive feedback for their participation in exchanging ideas.

Dr. Kim, how has earning a DNP degree impacted your practice as a nurse practitioner? Do you feel that having earned a DNP degree along with a specialty (nurse practitioner) has helped or hindered your practice?

I have been working as an advanced nurse practitioner for 7 months since I graduated from the DNP program. For the past 7 months I have put all my efforts in settling in to my new role as an advanced nurse practitioner in a busy clinic. As a novice in the new role, my priority in the job is to become at least proficient or competent in a year. While I am learning new roles in my current job, I have not yet perceived my DNP roles as a leader or a change agent in the field. While I am working in the field, however, I am seeing clinical situations with a DNP perspective by identifying gaps between quality care and current care. These identifications of gaps or problems are triggering my learning experiences as to how we can develop and form plans to produce quality care. I may not be able to perform and implement new processes while I am learning my new role, but I will be able do so in the near future when I am more confident with the DNP role. To conclude, I feel that a DNP degree will help my practice toward improving quality care with advanced nursing perspectives in the near future.

Dr. Kim, what advice do you have for others who may be considering, or who are already enrolled in, a BSN-to-DNP program?

I would like to recommend two things to BSNs who wish to pursue a BSN-to-DNP program. First of all, I believe clinical experience as a BSN in the field where they would like to pursue their specialty area is necessary before or while the student is enrolled in a BSN-to-DNP program. While the students are going through the DNP program, they will learn how to identify problems in the field and how to apply evidence-based practice. Furthermore, the students will earn hands-on experience in terms of implementing evidence-based practice to promote quality care in the field. Therefore, the students will need to go to the field and implement the proposed changes in the area. If students are not familiar with nursing in the field, it might be difficult to accomplish evidence-based practice and quality improvement projects. Hence, I personally believe that BSNs should have some experience in the field that they would like to pursue in their professional career.

Secondly, BSN-to-DNP students should be ambitious and self-motivated. When BSN-to-DNP students are studying with MSN-to-DNP students, it is easy to be intimidated because of lack of experience and lack of confidence in nursing. Self-motivation will encourage the individual and will expand their experiences in the field. Personally, being part of a new degree and in a new role as a DNP, it was difficult to find a good role model and to observe the new roles before I graduated. I contacted DNPs who are working in the field, although I did not have any acquaintance with them. I even found a DNP who published an article in the area of my interest. The DNP was working at a renowned cancer center in Boston. I contacted her by email and flew to Boston to spend a week with her. I observed her DNP roles and discussed my CIP with her. I had to have great courage and ambition to accomplish these projects.

Finally, I would like to support BSN-to-DNP programs and would like to encourage nurses to pursue BSN-to-DNP programs. While the roles of DNPs are not exactly visible yet because it is a new degree, this program will assist nurses to be fully equipped with useful information, such as leadership, systems thinking, policy changes, evidence-based practice, and quality improvement, as well as practicum in the APRN specialty area. The students excel in confidence as advanced nurses who can play a role at the doctoral level.

BOX 10-1

Tips for the BSN-to-DNP Student or Graduate

- BSN-to-DNP students and graduates should prepare their elevator speeches to include clarifying that the DNP is a doctorate degree, not a role. Further, they should clarify that the BSN-to-DNP path integrates the advanced nursing practice roles into the BSN-to-DNP program of study.

- BSN-to-DNP students and graduates should acquaint themselves with the seminal works from major nursing organizations, including NONPF's Practice Doctorate Task Force, the AACN Task Force position statement, the AACN *Essentials of Doctoral Education for Advanced Nursing Practice*, and the AANP white paper on the DNP degree.

- Potential BSN-to-DNP students should consider numerous variables regarding program delivery format. Networking with fellow students and faculty in an effort to create a community of scholars may be difficult with online programs.

- Develop relationships with mentors in the BSN-to-DNP program to ensure guidance and advanced-practice role actualization and clarification.

- BSN-to-DNP students should consider programs that offer a master's degree exit as part of the BSN-to-DNP sequence as a desired option. This option allows graduates to complete the specialty certification exam and begin practicing as advanced-practice nurses prior to completion of their DNP program.

- BSN-to-DNP students should assess available resources within individual DNP programs, recognize the need to identify strengths, and obtain guidance in developing meaningful projects that can be implemented within a realistic time frame.

- BSN-to-DNP students most likely will require additional semesters of clinical supervision and closer oversight of their projects and therefore should explore programs that are most suited to their learning styles (e.g., face to face or hybrid).

- BSN-to-DNP students should carefully consider clinical placements with expert preceptors and additional clinical experiences.

- BSN-to-DNP students who aspire to teach should consider taking education electives that are over and above the required course work. Identifying a faculty mentor who can facilitate appropriate teaching experiences is encouraged.

- BSN-to-DNP students and graduates should be familiar with the APRN Consensus Model as it relates to the BSN-to-DNP path of advanced-practice specialization.

SUMMARY

- The evolution of the BSN-to-DNP degree occurred within the context of burgeoning knowledge, changes in healthcare delivery, escalating demands of chronic illness care, diverse patient populations, and globalization.
- Core competencies within seminal documents were noted by the IOM, particularly to provide patient-centered care, work within interdisciplinary teams, employ evidence-based practice, apply quality improvement, and utilize informatics.
- By definition, indirect care broadens the applicability of the DNP degree beyond advanced-practice nurses to include master's-prepared nurse administrators and informatics nurses.
- The practice doctorate, with its focus on direct care of populations and leadership, responds to evaluating the evidence base for care, delivering the care, setting healthcare policy, and leading and managing clinical units and healthcare systems.
- Enhanced knowledge and leadership skills are needed to strengthen practice and healthcare delivery.
- The DNP as the terminal degree for APRNs has not been accepted by all disciplines, including nursing.
- There are many challenges in the transition to a BSN-to-DNP degree, including program variability, economic challenges, variability in the DNP project, and differences in rigor.
- Issues have surfaced regarding the BSN-to-DNP scholarly project because students are new to advanced-practice nursing roles, compared to expert practitioners who enter as postmaster's DNP students.
- Potential students should explore programs that are suited to their learning needs.
- The purpose of the final DNP project is to demonstrate a synthesis of the student's work and lay the groundwork for future scholarship, including mastery of specialty content.
- Doctoral education in nursing is designed to prepare nurses for the highest level of leadership in practice and scientific inquiry.
- The DNP graduate is an evolving practice scholar and practice expert.

REFLECTION QUESTIONS

1. What are the challenges inherent in the BSN-to-DNP degree?
2. Do you think that indirect care should be part of the DNP degree since the DNP is considered a practice doctorate?

3. Do you think the DNP degree should be a post-BSN degree, or should the DNP degree follow a master's degree for expert clinicians?

4. What should a potential student look for when choosing a DNP program?

5. Reflect on the variability of programs and your perception of the scholarly project.

REFERENCES

Ahmed, S. W., Andrist, L. C., Davis, S. M., & Fuller, V. J. (Eds.). (2013). *DNP education, practice, and policy*. New York, NY: Springer.

American Academy of Nurse Practitioners. (2010). *American Academy of Nurse Practitioners: Celebrating 25 years as the voice of the nurse practitioner*. Tampa, FL: Faircount Media Group. Retrieved from issuu.com/faircountmedia/docs/aanp25/142

American Association of Colleges of Nursing. (2004). *AACN position statement on the practice doctorate in nursing*. Washington, DC: Author. Retrieved from http://www.aacn.nche.edu/publications/position/DNPpositionstatement.pdf

American Association of Colleges of Nursing. (2006a). *DNP roadmap task force report*. Washington, DC: Author. Retrieved from http://www.aacn.nche.edu/publications/position/DNPpositionstatement.pdf

American Association of Colleges of Nursing. (2006b). *Essentials of doctoral education for advanced nursing practice*. Washington, DC: Author.

American Association of Colleges of Nursing. (2012). Frequently asked questions. Retrieved from http://www.aacn.nche.edu/dnp/about/frequently-asked-questions

American Association of Colleges of Nursing. (2014a). DNP fact sheet. Washington, DC: Author. Retrieved from http://www.aacn.nche.edu/media-relations/fact-sheets/dnp

American Association of Colleges of Nursing. (2014b). DNP tool kit. Retrieved from http://www.aacn.nche.edu/dnp/dnp-tool-kit

APRN Consensus Work Group & National Council of State Boards of Nursing APRN Advisory Committee. (2008). *Consensus model for APRN regulation: Licensure, accreditation, certification & education*. Retrieved from https://www.ncsbn.org/7_23_08_Consensus_APRN_Final.pdf

Brooten, D., Youngblut, J., Brown, L., Finkler, S. A., Neff, D. F., & Madigan, E. (2010). A randomized trial of nurse specialist home care for women with high-risk pregnancies: Outcomes and costs. *American Journal of Managed Care, 7*(8), 793–803.

Brown, M. A., & Crabtree, K. (2013). The development of practice scholarship in DNP programs: A paradigm shift. *Journal of Professional Nursing, 29*(6), 330–337.

Buerhaus, P. (2010). Have nurse practitioners reached a tipping point? Interview of a panel of NP thought leaders. *Nursing Economic$, 28*(5), 346–349.

Case Western Reserve University. (2013). Post-master's doctor of nursing practice (DNP) program. Retrieved from http://fpb.case.edu/DNP/

Chism, L. A. (2012). BSN-to-DNP education. Retrieved from http://nurse-practitioners-and-physician-assistants.advanceweb.com/Column/DNP-Perspectives/BSN-to-DNP-Education.aspx

Chism, L. A. (2013). *The doctor of nursing practice: A guidebook for role development and professional issues.* Burlington, MA: Jones & Bartlett Learning.

Christenbery, T. L. (2012). Preparing BSN students for the doctor of nursing practice (DNP) application process: The faculty role. *Nurse Educator, 37*(1), 30–35.

Committee on DrNP Competencies. (2003). *Competencies for a doctor of clinical nursing.* New York, NY: Columbia University School of Nursing.

Cragin, L., & Kennedy, H. P. (2006). Linking obstetric and midwifery practice with optimal outcomes. *Journal of Obstetric, Gynecologic, & Neonatal Nursing, 35*(6), 779–785.

Cronenwett, L., Dracup, K., Grey, M., McCauley, L., Meleis, A., & Salmon, M. (2011). The doctor of nursing practice: A national workforce perspective. *Nursing Outlook, 59,* 9–17.

Graff, J. C., Russell, C. K., & Stegbauer, C. C. (2007). Formative and summative evaluation of a practice doctorate program. *Nurse Educator, 32*(4), 173–177.

Institute of Medicine. (1999). *To err is human: Building a safer health system.* Washington, DC: National Academies Press.

Institute of Medicine. (2001). *Crossing the quality chasm: A new health system for the 21st century.* Washington, DC: National Academies Press.

Institute of Medicine. (2003a). *Health professions education: A bridge to quality.* Washington, DC: National Academies Press.

Institute of Medicine. (2003b). *Keeping patients safe: Transforming the work environment of nurses.* Washington, DC: National Academies Press.

Institute of Medicine. (2010). *The future of nursing: Leading change, advancing health.* Washington, DC: Author.

Magyary, D., Whitney, J. D., & Brown, M. A. (2006). Advancing practice inquiry: Research foundations of the practice doctorate in nursing. *Nursing Outlook, 54,* 139–151.

Mancuso, J. M., & Udlis, K. A. (2012). Doctor of nursing practice programs across the United States: A benchmark of information. Part II: Admission criteria. *Journal of Professional Nursing, 285,* 274–283.

Marion, L., Viens, D., O'Sullivan, A., Crabtree, K., Fontana, S., & Price, M. (2003). The practice doctorate in nursing: Future or fringe? *Topics in Advanced Practice Nursing eJournal.* Retrieved from http://www.medscape.com/viewarticle/453247

McArthur, D. B. (2014). The journey to the doctor of nursing practice degree. In K. Moran, R. Burson, & D. Conrad (Eds.), *The doctor of nursing practice scholarly project: A framework for success* (pp. 15–32). Burlington, MA: Jones & Bartlett Learning.

Moran, K., Burson, R., & Conrad, D. (Eds.). (2014). *The doctor of nursing practice scholarly project: A framework for success.* Burlington, MA: Jones & Bartlett Learning.

Mundinger, M. O., Kane, R. L., Lenz, E. R., Totten, A. M., Tsai, W. Y., Cleary, P. D., . . . Shelanski, M. D. (2000). Primary care outcomes in patients treated by nurse practitioners or physicians: A randomized trial. *Journal of the American Medical Association, 283,* 59–68.

Murphy, M. J., & Magdic, K. S. (2013). Measuring outcomes of doctor of nursing practice. In R. Kleinpell (Ed.), *Outcome assessment in advanced nursing practice* (3rd ed., pp. 291–312). New York, NY: Springer.

National Task Force on Quality Nurse Practitioner Education. (2012). *Criteria for evaluation of nurse practitioner programs.* Retrieved from http://www.aacn.nche.edu/education-resources/evalcriteria2012.pdf

Newhouse, R. P., Stanik-Hill, J., White, K. M., Johantgen, M., Bass, E. B., Zangaro, G., . . . Weiner, J. (2011). Advanced practice nurse outcomes 1990–2008: A systematic review. *Nursing Economics, 29*(5), 230–250.

Pine, M., Holt, K. D., & Lou, Y. B. (2003). Surgical mortality and type of anesthesia provider. *AANA Journal, 71*(2), 109–116.

Stoeckel, P., & Kruschke, C. (2013). Practicing DNPs' perceptions of the DNP. *Clinical Scholars Review, 6*(2), 91–97.

Udlis, K. A., & Mancuso, J. M. (2012). Doctor of nursing practice programs across the United States: A benchmark of information. Part 1: Program characteristics. *Journal of Professional Nursing, 28*(5), 265–273.

Zaccagnini, M. E., & White, K. W. (2011). *The doctor of nursing practice essentials: A new model for advanced practice nursing.* Sudbury, MA: Jones & Bartlett Learning.

CHAPTER 11

The Doctor Nurse: Overcoming Title Issues

Lisa Astalos Chism

With the novelty of being a pioneer, one has the responsibility to lead the way. As more nurses graduate with doctoral degrees, the dilemma of what title to use remains an issue. The dilemma associated with the use of the title *doctor* is not necessarily new in nursing, but now it is most definitely at the forefront due to the advent of the doctor of nursing practice (DNP) degree. Previously, PhD-prepared nurses struggled to be recognized for their educational preparation outside the academic setting. Most certainly this issue is not unique to nurses who hold doctorate degrees. All nonphysician healthcare professionals who are prepared at the doctorate level will potentially be faced with this issue. Further, the way in which DNP graduates manage this issue will affect how it develops in the future.

As part of her DNP curriculum, this author attended a leadership seminar in which a panel of DNP graduates was available for questions. The most frequently asked question of the panel was, are you referred to as doctor? The literature also reflects the pertinence of this topic (Klein, 2007; O'Grady, 2007; Reeves, 2008; Royeen & Lavin, 2007. The Institute of Medicine has recommended enhanced educational preparation of healthcare professionals (Greiner & Knebel, 2003). Moreover, parity among multiple healthcare professionals has also instituted an evolution of education preparation to include the doctoral degree (Griffiths & Padilla, 2006; Pierce & Peyton, 1999; Roeser, Thibodeau, & Cokely, 2005). As this evolution unfolds, the use of the title *doctor* by others outside of medicine will continue to be debated. Therefore, a discussion that includes relevant topics, such as the history of the title *doctor*, parity among healthcare professionals, review of the states' status regarding title protection, the debate in the literature, and a university's response to this issue, is provided in this chapter. An unfortunate case study, along with relevant interviews regarding this issue, are also included. Finally, advice for DNP graduates regarding the most appropriate ways in which to transition to the title *doctor* is reviewed.

The History of *Docere*: The First Teachers

The term *doctor*, derived from the Latin *docere*, originated in Bologna, Italy, during the 12th century (Skinner, 1970). The English translation for *docere* is "to teach," with "doctrine" being what is taught (Skinner, 1970). Merriam-Webster's Online Dictionary defines the term *doctor* as "a learned or authoritative teacher; a person who has earned one of the highest academic degrees conferred by a university; a person skilled in the healing arts, especially one who holds an advanced degree and a license to practice" (Doctor, 2014). Bailey (2003) related that the term *doctor* referred to a religious teacher, scholar, and father of the Christian church; *doctor* also took on the meaning, in the 13th century, "to make to appear right" and "a shower of the way" (Bailey, 2003, p. 490).

The first doctorate was conferred in Bologna and applied to masters who teach (Skinner, 1970). Universities were a community or guild, and the doctorate degree was actually a certificate of admission for professors (Marriner-Tomey, 1990). Additionally, licensing men to teach became the responsibility of clergy and professors (Marriner-Tomey, 1990). By the second half of the 12th century, the demand for learned men in the community increased, and men began earning professional doctorates without the intention to teach (Marriner-Tomey, 1990). As education developed in English universities, the doctorate degree was granted only for law, medicine, and divinity (Skinner, 1970). As universities grew and more men received professional doctorates, those prepared in medicine moved into the communities and among the people. It has been speculated that because of this, the general public began to associate the doctoral degree with medicine (Skinner, 1970). In reality, *doctor* refers to any person with a doctoral degree in any field (Bailey, 2003), not a specific profession. This is an important point for both DNP graduates and other professionals to remember when they are questioned about their title or educational preparation.

Parity Among Healthcare Professionals: One of the DNP Drivers Revisited

It is clear in the literature that one of the drivers of the DNP degree is parity in the healthcare setting (Clinton & Sperhac, 2006; Marion, O'Sullivan, Crabtree, Price, & Fontana, 2005; Newman, 1975; Olshansky, 2004). Arguments for parity have also made the point that current nursing master's degrees already have more requirements than many other professional doctoral degrees (Clinton & Sperhac, 2006). Hence, with the adoption of a doctoral degree, parity with other professionals occurs, and nurses finally gain the recognition for their educational accomplishments that they deserve. Olshansky noted that nurses "who earn a DNP will be on par with our practicing health care colleagues facilitating easier interdisciplinary collaboration on an equal playing field" (2004, p. 211).

As the DNP degree gains momentum, it is interesting to note that other health-care professions have adopted the doctoral degree as the terminal degree or as entry into practice. Pharmacy was one of the earlier adopters of a doctorate degree for entry into practice (Upvall & Ptachcinski, 2007). Physical therapy also requires a doctorate for entry into practice. Occupational therapy and audiology have followed suit and are moving toward doctoral preparation both as an option and as entry into practice (Griffiths & Padilla, 2006; Pierce & Peyton, 1999; Roeser et al., 2005). Reviewing other healthcare professions' transition to a doctoral degree, including their reasons for adopting doctoral preparation, provides a rationale for this evolution and parity across the healthcare team.

Upvall and Ptachcinski (2007) compared pharmacy's transition to doctoral preparation (PharmD) to nursing's adoption of the DNP degree. The PharmD was developed as a response to societal needs for increased clinical services, similar to the need for nursing to increase its educational preparation. Pharmacy identified the need for increased preparation in pharmacotherapy in health care and, as a result, parity and advancement of the profession were secondary benefits (Upvall & Ptachcinski, 2007). Further, pharmacy recognized that the 5-year under-graduate degree did not provide a sufficient time frame for the biomedical sciences and clinical component that are necessary to meet expectations in practice (Upvall & Ptachcinski, 2007). This is similar to nursing in that a nursing master's degree may not efficiently accommodate the changing needs for preparation of advanced nursing practice (Clinton & Sperhac, 2006). Although this preparation was met with resistance at first (two failed attempts), advocates argued that doctoral preparation in pharmacy met the needs of a changing healthcare environment (Upvall & Ptachcinski, 2007). An evaluation of healthcare outcomes has also shown improvement and a reduction in medical errors as a result of the services from clinical pharmacists (Bond, Raehl, & Franke, 2002). It has also been noted that healthcare outcomes are improved by advanced-practice registered nurses (APRNs) (Brooten & Naylor, 1995). It is safe to assume, therefore, that the additional preparation provided by the DNP degree will continually improve healthcare outcomes.

Physical therapy has adopted the doctoral degree for entry into practice, and occupational therapy is in the process of adopting doctoral preparation. The incentives for this transition have been cited to parallel pharmacy, medicine, and dentistry in that advanced education, higher standards for entry into practice, and extended clinical experience will provide educational preparation that is necessary to facilitate change (Pierce & Peyton, 1999). Further, these two professions have noted comparable drivers toward doctoral preparation, which include advanced preparation to meet the changing needs of health care and parity with other health-care professionals (Pierce & Peyton, 1999).

Audiology is currently offering doctoral preparation as well, which combines both didactic learning and extensive clinical experiences. Roeser and colleagues (2005) described an emerging doctor of audiology program that combines academic course work, clinical experiences, a research experience, and mentoring. This program is 4 years long and is offered as a postbaccalaureate degree. The format mirrors that of a postbaccalaureate DNP degree, integrating academic course work, clinical specialization, and research. This degree is yet another example of how the education of healthcare professionals is evolving to meet the demands of society and the healthcare environment.

In summary, understanding the evolution toward doctoral preparation of various healthcare professionals provides further explanation regarding the importance of recognition of all healthcare professionals' educational preparation. The advanced educational preparation of all members of the interprofessional team should be celebrated, not hidden. Indeed, it is this advanced educational preparation that will serve to improve healthcare outcomes and quality of care. Moreover, it is envisioned that someday soon the entire healthcare team will be doctors. This team of doctors may include pharmacists, physical therapists, occupational therapists, nurses, and physicians who all strive toward the same goal, each with valuable knowledge and expertise that should be acknowledged equally. Diminishing this in any way seems counterproductive to the goals of health care today.

Review of *The Pearson Report* Regarding Title Protection

Each year Dr. Linda Pearson publishes a state-by-state national overview of nurse practitioner legislation and healthcare issues (Pearson, 2014). Dr. Pearson has been recapping the latest legislative information from each state's nurse practice act and rules and regulations, along with pertinent government, policy, and reimbursement information for several years.

It is interesting that in recent years Dr. Pearson has included legislation and regulations regarding the use of the title *doctor* by nurses who hold doctoral degrees. Moreover, in the 2008 report, Dr. Pearson included comments in her "My Impressions" section regarding this legislation and listed it as "Impression #1." Dr. Pearson specifically states, "We need to legislatively remove NP-degrading discrimination" (Pearson, 2008, p. 10). Dr. Pearson further commented that "NPs must remove any and all statutory restrictions prohibiting those of us with university earned doctorates from being addressed as doctor" (2008, p. 10). In her 2014 report, Dr. Pearson noted that 21 states (Alabama, Arizona, California, Florida, Georgia, Illinois, Kentucky, Maryland, Minnesota, Mississippi, New York, Ohio, Oklahoma, Oregon, Pennsylvania, South Carolina, South Dakota, Texas, Utah, Virginia, and Wyoming) have legislatively allowed qualified nurse practitioners to be addressed as *doctor* as long as they clarify that they are nurse practitioners (Pearson, 2014). Dr. Pearson related that this is appropriate because nurse practitioners are proud to be nurses and have no interest in being confused with physicians. Unfortunately, five states (Arkansas, Connecticut, Maine, Michigan, and Vermont) currently prohibit nurses with earned doctorates from being addressed as *doctor* (Pearson, 2014). Dr. Pearson related that "a quietly emerging trend in health care [is] likely to have a major effect on who will diagnose and treat illness in the coming years. Rather than a physician, a comprehensive-care provider may very well be a nurse—who also happens to be a doctor" (Pearson, 2008, p. 10). Dr. Pearson's comments and synopsis on this topic are timely and reflect the urgency to protect the right of nurses, and other doctoral-prepared professionals, to be appropriately recognized for their credentials, knowledge, and expertise.

The Debate

A debate previously unfolded in the literature in response to the American Medical Association (AMA) resolutions, which attempted to restrict the use of the title *doctor* by nurses with doctoral degrees. Nursing organizations have responded to this issue with arguments against such regulations that would restrict nurses from appropriately identifying their credentials. In addition, universities are also responding to this impending issue with ideas for a proactive, solution-based response.

American Medical Association Resolution

The AMA House of Delegates identified Resolution 211 (A-06) in May 2006, titled "Need to Expose and Counter Nurse Doctoral Programs (NDP) Misrepresentation" (AMA, 2006). This resolution states, "The quality of care rendered by individuals with nurse doctoral degrees is not equivalent to that of a physician" (AMA, 2006). Additionally, this resolution states that "Nurses and other nonphysician providers who hold doctoral degrees and identify themselves as doctors will create confusion, jeopardize patient safety, and erode the trust inherent in the true patient–physician relationship" (AMA, 2006). The resolution further states that "patients led to believe that they are receiving care from a doctor, who is not a physician, but who is a DNP may put their health at risk" (AMA, 2006). Therefore, the following resolutions were adopted:

- That it shall be the policy of our AMA that institutions offering advance education in the healing arts and professions shall fully and accurately inform applicants and students of the educational programs and degrees offered by an institution and the limitations, if any, on the scope of practice under applicable law for which the program prepares the student; and it be further
  - resolved that our AMA work jointly with state attorneys general to identify and prosecute those individuals who misrepresent themselves as physicians to their patients and mislead program applicants as to their future scope of practice; and it be further

- resolved that our AMA pursue all other appropriate legislative, regulatory and legal actions through the Scope of Practice Partnership, as well as actions within hospital staff organizations, to counter misrepresentation by nurse doctoral programs students and graduates, particularly in the clinical setting. (AMA, 2006)

It should be noted that if nurses identify themselves appropriately by their earned degree and professional designation, none of these resolutions apply. If nurses identify themselves as "Dr. Smith, nurse–midwife" or "Dr. Jones, chief nursing officer," it should be quite obvious what discipline these professionals subscribe to. Further, it is safe to assume that when nurses apply to a DNP program they are well aware of the discipline in which they are getting their degree. After all, nurses went to college, too.

The Literature

This issue has also been discussed and debated in the literature in response to the AMA Resolution 211 (A-06). Royeen and Lavin (2007) wrote a commentary on the analysis of healthcare professionals who earn doctorate degrees and responded to the issues regarding the title *doctor*. It was acknowledged that the public commonly associates the term *doctor* with physicians. However, Royeen and Lavin stated the following:

> That does not mean that others may not be referred to as doctor when holding a professional degree. It does mean that the nature of the degree needs to be clearly communicated to the public for whom they care and that professionals identify themselves [as] physicians, nurse practitioners, physical therapists, occupational therapists, and so on instead of using the term doctor as if it were synonymous with one professional group. (2007, p. 102)

Reeves (2008) also responded to AMA Resolution 211 (A-06) and highlighted the fact that APRNs do not wish to be confused with physicians, and, in fact, APRNs capitalize on the different type of care they provide. Explaining further, Reeves stated, "It is essential that health care professionals and the public be taught the differences between the disciplines of nursing and medicine. Nurses do not want to misrepresent themselves. We understand that health care often involves working together with an interdisciplinary team to provide optimal patient care" (2008).

O'Grady (2007) shared a similar response to the current debate regarding this issue and reinforced the notion that the public and other healthcare professionals need to be educated regarding this issue. The author noted that it is the public's right to know who is caring for them and what credentials those individuals hold: "To require health professionals other than physicians to hide their credentials is directly contrary to health care transparency and consumer empowerment" (2007, p. 8). Moreover, O'Grady related that "the truth—letting patients know in the clearest possible way who is caring for them—should be the foundation for sound policymaking" (2007, p. 8). Nursing as a whole is responsible to respond to this issue. The belief that the DNP degree results in social good as a consequence of more educated nurses, along with the belief that nurses have power over their practice, means that nurses must work together to be freed from illogical and oppressive policies that force nurses to hide their credentials (O'Grady, 2007).

Nursing's Response

Nursing responded collectively to this issue by addressing the AMA directly. Major nursing organizations drafted a unified statement and published "DNP Talking Points" specific to this issue (American Association of Colleges of Nursing [AACN], 2014). In June 2008 the American Nurses Association (ANA) sent a letter to the director of the AMA House of Delegates. This letter specifically addressed protection of the title *doctor*. In the letter, Rebecca Patton, MSN, RN, CNOR, ANA president and Linda J. Stierle, MSN, RN, CNAA-BC, ANA CEO summarized the origin of the title *doctor* and further explained that a doctor is one who has earned a doctoral degree in any field. Ms. Patton and Ms. Stierle also addressed the issue of patient confusion and stated, "If patient confusion is really the concern, the nursing community would welcome the efforts to communicate to patients just who—and what type—of healthcare professionals are examining and treating them" (ANA, 2008, p. 2). Further, the notion of restraint of trade was brought to Dr. David Lichtman's (Chair, AMA Reference Committee C, Medical Education) attention. In previous situations, the U.S. Court of Appeals ruled that the AMA could not boycott another's healthcare profession because this would violate the Sherman Act, which pertains to antitrust. This communication from the ANA to the AMA exemplifies the proactive, united stance that nursing must take when confronted with this issue.

Another example of collectively addressing this issue occurred when several nursing organizations drafted a unified statement regarding nurse practitioner DNP education. This statement was written collaboratively by the American Academy of Nurse Practitioners, the American College of Nurse Practitioners, the National Association of Pediatric Nurse Practitioners, the Association of Faculties of Pediatric Nurse Practitioners, the National Organization of Nurse Practitioner Faculties, the National Conference of Gerontological Nurse Practitioners, and the National Association of Nurse Practitioners in Women's Health, collectively referred to as the Nurse Practitioner Roundtable. This statement addresses certification and titling issues and specifically outlines the utilization of the title *doctor* by nurse practitioners. The recommendations of this statement are as follows:

1. The title doctor represents an academic credential and is not limited to professional programs. Graduate educational programs in colleges and universities in the United States confer academic degrees, which permit graduates to be called doctor. No one discipline owns the title "doctor."

2. In the healthcare field, the term doctor is not limited to medical doctors. Other health professions use their academic title: e.g., Doctor of Osteopathy, Doctor of Pharmacy, Doctor of Podiatry, Doctor of Psychology, Doctor of Physical Therapy, and others.

3. While the titles "Medical Doctor" or "Doctor of Osteopathy" may be protected by statute in a given state, the term "doctor" alone is not.

4. Recognition of the title "doctor" for doctoral-prepared nurse practitioners facilitates parity within the healthcare system. (Nurse Practitioner Roundtable, 2008, p. 2)

Finally, the AACN developed a "DNP Talking Points" document that describes the rationale for the DNP degree, which was developed to provide valuable, factual information for nurse educators, DNP graduates, nurses, and other healthcare professionals. The talking points include the following statements:

- "The rapid expansion of knowledge underlying practice; increased complexity of patient care; national concerns about the quality of care and patient safety; shortages of nursing personnel, which demands a higher level of preparation for leaders who can design and assess care; shortages of doctorally prepared nursing faculty; and increasing educational expectations for the preparation of other health professionals contribute to the momentum of nursing graduate education" (AACN, 2014).

- "The Institute of Medicine, Joint Commission, and other authorities have called for reconceptualizing health professions education to meet the needs of the healthcare delivery system. Nursing is answering that call by moving to prepare APRNs for evolving practice" (AACN, 2014).

- "In a 2005 report titled 'Advancing the Nation's Health Needs: NIH Research Training Programs,' the National Academy of Sciences called for nursing to develop a nonresearch clinical doctorate to prepare expert practitioners who can also serve as clinical faculty. The AACN's work to advance the DNP is consistent with this call to action." (AACN, 2014)

- "Nursing is moving in the direction of other health professions in the transition to the DNP. Medicine (MD), Dentistry (DDS), Pharmacy (PharmD), Psychology (PsyD), Physical Therapy (DPT), and Audiology (AudD) all offer practice doctorates." (AACN, 2014)

- "Historically, advanced practice nurses, including nurse practitioners, clinical nurse specialists, nurse–midwives, and nurse anesthetists, are typically prepared in master's degree programs, some of which carry a credit load equivalent to doctoral degrees in the other health professions." (AACN, 2014)

- "Transitioning to the DNP will not alter the current scope of practice for APRNs. State Nurse Practice Acts describe the scope of practice allowed, and these differ from state to state. The transition to the DNP will better prepare APRNs for their current roles given the calls for new models of education and the growing complexity of health care." (AACN, 2014)

- "The title of doctor is common to many disciplines and is not the domain of any one health profession. Many APRNs currently hold doctoral degrees and are addressed as doctors, which is similar to how clinical psychologists, dentists, podiatrists, and other experts are addressed. Like other providers, DNPs would be expected to display their credentials to insure that patients understand their preparation as a nursing provider." (AACN, 2014)

- "Nursing and medicine are distinct health disciplines that prepare clinicians to assume different roles and meet different practice expectations. DNP programs will prepare nurses for the highest level of nursing practice." (AACN, 2014)

The Emergency Nurses Association also drafted a position statement, titled "Appropriate Credential Use/Title Protection for Nurses with Advanced Degrees," to address title issues. It states the following:*

1. Nurses are entitled to have their professional degree recognized and acknowledged in the same manner as other professions.

2. The proper title protection and use of accurate credentials is appropriate in the clinical setting.

3. When being addressed or introduced in the clinical environment, it is the responsible practice for all healthcare providers to clarify their professional role.

4. Patients, families, and the general public have a right and expectation to be informed regarding the credentials of their caregivers, including the use of the title "doctor."

DNP graduates may use documents such as these to educate themselves, nurses, and other healthcare professionals so they can effectively respond to questions and debate title issues.

A University's Response

Oakland University in Rochester, Michigan, graduated the first DNP program in the state in December 2007 and May 2008. Twenty-two nurses with DNP degrees returned to their settings, both academic and clinical, and began to proudly display

---

*Used with permission of the Emergency Nurses Association, ENA Position from "Appropriate Credential Use/Title Protection For Nurses With Advanced Degrees" Position Statement. © 2013 http://www.ena.org/SiteCollectionDocuments/Position%20Statements/AppropriateCredential.pdf, p. 1.

their new credentials. Most were met with support, but unfortunately, as with many pioneers, some graduates were faced with resistance to change. One case in particular, which will be described later in the chapter, resulted in the DNP graduate being threatened with a misdemeanor charge if she used the title *doctor*. Fortunately, Oakland University supported its DNP graduates and responded to this oppressive, irrational behavior. Consequently, Dr. Frances Jackson, director of Oakland University's DNP program, organized a coalition meeting. This meeting was attended by various university deans; nursing political organizations; Michigan's chief nurse executive, Ms. Jeanette Wrona Klemczak; physical therapy organizations; and various DNP program directors. Dr. Jackson moderated the meeting, and overall it established a unified stance between nursing and physical therapy as an early response to title issues.

American Medical Association Resolution Rejected

In June 2008 the AMA House of Delegates officially rejected the resolution that would limit the use of the titles *doctor*, *resident*, and *residency* to physicians, dentists, and podiatrists. Mason commented on this in an editorial and stated, "Somehow, the group realized that the term doctor applies to anyone who has earned a doctoral degree" (2008, p. 7). Incidentally, if the resolution would have progressed further, it would have supported making it a felony for a nonphysician to represent her- or himself as a physician by using the title *doctor* (Mason, 2008). It should be noted, however, that despite the rejection of this resolution, individual states may still mandate the use of the title *doctor*. These mandates range from prohibiting the use of the title *doctor* by those not specified within the mandate to requiring that the professional designation follow the title *doctor*. Nursing has long supported making sure that patients know who is providing their care and will continue to educate the public regarding their educational preparation and professional role.

Most Recent Legislative Action Regarding Title Restriction

In 2013 two proposed bills in the Florida State Senate asserted that it was a third-degree felony for nurses with doctorates to use the title *doctor* when introducing themselves to patients (Florida House of Representatives, 2013). Nurses would be required to immediately qualify their use of the title with a statement explaining they are not medical doctors (Waldrop, 2013). The American Association of Nurse Practitioners responded by formally asking its members to contact their Florida legislators and request that they vote no on this bill. Fortunately, it died in Health Quality Subcommittee on May 3, 2013 (Florida Senate, 2013). Interestingly, an existing Florida law already states that healthcare professionals must identify their professional designation orally or in writing (on a name badge), and misrepresenting themselves as a physician will result in a misdemeanor charge (Waldrop, 2013).

In 2011 the New York State Senate proposed a bill that would limit nurses from advertising themselves as doctors, regardless of their educational preparation (Waldrop, 2013). Fortunately this bill also died in the 2011–2012 session. Currently, in Arizona and Delaware, nurses, pharmacists, and other nonphysician providers are restricted from using the title *doctor* without immediately identifying their professional designation (Waldrop, 2013).

Case Scenario: A Doctor Nurse's Story

Unfortunately, despite the realization that all professionals may earn doctorate degrees and use the title associated with the degree, some recent DNP graduates are experiencing significant resistance to using the title of *doctor*. This case scenario is a true account of a DNP graduate clinician who is a nurse practitioner in rural Michigan. Her interview follows the highlights of her story, which are provided in this case scenario.

Dr. O. was welcomed back after graduation from her DNP program with a congratulatory advertisement in her local newspaper, which addressed her as Dr. O., FNP, Doctor of Nursing Practice; Family Nurse Practitioner. Shortly after this, the RN Staff Council of her hospital organization received a letter from the hospital's attorney stating that Michigan Public Act 368 of 1978 strictly limits the use of the term *doctor* by anyone licensed under the Public Health Code. It further stated that by specifying the professions licensed under the Public Health Code that are entitled to use the term *doctor*, the legislation implicated the limited use of the term to those listed healthcare professionals. The letter surmised that the limitation on the term *doctor* was related to the "high likelihood of confusion among consumers/patients and not an indictment against the degree holder" (personal communication). The letter went on to say that use of the term *doctor* by a healthcare professional not listed in Public Act 368 was a misdemeanor. Dr. O. was notified that the case was apparently discussed with the local prosecuting attorney's office, and they would not take action provided any further use of the designations be in compliance with Public Act 368.

The action from the hospital administration did not change Dr. O.'s title in the clinical setting. The clinic did not have any interaction with hospital administration, and Dr. O. has never heard directly from the hospital attorney's office. Therefore, in her practice setting Dr. O. has continued to use her appropriate title.

Dr. O.'s next actions were very insightful and proactive. She started to write multiple emails to hospital administration purporting the benefit of supporting DNPs in the use of the *doctor* title in clinical practice. She also began educating colleagues, patients, and the community regarding the doctorate of nursing practice and the use of the title *doctor* in clinical practice. In an effort to educate her hospital organization directly, Dr. O. personally presented before the RN Staff Council and explained the DNP and use of the title.

To date, Dr. O. continues to write numerous letters and communicate with multiple nursing organizations regarding the controversial use of the *doctor* title for DNPs. She has also attended state and national meetings to discuss the use of the *doctor* title for DNPs in Michigan and nationally. In addition, she has made personal contacts with the president and president-elect of the Michigan Council for Nurse Practitioners (MICNP). Dr. O. has also been in personal contact with the chief nurse executive of Michigan, Ms. Jeanette Wrona Klemczak. She contacted the legal council for the American Academy of Nurse Practitioners. Dr. O. also gained support from the university from which she earned her DNP degree. In response to her situation, a coalition meeting was organized to begin addressing this issue in Michigan. This meeting demonstrated the support of other professionals regarding this issue. Finally, Dr. O. has become a member of the Coalition of Michigan Organizations of Nursing, a representative of MICNP, to pursue the issue with nursing organizations throughout Michigan. Dr. O. continues to be proactive and use the leadership and interprofessional collaboration skills she garnered in the DNP program to educate others regarding this very controversial and pertinent issue.

Interview with a Doctor Nurse Champion: Then and Now

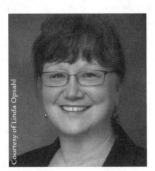

Courtesy of Linda Opsahl

LINDA OPSAHL, DNP, APRN, BC, is a family nurse practitioner who works in rural Michigan. Her story was told in the preceding case scenario.

THEN . . . 2008

Dr. Opsahl, could you please describe your position?

I am a family nurse practitioner working in the rural Upper Peninsula of Michigan. I work for a hospital organization with several satellite clinics as well as the typical hospital setting. I work in two rural health clinics, and I also fill in for several other clinics on my days off. I am busy. I have a productive and growing practice. I am associated with a physician who is well liked and very knowledgeable. I love being a nurse practitioner. I consider it my calling.

Dr. Opsahl, what was the motivation for you to return to school for a DNP?

What motivated me to spend less time with my family, increase pressures and stressors in my life, and pull all-nighters at the ripe age of 52?

It wasn't that I would gain financially by going back to school. When I told my employer that I would be going back to school, they told me there would be no monetary increase because of the degree. They informed me that the degree would not change the way I practiced in the clinics; therefore, there would be no wage increase. Sadly, I also would not gain financially if I were to become a nursing professor. In fact, I would take a very large pay cut to teach in a university. The wage discrepancy for nursing instructors as compared to other university instructors such as engineers and medical doctors is something our profession must address.

It wasn't that I desired the prestige and recognition that the DNP degree would bring. When I told my physician partner I was going back to school, he told me I should go to medical school rather than obtain a nursing doctorate. Those same thoughts were echoed by family, friends, and patients who wondered just what a nurse doctor was. Many did not have a clear understanding of just what a nurse practitioner was. Some asked, "Will a doctorate in nursing make you equal to a PA?" I was also surprised by the negative responses of some PhD nurses toward the DNP. Their "my degree is better than your degree" attitude is proof that the theory–practice gap in nursing continues to plague our profession.

My motivation was higher education and the opportunities a doctorate degree could bring to my professional practice and the nursing profession in general. I've wanted to be a doctor since I was in grade school. I love the philosophy and foundation of nursing. A nurse doctor fits my personal and professional philosophy of holism and caring as compared to that of a traditional medical doctoral education. I was also motivated by the shortage of nursing instructors and made a personal and professional commitment to help fill that gap in the future.

Dr. Opsahl, how has your role evolved since earning your DNP degree?

My role as a family nurse practitioner has been markedly enhanced by the degree. I use more evidence-based practice. I collect more practice information and study quality indicators more closely. I use the quality indicators to show that nurse practitioners provide quality care with exceptional results. I am much more politically active in regard to health-care issues affecting nurses, patients, the local community, and the nation. If you asked my employer if my role has changed, they would say no. To most people, the changes in my role are unseen. I think they would not be understood by others unless they were to truly appreciate, understand, and commit to the methods and importance of quality care and patient advocacy in the health of patients.

In the best of worlds, I hope to gain equal standing and respect with other doctorate degrees in health care. In reality, representatives of the administration and medical staff of the hospital where I am employed take a different view. I am told that the doctor designation for a nurse practitioner would be too confusing to the public and therefore should not be associated with the DNP in my current employment.

In my actual clinic sites, patients are proud that I have now become a nurse doctor. Many of them call me doctor, *and all of them understand that I am a doctor of nursing practice rather than a doctor of medicine. I do not stop them from calling me* doctor. *There are also many patients that continue to call me by my first name. I don't correct them. Many of them have been calling me Linda for over 10 years.*

Dr. Opsahl, how have your colleagues in your immediate clinical setting responded to your new degree?

My physician partner and the office staff in my clinical settings have been supportive of the DNP educational process and the new degree. I had no trouble getting time off when needed. I maintained my schedule and actually saw more patients in the one and a half years of the DNP program than in previous years. My physician partner continues to have difficulty understanding why I would choose to be a nurse doctor over a medical doctor. Initially, he felt that physicians held sole rights to the title of doctor *in the healthcare environment. After I explained the origin and meaning of the word* doctor *and described and stated the numerous professions that also hold the title, he understood my reasoning and changed his mind a bit. Professionally, he now introduces me as Dr. Linda Opsahl.*

Dr. Opsahl, have you found nursing to be supportive in your clinical setting?

The LPNs in my immediate clinical setting have been supportive. The RNs in my immediate clinical setting have been very supportive. The RNs in the hospital setting and in the community have been very supportive. The office staff in my immediate clinical settings threw me a party at the office and gave me an engraved name pin with the title Dr. *before my name. RNs in the local council of the state nursing organization took out an ad in the local newspaper congratulating me on my accomplishment and recognized me as "Dr. Linda Opsahl, Family Nurse Practitioner." They sent letters of support to the hospital administration for the use of the title* doctor *with nurse practitioners or any nurse achieving a doctorate degree.*

Dr. Opsahl, how have you educated your colleagues and patients about your DNP degree?

As a family nurse practitioner, I am very familiar with addressing the question of why I am a nurse practitioner rather than a PA or physician and how my role as a nurse practitioner will affect the care I give to patients. Now I just modify the statement to tell them why I chose to become a nurse doctor. The answer is very similar. I chose to become a nurse practitioner with a doctorate in nursing practice because I love the holistic, caring, all-encompassing philosophy of nursing toward patients, their health, and their environment. As a nurse doctor, I can use the philosophy of nursing to guide my practice and enhance the care I give and patients receive. I tell patients and colleagues that I view multiple issues of a person or patient simultaneously. Each perspective or issue (emotional, financial, personal views, religious views, social, etc.) adds crucial information to the care and treatment plan for that patient. As a nurse, I am a health partner with the patient, developing and providing the necessary information and treatment plan in partnership with each individual.

I tell patients that I have a doctorate degree in nursing, not medicine. I tell them I am a nurse doctor. I combine the philosophy of nursing with the clinical and diagnostic perspective of medicine, integrating both with old and new evidence-based practice for their benefit. I provide the best of both worlds.

Dr. Opsahl, could you describe what happened when the hospital administration realized you were using the title *doctor*?

I was reviewing an article from the public relations department of my organization with regard to my recent DNP degree. The article was wonderful, explaining what a nurse practitioner was and what the new degree entailed. In editing the article, I added the title Dr. in front of my name. Not only did I deserve the title through my degree acquisition, but I also felt that because this article would be sent to all my patients and other members of the community, it would be respectful and professionally appropriate to use the title. The article then went for review to the physician services department where a nurse manager evaluated the article and, under the direction of administration, removed the title Dr. from the article. Their rationale was that the designation of Dr. for a nurse practitioner would be too confusing to the public when associated with a DNP.

Dr. Opsahl, could you describe the legal action that took place as a result of administration restricting your use of the title *doctor*?

When the hospital RN staff council placed a congratulatory advertisement in the paper addressing me as "Dr. Linda Opsahl, FNP; Doctor of Nursing Practice; Family Nurse Practitioner," the RN staff council received a letter from the hospital attorney stating that Michigan Public Act 368 of 1978 strictly limits the use of the term doctor *by anyone licensed under the Public Health Code. It further stated that by specifying the professions licensed under the Public Health Code entitled to use the term* doctor*, the legislation implicated the limited use of the term to those listed healthcare professionals. The letter surmised that the legislative history suggests that the limitation of the use of the term* doctor *was* related to the *"high likelihood of confusion among consumers/patients and not an indictment against the degree holder."* The letter went on to say that use of the term doctor by a healthcare professional not listed in Public Act 368 was a misdemeanor. The case was apparently discussed with the local prosecuting attorney's office, and they would not take action provided any further use of the designations be in compliance with Public Act 368.

Dr. Opsahl, what has been the reaction in your immediate clinical setting to this?

This issue has not been addressed in my immediate clinical setting. I did not hear directly from the hospital attorney. I have not changed my practice or title in the clinical setting.

Dr. Opsahl, what steps have you taken at this point to be proactive regarding your earned degree title?

I have written multiple emails to hospital administration purporting the benefit of supporting DNPs in the use of the doctor *title in clinical practice. I educate colleagues, patients, and the community regarding the doctorate of nursing practice and the use of the title* doctor *in clinical practice. I explain that there is currently controversy over title use. I went before the RN Staff Council to explain the DNP and title use. I have written numerous letters and communicated with multiple nursing organizations regarding the controversial use of the* doctor *title for DNPs. I attended state and national meetings to discuss the use of the* doctor *title for DNPs in Michigan and nationally. I have made personal contacts with the president and president-elect of the nurse practitioner council in Michigan. I have made personal contact with the chief nurse executive of Michigan. I have made personal contact with legal council for the American Academy of Nurse Practitioners. I have become a member of COMON as a representative of MICNP to pursue the issue with nursing organizations throughout Michigan.*

Dr. Opsahl, how do you feel about Oakland University's response and support regarding this issue?

I was very impressed by the response of Oakland University toward the titling issue. Dr. Jackson did an excellent job in bringing nurses across Michigan together to resolve this issue.

Dr. Opsahl, how do you feel this issue should be dealt with by other DNP graduates and healthcare professionals?

I think we are making a mistake by stepping or treading quietly regarding this issue and many issues in nursing. As nurse practitioners in Michigan, we are essentially a very small group. With the current situation in our state nurses' organization (MNA), we are left to fight on our own. Nursing in Michigan, the United States, and internationally must unite for common purposes, one of which is to enhance the profession for all nurses regardless of education. As it sits now, the staff nurses have their group, the nurse practitioners have their group, academia and PhD nurses have their group, and little is being done to bring us all together. By walking softly, there exists a communication gap between nursing organizations. By walking softly, the public is not aware of the controversies between nursing, administration, and medicine that ultimately affect patient care.

We have this attitude in Michigan right now. Nurses are saying that we can't get anything passed or accomplished until so and so is out of office. I don't believe that to be true. I think there are plenty of back doors in many situations. If the public is made aware that their nurse practitioner is being discriminated against, they will also stand up and fight. The DNP titling issue is discrimination. We are being crimped by administrators and the AMA because we are nurses and because we are women, and because we tend to walk softly.

Dr. Opsahl, despite what has occurred regarding your title, do you feel it was a good decision to return to school for a DNP degree?

Oh, yes. I would do it again and again. It was a wonderful opportunity. It has motivated me to become a better practitioner, a better patient advocate. I have become more verbal about important issues in practice because of it. I feel more confident. I feel it has given me the tools to fight discriminatory practice toward nurses.

NOW . . . 2014

Dr. Opsahl, upon graduating with a DNP degree in 2007, you experienced significant resistance regarding using the title *doctor* from a large hospital organization. How has this situation evolved over time?

The organization is essentially avoiding any controversial discussion in regard to the use of the doctor *title.*

Dr. Opsahl, are you still feeling supported to use the title *doctor* by your colleagues in your immediate clinical setting?

Yes, but I have recently added another clinic to my workload and am at square one again in that I have a whole new group of colleagues and patients to educate regarding the doctor of nursing practice degree and title. It's all about educating the public to the point where they feel comfortable and satisfied with your explanation of who you are and the care you give. I feel I have earned the title in the eyes of my patients (as well as with the diploma on my office wall).

Dr. Opsahl, do you continue to use the title *doctor* in your clinical setting? If so, how do you introduce yourself?

To new patients, I introduce myself as follows: I am Dr. Linda Opsahl, a family nurse practitioner with a doctorate degree in nursing practice. I am not a medical doctor. I am a nurse doctor. There are many types of doctors: doctor of dentistry, doctor of psychology, doctor of osteopathy, doctor of chiropractic, doctor of medicine . . . like them, I graduated with a doctorate degree. My degree is in nursing practice. I am able to evaluate and treat your healthcare issues and needs similar to a physician. Doctors of nursing have a different philosophy than doctors of medicine. We see you as a holistic or whole being and include all your psychosocial needs in our decision making, as well as your physical needs. We want you to be an involved and educated member of your healthcare decision-making process.

Dr. Opsahl, in 2013 the Florida State Senate introduced a bill that would allow charging nurses using the title *doctor* with a felony. In 2011 the New York State Senate introduced a similar bill placing restrictions on use of the title *doctor*. Both of these bills died in legislation. What do you think about recent state legislation restricting use of the title *doctor* by nurses who have an earned doctorate degree?

According to a New York Times article in 2011 in regard to these legislative bills (Harris, 2011), the moving force behind the legislation to restrict the use of the doctor title is physicians and their allies. The article cited Dr. Roland Goertz, the board chairman of the American Academy of Family Physicians at that time, as saying "physicians are worried that losing control over 'doctor,' a word that has defined their profession for centuries, will be followed by the loss of control over the profession itself" (2011, para. 8). Physicians are concerned that doctorate degrees in nursing, pharmacy, and physical therapy will persuade more state legislators to pass legislation allowing these groups to treat patients without physician supervision. There is concern among physician groups that the use of the word doctor by professions other than physicians will be confusing for patients. These groups insist that nurses are obtaining doctorates for selfish gains including money, power, and prestige.

Legislation to restrict use of the doctor title is being driven by fear of loss of control by physician groups. Somehow physician groups are convincing legislators that to allow professions other than medical doctors to use the title doctor is harmful and confusing to society—so harmful that to do so should be considered a felonious criminal offense! Publicists are printing irrational articles giving false credence to their concerns.

I see this as an act of intimidation and basic bullying by these physician groups and their allies. Their allies are a large group that we must pay attention to, including healthcare administrations, legislators, legal systems, and publication sources. Nursing has been intimidated by physicians and their allies for decades. To consider felonious legislation against a doctor of nursing practice is an injustice against nursing. The doctor title in nursing is a nursing profession issue, a feminist issue, an academic issue, and a constitutional issue. This issue will be solved only when groups of supporters, including all nursing organizations, feminist organizations, and most importantly, academic institutions, come together to educate legislators, the public, and physicians regarding the appropriate use of the title doctor with any doctoral degree. Where are these organizations? Where are the academic institutions that award these degrees?

Dr. Opsahl, what advice do you have for others graduating with a DNP degree regarding using the title *doctor*?

Ask yourself what motivated you to go the extra mile to obtain your doctorate. For me, it was to improve my education, and the profession that I am so proud of, so that I am able to provide the best care I can to the patient. It wasn't about prestige, power, and certainly not about money. We need to advertise the fact that we are doing this to improve patient care and the profession of nursing, not for financial gains or the prestige of being called doctor.

Nurses in doctorate programs, and graduates of other doctorate programs, should be writing to their universities insisting that they offer support in solving this. The doctor title is an academic matter.

Don't be intimidated by the big guys. If you are told that you cannot use the title in your practice, engage your resources such as nursing organizations and supportive colleagues to help you resolve the conflict. Be proactive. Don't feel victimized. Hierarchy, inequality, and disparity have always been a part of our social structure. For me, these injustices are a cause for a response, sometimes a battle, not a retreat.

Use the title as you introduce yourself to patients and colleagues. Always explain that you are a doctor of nursing practice. Use it as an opportunity to engage the patient in a conversation regarding the scope of practice of a nurse practitioner and the positive, evidence-based outcomes that we can provide to patients.

Interview with a Doctor Nurse Advocate and DNP Program Director: Then and Now

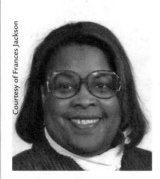

Courtesy of Frances Jackson

FRANCES JACKSON, PHD, RN, is associate professor and previous director of the doctor of nursing practice program at Oakland University School of Nursing in Rochester, Michigan.

THEN . . . 2008

Dr. Jackson, could you please describe your background, including why you pursued a career in nursing?

I came from a family of schoolteachers, so initially my interest in nursing was met with some resistance. My original interest in nursing stemmed from watching the soap opera Another World. *I used to like the character Alice; she was a nurse and all she did was visit with friends in the cafeteria, hold patients' hands, wipe their brow. I thought, I could do that. When I started nursing school and experienced my first clinical rotation at Wayne State University School of Nursing, I was in for a big surprise. I thought immediately, "This is fantastic!" I still feel blessed to be in a profession that gives you a front-row seat of people's lives—the good, the bad, and the ugly. In nursing, you see people at their best and at their worst. I feel it is a privilege to do so and a privilege to say that I am a nurse. After graduation from Wayne State University with a bachelor's in the science of nursing, I worked at Harper Hospital in Detroit, Michigan, in substance abuse and home care.*

I then returned to graduate school and earned a master's degree in counseling. I worked at Oakland University as a counselor in the School of Nursing. I wanted to give students someone to talk to while they were going through the nursing program. My position was later phased out, and I was faced with a decision. I had an epiphany conversation with my dean at the time. She asked me, "Are you a nurse, or a counselor?" If I was a counselor first, she suggested I do that. If I was a nurse first, she said I needed to return to graduate school. When I asked myself this question, without hesitation I answered that I am a nurse, first, last, and always. I then went back to graduate school at the University of Michigan in Ann Arbor, Michigan, and earned a master's in medical–surgical nursing. I worked in hospice care to try to improve end-of-life care and as a medical–surgical clinical nurse specialist. I also began teaching part time at Oakland University. I then returned to Wayne State University and earned a PhD in counseling. During this time I remained on faculty at Oakland University and also worked at Harper Hospital in medical–surgical nursing. I refer to working in med–surg as the call of the wild for me. I was successfully able to integrate my nursing background with counseling, and my PhD dissertation was based on the burnout of hospice nurses. Today I am still on faculty at Oakland University. I am the most senior faculty here. I am also the director of the DNP program.

Dr. Jackson, could you please describe your position as the director of the DNP program at Oakland University?

I am responsible for recruitment, understanding how classes work and how they will be scheduled, selection of faculty for the DNP program, interviewing and admission of students, and the DNP student handbook.

Dr. Jackson, do you believe the DNP is gaining momentum in enrollment, and if so, why?

Yes, it is definitely gaining momentum. The role of the APRN has expanded beyond anything we envisioned. APRNs need other kinds of skills that the master's in nursing does not sufficiently provide. The DNP gives APRNs more skills than the master's degree in nursing and allows APRNs to function more effectively in a 21st century healthcare environment.

Dr. Jackson, could you please describe any challenges you are facing as director of the DNP program?

The challenge is keeping true to the purpose of the degree. People who don't want a PhD but are on faculty at a school of nursing and need a doctorate sometimes feel the DNP is a good degree for them. But this degree is for clinicians. It is not the stepsister of the PhD. Some feel the DNP is a mini-PhD. It is not. It is for nurses whose interest, passion, and priority is patient care.

The second issue I have been surprised about is that I did not envision Oakland University's program to be a national program. I am surprised by the enrollment and interest of individuals from all over the country. This is probably due to the delivery of much of the course work being distance-learning oriented. However, even when classes require a student to be on campus, they are making arrangements to be here.

Dr. Jackson, what is your opinion regarding the reaction we are seeing to nurses using the title *doctor*?

I feel the reaction is a smoke screen for the real issues. APRNs are viewed as competitors and an economic threat to physicians. Hospitals have had problems with nurses using the title doctor because doctors have a problem with it. Doctors are considered the hospital's customers and nurses are employees. If doctors were okay with it, hospitals would be okay with it. Look at pharmacy: hospitals and physicians have no problem acknowledging their title when pharmacists have a PharmD. This could be because pharmacists have limited patient contact. Also, pharmacists have an extensive science background. They are identified with science and are therefore more respected by the medical community. They are viewed as a resource for physicians and others in health care, not as one trying to invade physicians' turf.

Dr. Jackson, as a PhD-prepared nurse, how have you dealt with title issues in the past?

I tend to be quite confrontational. I was asked to join a hospital-based hospice committee, and when I attended the first meeting I noticed only the physicians' credentials were listed in the meeting agenda. I asked immediately, "Is it the culture of this hospital that only physicians went to college?" They responded yes, to which I responded, "Well, aren't you glad I am here to help you change that! I believe it is safe to say that everyone here went to college and therefore, everyone's credentials should be listed." By the next meeting, all of the credentials were listed for all members of the committee. I further explained at this meeting, "I don't mind being 'Frances' if he is 'John,' but if he is 'Dr. Smith,' then I am 'Dr. Jackson.'" This continues to be a problem outside the academic environment. In the clinical setting, when I have students on a floor in the hospital, the physicians stumble when they read my name badge that clearly displays "Frances Jackson, RN, PhD, Oakland University School of Nursing." I help them out and say, "Hi, I am Dr. Jackson, professor at Oakland University School of Nursing." Then they struggle less and call me "Dr. Jackson." Let me also say, I always tell patients, physicians, and family members in the clinical setting that I am a nurse. I am proud to be a nurse, and the very last thing I would do is hide that fact.

Dr. Jackson, do you feel this is an issue for all nurses who hold doctoral degrees?

No, not as much so in academia. Those of us in this setting are not an academic threat.

Dr. Jackson, could you describe what the catalyst was for you to call the coalition meeting at Oakland University to bring some leadership to this issue?

Well, Oakland University had the first DNP program in Michigan and the first DNP graduates who graduated from a program in Michigan. My students have been generous in keeping up with me regarding their evolving roles, publications, and reactions to the DNP degree. I was deeply disturbed by the response of Dr. Linda Opsahl's hospital administration. This was a clear attempt to squash any kind of acknowledgement of the accomplishment of the nurses who graduated from our program and went back to practice in this setting. What was really disappointing was that so often in nursing we don't celebrate each other's accomplishments. The nurses in this setting were very supportive and wanted to share these students' accomplishments. This is, I am afraid, the tip of the iceberg—the absurdity that nurses being addressed as doctor is against the law.

The deeper issue here is that there is a continual assault by physician lobbyists in the state of Michigan on APRNs—prescriptive authority, limiting what APRNs can do. We know that our doctoral preparation—and the title that comes with this—will be under attack as well. I decided that rather than wait for the attack we would be proactive by having a coalition meeting. Further, we invited physical therapy representation—we will surely not be the only healthcare professionals dealing with this issue.

Dr. Jackson, what do you feel nursing must do to be proactive regarding this issue?

We can't sit back and wait for others. We need to fight our own battles. We need to recruit other professions; there is power in numbers. We can't just sit back and talk about it in nursing, we have to have the numbers. Secondly, we need to ask for help from other organizations with political connections. We need to use the resources we have so we don't create problems. We need to inform and get feedback from our large nursing organizations and garner support from them as well. Third, we need to share successful strategies with other states that are facing similar issues. And fourth, we [need] to respond to threats and answer back, even if it's just a letter to the AMA or to an editor.

Dr. Jackson, do you have any advice for new PhD or DNP graduates who are met with resistance to the title *doctor*?

It is very important to educate yourself about your degree so you can respond appropriately when questioned regarding your title. It is also critically important to educate other nurses. Finally, my advice is don't let other people and their ignorance diminish your accomplishments.

UPDATE . . . 2011

Dr. Jackson, we discussed your nursing background and education last time we spoke. Could you please describe your current position?

I am the director of Graduate Programs in the School of Nursing. That includes the MSN and DNP programs.

Dr. Jackson, as a DNP program director, could you describe the progress of your program at Oakland University?

It has simply been amazing. As the first DNP program in the state of Michigan, we have enjoyed tremendous success in attracting and graduating DNP students. We have developed a BSN-to-DNP program, and that will be reviewed by the Graduate Council in the fall. We have also developed a DNP track for nurse anesthetists. They will be required to earn the DNP, I believe by 2025, to take the certification exam for CRNA [certified registered nurse anesthetist].

Dr. Jackson, could you please describe your perception of the progress of the DNP degree in general?

It is clear from the number of new DNP programs listed by the Commission on Collegiate Nursing Education (CCNE) that this degree is enjoying phenomenal success. However, it is also clear that there are many barriers for nurses who earn a terminal degree. The use of the title doctor continues to be a source of controversy. One major unresolved issue is whether the organizations that administer the certification exams for nurse practitioners will indeed require the DNP as the credential to take those exams. If they do require the DNP, then the success of the DNP will be assured. Even without it, students see the DNP course work as value added for their career plans.

Dr. Jackson, do you think the momentum of enrollment has increased over time? If so, why?

I believe it has increased. Some of the momentum, as stated previously, is directly related to the expectation that the organizations that administer the certification exams will require the DNP in order to take the exam. However, healthcare reform is also a driving force behind this degree. Never in my memory have nurse practitioners enjoyed such high employability. Almost every student I interview for admission to our DNP program has an interest in teaching at some point in the future. Most believe that possessing the DNP will enhance their ability to step into that role, even if it's only on a part-time basis.

Dr. Jackson, how has Oakland University benefitted from having a DNP degree program?

As the first DNP program in the state of Michigan, we naturally led the way with implementing this new degree. We also have had a longer time to evaluate what works and what isn't working. There will be some changes to the program starting in 2012. Starting the DNP expanded our visibility in the state but also nationally and even internationally. We have been privileged to attract students from 15 states and Canada. We are also attracting cohorts as hospitals and other agencies are sending groups of students to our program.

Dr. Jackson, what are some of the new challenges you face as a DNP program director?

We have been approached by nursing programs in foreign countries about offering the DNP abroad. Given the world situation, that is going to require very careful planning. Secondly, I see an increased need for financial aid at a time when the state is cutting back support for public universities.

Dr. Jackson, how do you think the DNP degree has affected nursing education since you became a DNP program director?

The CCNE requires that the director of the DNP program is someone who has a DNP. We have several faculty who have a DNP degree, something that was unheard of even 3 years ago. Faculty who are practicing clinicians bring a richness and depth to course work that is unique and special.

Dr. Jackson, do you agree with the AACN's recommended target date of 2015 for the DNP degree as entry into practice for APRNs? If so, how do you recommend we continue to strive toward this goal?

I agree with it. I'm not sure there is much more to be done than what is already being done. Many organizations are working very hard to enhance and support the DNP as the terminal degree for APRNs. If there is one issue on which we must have a united front it is the titling of DNP graduates. We cannot be silent and allow them to be treated as second-class citizens, subject to terrorist tactics by some physicians (not all!) who seem to believe that the title doctor is their exclusive domain.

Dr. Jackson, what is your advice to nurses and potential students regarding the DNP degree?

It is very important to understand the differences between the PhD and the DNP. Make sure you are applying for the degree that matches your future plans. If I ask you about your future plans and your response reflects more of a PhD trajectory, that could be enough to stop or delay your admission.

Dr. Jackson, do you think nurses have made any progress regarding using the title *doctor*? Why or why not?

If they have, it's not apparent to me. I think the powerful physician lobby has successfully blocked this issue. It's disheartening.

Dr. Jackson, what is your opinion regarding certain states' continued attempts at legislature mandating against nurses using the title *doctor*?

From what I've read, most of those states have forgotten that people like myself, nursing faculty who have an earned PhD, are also entitled to be called doctor. Nurses have been earning PhDs for decades and there was no legislative push to prohibit the title of doctor for nurses with PhDs. However, the amount of time and money physicians have spent on blocking the use of this title for nurses borders on the absurd. Where were these legislators when PharmDs graduated? What about dentists? They also have a professional doctoral degree.

Dr. Jackson, what advice do you now have for nurses who are graduating with a DNP degree and using the title *doctor* in the clinical setting?

Introduce yourself as "Dr. X," then say "I'm a nurse practitioner," or whatever you are. Make sure they understand your role and the limitations, if any, of your practice. I also think it is important to insist on what you've earned, where appropriate. I'm on several advisory boards, one of which is part of a major medical center. Years ago when we received the minutes of the first meeting, I noted that my credentials were omitted, but not the credentials of the physicians. I told the group that I had 15 years of college and four earned degrees, including PhD, and that I was Dr. Jackson. Either include everyone's credentials, or no one's credentials, but doctors weren't the only people in the room who had been to school. From that day on, everyone's credentials were included. Sometimes it's something as simple as that to make a difference.

Editor's note: Since publication of this text, Dr. Francis Jackson has retired from Oakland University. Her contributions to nursing education and research are greatly appreciated.

Tips for Using the Title *Doctor*

First and foremost, DNP graduates, and others, need to be educated about their degree. Royeen and Lavin noted the need to clear up misconceptions of the practice doctorate and "place the doctorate in context of larger educational change and innovation and share summary judgments about the nature and course of the newer doctoral degrees" (2007, p. 101). Further, these authors predicted that "within less than a generation, the majority of health care practitioners in allied health and advanced practice nursing will be degreed at the level of the clinical doctorate" (2007, p. 105). It is imperative that DNP graduates become familiar with the purpose and goals of their degree, the arguments against their title, the issues associated with their title, the history of the title *doctor*, and, as Dr. Frances Jackson emphasized, the true meaning of a practice doctorate. Moreover, DNP graduates must have the courage to stand up for their degree, expertise, and accomplishments. During the first day of this author's DNP Advanced Nursing Theory course, Professor Morris Magnan asked the question, "Are you going to stand for something or fall for everything?" This further emphasizes the point made in the beginning of the chapter. As pioneers, DNP graduates have the responsibility to know their degree and role in health care, lead the way, and stand for their educational achievements and value. The value and educational achievements that DNP graduates bring to the healthcare setting should be celebrated and not diminished in any way.

Please refer to **Box 11-1** for a list of tips for using the title *doctor*.

BOX 11-1

Suggested Tips for DNP Graduates Using the Title *Doctor*

- Educate yourself expansively about the history of the title *doctor*, including its true meaning and origins.

- Educate yourself about practice doctorates in other fields and become familiar with their issues and title use.

- Take a proactive stance when confronted with these issues and use the literature, comparable practices of others with the title of *doctor* (PharmD, DPT, PhD), and knowledge about your practice doctorate to support your position.

- Maintain a professional demeanor at all times despite conflicts. The ways in which DNP graduates deal with this issue will set the precedent for others in similar circumstances.

- Form coalitions with other organizations that are possibly confronted with this issue, such as physical therapy, occupational therapy, audiology, and others. A unified stance is always best.

- Educate other nurses and nursing organizations to garner support now and in the future. Our own profession must understand the importance of nursing's evolving academic preparation and the value this has for the entire profession.

- Use every opportunity to educate others about your title and degree, in and out of the practice setting.

- Always and without exception, use the title *doctor* followed by your professional title, such as nurse practitioner, nurse–midwife, nurse educator, clinical nurse specialist, or chief nursing officer, to prevent any misrepresentation and to advertise that you are a nurse.

- Ease others into the transition if you reenter a practice position where you were referred to differently in the past. Take the time to educate staff members, other nurses, and physicians in your setting regarding your title change, and allow time for adjustment. Be sure to provide resources to others regarding your title and degree preparation to reinforce the importance of the transition.

A Personal Note: My Experiences Using the Title *Doctor*

My experience using the title *doctor* has been a journey of sorts. Upon graduation I was a proud doctoral-prepared nurse, filled with conviction regarding my title. My previous place of employment was a small private practice with a very supportive collaborating physician. He greeted me immediately after graduation and asked if I was going to be "Dr. Chism" or "Dr. Astalos." I had previously practiced under my maiden name (Astalos), but during my DNP program I began using my married name, Chism. The front desk staff began scheduling patients for Dr. Chism but had trouble remembering to explain that I was a nurse practitioner. It seemed that others' use of my title had gone to the extreme.

About 2 years after graduation I began working within a large academic setting in a comprehensive breast center. It is a wonderful, collaborative group of nurse practitioners, clinical nurse specialists, physician assistants, surgeons, medical oncologists, radiologists, radiation oncologists, and pathologists. Some of the providers are also PhD-prepared researchers. Within our group, we all use our first name. In addition, no one in this setting understood or knew what a DNP degree was. Although I was respected as a nurse practitioner, the fact that I had a doctorate was either not noted or not understood. Instead of pushing the issue, I followed my colleagues' lead and used my first name and did not use the title *doctor*.

I am sure that some of you are surprised; allow me to explain. The skill termed "emotional intelligence" (Goleman, 1995) is useful in any setting, and I used my emotional intelligence to guide me regarding this situation. I knew I was practicing with some of the most accomplished and educated practitioners and researchers in the country, yet no one was concerned with titles. I made a decision to quietly educate others about my degree and lead by example.

After about a year in this setting, I became certified as a menopause practitioner through the North American Menopause Society (NAMS). I then developed a patient education booklet on menopause for patients with and without cancer that is now used throughout the center. Throughout this experience, my credentials became known. Others frequently commented on my degree and preparation. I had used my leadership skills to become certified as a menopause practitioner, develop a patient education booklet that is widely used within a certified cancer center, and develop a menopause consultant role within my practice. I then was selected as Menopause Practitioner of the Year through NAMS in 2011. My emotional intelligence skills had shown me that in this setting I would become more credible after I had exemplified my DNP skill set through my contributions to patient care and education.

Today many of my colleagues in this setting refer to me as Dr. Chism when I am introduced. I recently was at a work-related function, and a nursing colleague I had not yet met said, "Hello Dr. Chism, it's nice to finally meet you." Many colleagues have also become more aware of my DNP degree after I was inducted as a fellow of the American Academy of Nurse Practitioners. It was in that moment that I realized how important it is that after graduation we exemplify leadership through our contributions to establish our credibility. Although our title is earned and well deserved, it is through our contributions that we will have an impact on our profession. As DNP graduates' contributions are disseminated, perhaps our title will no longer be questioned.

SUMMARY

- The issues with use of the title *doctor* are not new but are now at the forefront of the debate about the DNP degree.

- The root of the term *doctor* is *docere*, which is Latin for *to teach* (Skinner, 1970).

- The first doctorate degrees originated in Bologna in the 12th century and were conferred to masters who teach (Skinner, 1970).

- The first doctorally prepared men exposed to the public were physicians, which may explain why the public associates this title with medicine (Skinner, 1970).

- Several other allied health professionals are adopting doctoral preparation, such as pharmacy, physical therapy, occupational therapy, and audiology.

- Doctoral preparation provides parity for nurses within the healthcare setting and places nurses "in an equal playing field" (Olshansky, 2004, p. 211).

- *The Pearson Report* is published each year and provides an update regarding legislative and regulatory issues for APRNs (specifically nurse practitioners). In 2014 Dr. Pearson reported that five states have regulations against the use of the title *doctor* by a nurse, despite academic preparation (Pearson, 2014).

- The AMA introduced Resolution 211 (A-06) in 2006, which suggests that nurses with DNP degrees are at risk for misrepresentation as physicians if they use the title *doctor* (AMA, 2006).

- Nursing responded to Resolution 211 (A-06) with letters to the AMA, responses in the literature, and talking points specifically developed to address this resolution.

- Oakland University responded to Resolution 211 (A-06) by forming a coalition with stakeholders who are taking a proactive stance against restrictive regulation regarding the title *doctor*.

- All DNP graduates need to educate themselves regarding the title *doctor*, the meaning of a practice doctorate, and their degree to formulate proactive, informed, and professional responses when faced with using the title *doctor*.

- All DNP graduates need to educate others, including patients, nurses, and other healthcare professionals, regarding their degree preparation in an effort to effectively and proactively respond to disputes regarding the use of the title *doctor*.

REFLECTION QUESTIONS

1. Before reading this chapter, did you know the origin of the title *doctor*? If not, what meaning did you associate with the title?

2. Do you think that DNP graduates, and others prepared with practice doctorates, should use the title *doctor*? Why or why not?

3. What is your response to the AMA's Resolution 211 (A-06)? What do you think is really driving this response from the AMA to nurses being prepared at the doctoral level?

4. Do you agree with nursing's proactive stance? What other suggestions do you have to continue to respond to this issue?

5. Upon graduation, how will you refer to yourself in the clinical setting?

6. Do you think you will be intimidated by others with practice doctorates (medical doctors, pharmacists) when you begin to use the title *doctor*? If so, how will you deal with this?

7. If you are met with resistance to your appropriate title, what approach will you take to resolve this issue in your setting?

REFERENCES

American Association of Colleges of Nursing. (2014). DNP talking points. Retrieved from http://www.aacn.nche.edu/dnp/talking-points

American Medical Association. (2006). Resolution 211 (A-06). Retrieved from http://www.ama-assn.org

American Nurses Association. (2008, June 11). Letter to American Medical Association. **Retrieved from nursingworld.org**/.../PressReleases/2008PR/**AMA**LetterTitles.pdf

Bailey, J. (2003). The story of "doctor," "physician," and "surgeon." *Journal of the National Medical Association, 85*(6), 489–490.

Bond, C., Raehl, C., & Franke, T. (2002). Clinical pharmacy services, hospital staffing and medication errors. *Pharmacotherapy, 22,* 134–147.

Brooten, D., & Naylor, M. (1995). Nurses' effect on changing patient outcomes. *IMAGE: Journal of Nursing Scholarship, 27*(2), 95–99.

Clinton, P., & Sperhac, A. (2006). National agenda for advanced practice nursing: The practice doctorate. *Journal of Professional Nursing, 22*(1), 7–14.

Doctor. (2014). In Merriam-Webster's online dictionary. Retrieved from http://www.merriam-webster.com/dictionary/doctor

Emergency Nurses Association. (2013). Appropriate credential use/title protection for nurses with advanced degrees. Retrieved from http://www.ena.org/SiteCollectionDocuments/Position%20Statements/AppropriateCredential.pdf

Florida House of Representatives. (2013). HB 805. Retrieved from http://www.flsenate.gov/Session/Bill/2013/0805/BillText/__/PDF

Florida Senate. (2013). HB 805: Health care practitioners. Retrieved from http://www.flsenate.gov/Session/Bill/2013/0805

Goleman, D. (1995). *Emotional intelligence: Why it can matter more than IQ.* New York, NY: Bantam Dell.

Greiner, A. C., & Knebel, E. (Eds.). (2003). *Health professions education: A bridge to quality.* Washington, DC: National Academies Press.

Griffiths, Y., & Padilla, R. (2006). National status of the entry-level doctorate in occupational therapy. *American Journal of Occupational Therapy, 60*(5), 540–549.

Harris, G. (2011, October 1). When the nurse wants to be called "doctor." *The New York Times.* Retrieved from http://www.nytimes.com/2011/10/02/health/policy/02docs.html?_r=0

Klein, T. (2007). *Are nurses with a doctor of nursing practice called "doctor"?* Retrieved from http://www.medscape.com/viewarticle/563176

Marion, L., O'Sullivan, A., Crabtree, K., Price, M., & Fontana, S. (2005). Curriculum models for the practice doctorate in nursing. *Topics in Advanced Practice Nursing eJournal, 5*(1). Retrieved from http://www.medscape.com/viewarticle/500742_print

Marriner-Tomey, A. (1990). Historical development of doctoral programs from the middle-ages to nursing education today. *Nursing and Health Care, 3*(11), 132–137.

Mason, D. (2008). Resolved: The AMA is out of touch. *American Journal of Nursing, 8*(108), 7.

Newman, M. (1975). The professional doctorate in nursing: A position paper. *Nursing Outlook, 23*(11), 704–706.

Nurse Practitioner Roundtable. (2008). *Nurse practitioner DNP education, certification, and titling: A unified statement.* Washington, DC: Author.

O'Grady, E. (2007). Hiding the doctoral degree: Jettison this policy. *Nurse Practitioner World News, 12*(12), 1–8.

Olshansky, E. (2004). Are nurses at the table? A new nursing degree could help. *Journal of Professional Nursing, 20*(4), 211–212.

Pearson, L. (2008). The Pearson report. *American Journal for Nurse Practitioners, 12*(2), 9–80.

Pearson, L. (2014). *The Pearson report.* Retrieved from http://nursing.jbpub.com/pearsonreport/Login.aspx?ref=/pearsonreport/Default.aspx

Pierce, D., & Peyton, C. (1999). A historical cross-disciplinary perspective on the professional doctorate in occupational therapy. *American Journal of Occupational Therapy, 53*(1), 64–71.

Reeves, K. (2008). "Doctor" for physicians only? *MedSurg Nursing, 17*(1), 5–6.

Roeser, R., Thibodeau, L., & Cokely, C. (2005). The University of Texas at Dallas/Callier Center for Communication Disorders doctor of audiology program. *American Journal of Audiology, 14*(2), 151–160.

Royeen, C., & Lavin, M. (2007). A contextual logical analysis of the clinical doctorate for health practitioners: Dilemma, delusion, or de facto? *Journal of Allied Health, 36*(2), 101–106.

Skinner, H. (1970). *Medical terms* (2nd ed.). New York, NY: Hafner.

Upvall, M., & Ptachcinski, R. (2007). The journey to the DNP program and beyond: What can we learn from pharmacy? *Journal of Professional Nursing, 23*(5), 316–321.

Waldrop, J. (2013). State medical boards trying to limit who can be called "doctor." Retrieved from http://www.clinicaladvisor.com/state-medical-boards-trying-to-limit-who-can-be-called-doctor/article/284167/

CHAPTER 12

Why Didn't You Just Become a Doctor? Educating Others About the DNP Degree

Lisa Astalos Chism

It is probable that nurses at every level of educational preparation have been asked, why didn't you just become a doctor? This question is often posed by patients, family members, friends, and other healthcare professionals. Due to the increasing curiosity about the doctor of nursing practice (DNP) degree, this question may be posed by others, including nurses, even more frequently than in the past. Therefore, developing a well-formulated, knowledgeable, and accurate response has become the responsibility of all DNP graduates. Further, the responses provided to these types of questions will have implications for the continued education of all who may inquire about the DNP degree.

To provide appropriate responses to these types of questions, those representing nursing, especially those with a DNP degree, need to be very clear about their professional and educational preparation. Often the water becomes muddied by titles, roles, and other factors that may make it difficult to quickly respond when asked about one's profession or degree. Hence, this chapter reviews the definitions of nursing, nursing practice, advanced-practice nursing, medicine, physician, and doctor. Easily accessible definitions are provided in an effort to maintain consistency. The practice doctorate and the DNP degree are also discussed in an effort to provide clarity and enable nurses to develop the well-formulated, knowledgeable, and accurate responses necessary to effectively educate others about the DNP degree. This chapter also provides tips for educating patients, nurses, and healthcare professionals about the DNP degree. Finally, recommendations for speaking publicly about the degree are reviewed. As pioneers, DNP graduates will likely be expected to speak publicly about the degree. Expertise in this area will further promote the degree and nursing as a whole.

Definitions Revisited: Know Who You Are

Educating others about the DNP degree is largely dependent on DNP graduates' ability to define their profession and degree. It is therefore pertinent to develop a clear understanding of nursing and the DNP degree. The following information will allow DNP graduates to efficiently and accurately educate others about their degree.

Nursing

Nursing has been defined as the "autonomous and collaborative care of individuals of all ages, families, groups and communities, sick or well and in all settings. Nursing includes the promotion of health, prevention of illness, and the care of ill, disabled and dying people. Advocacy, promotion of a safe environment, research, participation in shaping health policy and in patient and health systems management, and education are also key nursing roles" (International Council of Nurses [ICN], 2014). According to the American Nurses Association (ANA), nursing is "the diagnosis and treatment of human responses to actual or potential health problems" (1995, p. 6). It should also be mentioned that nursing is an "essential part of the society from which it has grown and within which it continues to evolve" (ANA, 1995, p. 2). Further, nursing is dynamic rather than static and continues to reflect the changing needs of society (ANA, 1995). To summarize, nursing continually evolves to meet the societal needs of others by caring for individuals, families, and communities in an effort to maintain their health and well-being in various states of health and illness.

Nursing Practice

Nursing practice describes what nurses do when they provide nursing care (Bryant-Lukosius, DiCenso, Browne, & Pinelli, 2004). Nursing practice "includes direct care giving and evaluation of its impact, advocating for patients and for health, supervising and delegating to others, leading, managing, teaching, undertaking research and developing health policy for health care systems" (ICN, 1998). Hence, nursing practice includes both the act of caring for individuals, families, and communities in an effort to promote health and well-being and the relationship that develops between nurses and patients.

To further elaborate, the ANA asserted that "nursing is a scientific discipline as well as a profession" (1995, p. 7). Hence, to further develop the scope of nursing practice and "expand the knowledge base of the discipline of nursing, nurses generate and utilize theories and research findings that are relevant to nursing practice and fit with nursing's values about health and illness" (ANA, 1995, p. 7). It is therefore pertinent for nurses and DNP graduates to understand that nursing is a discipline, science, and profession. Nursing practice is derived from the science and discipline of nursing. In other words, the profession of nursing includes a knowledge base (discipline) and reproducible modes of inquiry (science) that purport to explain how, why, and what nurses do when providing care (nursing practice).

Advanced-Practice Nursing

Advanced-practice nursing describes the "whole field of a specific type of advanced nursing practice" (Bryant-Lukosius et al., 2004). Advanced-practice nursing may include several specialty roles in which nurses function at an advanced level of practice (ANA, 1995; Brown, 1998). The advanced-practice registered nurse "acquires specialized knowledge and skills through study and supervised practice at the master's or doctoral level in nursing" (ANA, 1995, p. 14). Advanced-practice registered nurses incorporate their advanced knowledge and skills within their specialty roles to care for individuals, families, and communities.

Medicine

Medicine is defined as "the science or practice of the diagnosis, treatment, and prevention of disease" (Medicine, 2007). Medicine has further been defined as the "science and art of dealing with the maintenance of health and prevention, alleviation, or cure of disease" (Medicine, 2014). Hence, medicine is focused on the diagnosis, treatment, and alleviation of disease and disease states.

Physician

The term *physician* is thought to have originated in ancient Greece. A group of philosophers called *physicos* were known for garnering their knowledge of nature from firsthand experience as opposed to studying from books (Bailey, 2003). From their experiences, these philosophers derived what they learned in nature as biology and medicine. They taught and hence were referred to as doctors; their students were referred to as *physicos*, which later evolved to the term *physician*. The modern definition of physician includes "a person skilled in the art of healing; educated, clinically experienced, and licensed to practice medicine" (Physician, 2014).

Doctor

The relevant history of this term includes its origination in the 12th century in Bologna (Bailey, 2003; Marriner-Tomey, 1990; Skinner, 1970). The term *doctor* is derived from *docere* in Latin, which is translated as "to teach" (Skinner, 1970). Although medicine was included in early doctoral professional degrees, along with divinity and law (Marriner-Tomey, 1990), the term refers to one who holds the highest degree awarded by a graduate school (Knowles, 2006). Bailey agreed that "today, the term 'doctor' is applied to both a person with a doctoral degree in non-medical subjects, as well as physicians and surgeons" (2003, p. 490).

Practice Doctorate

The terms *professional doctorate*, *clinical doctorate*, and *practice doctorate* have all been used somewhat interchangeably when referring to the highest or terminal degree in a field or profession (American Association of Colleges of Nursing [AACN], 2006a; Marriner-Tomey, 1990; Montoya & Kimball, 2006; Royeen & Lavin, 2007). For clarification, *practice doctorate* has been adopted as the term to describe the terminal degree in nursing (AACN, 2006a). A practice doctorate can be generally defined as an entry into practice degree, such as physical therapy or pharmacy (Griffiths & Padilla, 2006; Upvall & Ptachcinski, 2007), or the terminal degree awarded within a particular profession, such as nursing and occupational therapy (AACN, 2006a; Griffiths & Padilla, 2006). It should be mentioned, however, that the practice doctorate in nursing (DNP) has been adopted as both the terminal degree for nursing practice and the entry-level degree for advanced-practice nursing (AACN, 2006a). A practice doctorate differs from a research doctorate, or doctor of philosophy degree (PhD), in that the PhD degree is a research-focused degree with an emphasis on the development of new knowledge, and the practice doctorate is a practice-focused degree with an emphasis on the skills and expertise necessary for a particular discipline (Montoya & Kimball, 2006; Newman, 1975).

Doctor of Nursing Practice Degree

The DNP degree is a practice-focused doctorate that is the terminal practice degree for nursing. It is designed to prepare nurses to meet the changing demands of health care and healthcare delivery systems. The DNP degree curriculum is focused on, although not limited to, evidence-based practice, scholarship to advance the profession, organizational and systems leadership, information technology, healthcare policy and advocacy, interprofessional collaboration across disciplines of health care, and advanced-nursing practice (AACN, 2006b). The DNP degree is currently offered as a postmaster's degree and a postbachelor's degree. The AACN projects that by 2015 the DNP degree will replace master's degree programs, which prepare advanced-practice registered nurses (AACN, 2006a).

Go Forth and Teach

After graduates develop an understanding of the DNP degree, it is their responsibility to go forth and educate others about the degree. Discussion regarding others' perceptions of the DNP degree is limited. However, a study by Nichols, O'Connor, and Dunn (2014) describes chief nursing officers' perceptions and knowledge of DNP-prepared nurses. The literature regarding what is known about others' perceptions of advanced-practice registered nurses is reviewed in the following sections. This information may be used to guide DNP graduates when they educate others about the DNP degree.

Educating Patients: The Literature

To date, little is known about patients' perceptions of DNP graduates. However, discussion regarding patients' perceptions of advanced-practice registered nurses was noted in the literature and may be appraised to provide insights for DNP graduates. Although not all DNP graduates may be in advanced-practice nursing roles, understanding patients' perceptions of advanced-practice registered nurses will enable DNP graduates to develop strategies to educate patients about the DNP degree.

It is interesting that patient awareness regarding nursing was studied as early as the 1970s. Levine, Orr, Sheatsley, Lohr, and Brodie (1978) examined patient satisfaction and comfort level with nurse practitioners. This study found that patients were "generally satisfied with nurse practitioners and felt comfortable being treated by them" (Levine et al., 1978, p. 253). Further, patients who participated in this study "formulated highly complimentary opinions of nurse practitioners" (Levine et al., 1978, p. 253). Notably, 57% of the pediatric patients and 70.9% of the adult patients formulated highly complimentary opinions after seeing a nurse practitioner for the first time (Levine et al., 1978).

Whitemore and Jaffe (1996) evaluated patients' perceptions of nurse practitioners through surveys. The results were summarized, and it was found that "most of the respondents generally had knowledge about the scope and practice of nurse practitioners" (1996, p. 19). Further, the majority of these respondents described their quality of care as excellent. It was related that these respondents felt that the nurse practitioners were "more thorough, more attentive, spent more time with them, and was a better educator" (1996, p. 19). The patients' comfort levels were also noted to be high in all but two of the respondents ($n = 16$). Overall, the surveyed patients felt their quality of care was at least equal to that of other healthcare providers (1996).

Mitchell, Dixon, Freeman, and Grindrod (2001) surveyed 277 patients regarding their perceptions of nurse practitioners. The authors found that most patients (91.9%) were agreeable to nurse practitioners treating their illnesses. It was also noted that patients with higher education levels were more familiar with the nurse practitioner role. This suggests that familiarity with nurse practitioners could be fostered with increased education regarding nurse practitioners and their role (Mitchell et al., 2001). Further, the majority of the respondents in this study were from an academic clinical setting where patients were familiar with comprehensive, high-quality care from nurse practitioners. This may also lend support to the notion that with increased education and familiarity with nurse practitioners, the level of satisfaction is increased (Mitchell et al., 2001).

Brown (2007) studied consumer perspectives of nurse practitioners in independent practice. A large majority of this sample (90%) indicated that they were familiar with the role of a nurse practitioner and had seen a nurse practitioner for care (2007). This study also provided support that previous experience with an advanced-practice registered nurse (nurse practitioner) resulted in an increased intention to use a nurse practitioner's services and increased satisfaction with these services.

Sheer (1994) agreed with the notion that patients' perceptions of nurse practitioners were directly related to their exposure to nurse practitioners. Conversely, patients who have not had exposure to the nurse practitioner role may not have favorable perceptions of nurse practitioners. Sheer suggested that socialization of the nursing role must take place early on to enable nurses and nurse practitioners to influence public opinion and "take their place as equal and autonomous providers of health care" (1994, p. 216). Sheer related that through the socialization of nurses and nurse practitioners to be independent, strong leaders in health care, they will become empowered to impact the public's perceptions and act as strong role models for the profession (1994).

Edmunds (1988) discussed visibility of the nurse practitioner role and noted that the multiple titles used by nurses who practice in an expanded role may lead to patient confusion about the role of nurse practitioners. This lack of unity within nursing has hurt the profession's recognition in the healthcare setting. Edmunds further related that nurse practitioners remain largely unknown to many prospective patients and stated that "not enough people in the United States are aware of nurse practitioners' unique contributions to health care" (1988, p. 53). In an effort to change this, Edmunds offered some strategies to increase patient awareness about nurse practitioners. These strategies include using the media to gain visibility, such as calling local radio or television stations to volunteer for interviews, prepare public service announcements, or write health information spots (1988). Additional strategies suggested by Edmunds include effectively utilizing nurse practitioners' political power to garner support from legislators and establishing relationships within their professional communities. This strategy would include personally visiting local hospitals, nursing homes, retirement communities, and charity organizations in an effort to increase visibility of their unique role (1988). Finally, an increased effort to educate patients was mentioned. This could be done in the form of brochures or pamphlets distributed locally and kept in offices or exam rooms (1988). Overall, Edmunds reinforced that nurse practitioners should never miss an opportunity to hand out business cards and explain who they are and what they do. Similar strategies could be employed by DNP graduates to increase their visibility and educate patients regarding the DNP degree.

Educating Patients: Seize the Moment

Although the literature primarily discusses patients' awareness and perceptions of advanced-practice registered nurses, this information provides useful insights regarding educating patients about the DNP degree. First and foremost, it is supported by the literature that patients who are cared for by advanced-practice registered nurses (even through one experience) have favorable perceptions of them (Brown, 2007; Levine et al., 1978; Mitchell et al., 2001; Sheer, 1994). DNP graduates have likely already established trusting relationships with their patients and have established patient comfort and satisfaction. Therefore, patients are likely to be receptive to DNP graduates introducing the concept of a practice doctorate in nursing and what this means. The rapport DNP graduates have established with patients will enable open communication that is necessary to seize the moment during patient visits so DNP graduates can share what a DNP degree is and the impact they have on an ever-changing, complex healthcare environment.

For patients who are new to either a practice setting or advanced-practice registered nurses, or who may have limited knowledge regarding nursing in general, the research has shown that even limited experience with advanced-practice registered nurses usually results in patients having a favorable perception of them (Brown, 2007; Levine et al., 1978; Mitchell et al., 2001). Therefore, DNP graduates should use every opportunity with patients, regardless of the length or context of the relationship, to educate them about advanced-practice registered nurses' preparation, including defining for patients what a DNP degree is. This author has found that patients who are new to the practice setting are often eager to learn what it means to have a DNP degree and are impressed at the level of preparation DNP graduates have.

Finally, DNP graduates should utilize their knowledge base regarding nursing. What better time to promote nursing and educate patients about what nursing actually is? DNP graduates should also familiarize themselves with the terms presented in the beginning of the chapter. It seems the pertinent issues include clearly defining for patients the terms *nursing, nursing practice, medicine, doctor, physician, practice doctorate*, and *doctor of nursing practice*. This author has found that patients are receptive and appreciative when a DNP graduate takes time to explain his or her educational preparation, role, and degree. **Box 12-1** lists some tips for educating patients about the DNP degree.

BOX 12-1

Tips for Educating Patients About the DNP Degree

- Educate yourself and your patients about the meaning of *nursing*, *nursing practice*, and *advanced-practice nursing*.

- Educate yourself and your patients about the meaning and origins of the terms *physician*, *doctor*, and *medicine*.

- Seize every opportunity with patients to distinctly explain that you are a nurse with a doctorate in nursing practice.

- If a patient questions the term *doctor*, explain that you are a doctor and a nurse; you are a doctor of nursing practice.

- Use consistent language with patients when describing the DNP degree (e.g., use the terms *doctor of nursing practice* or *DNP*). Consistency will prevent patient confusion and promote unity (Edmunds, 1988).

- Develop a brochure or pamphlet explaining your role and degree preparation, and leave it in your practice setting lobby and exam rooms.

- Clearly display your degree and title on your name tag.

- Educate the staff in your practice setting to ensure that your preparation is appropriately communicated (e.g., "Dr. Smith has a doctorate in nursing practice").

- Educate receptionists that when they make patient appointments, your appropriate degree and title should be used (e.g., Dr. Smith, nurse practitioner).

- Volunteer to provide in-service training to the staff and patients regarding your degree and preparation.

- Volunteer to provide patient education presentations with a quick introduction about your title and your educational preparation.

- DNP graduates in the nurse educator role, including those who precept students in the clinical setting, should begin socializing students (in all nursing degree programs) to be strong, autonomous, independent practitioners of nursing practice. This will encourage empowerment when communicating with patients regarding their roles as nurses, advanced-practice registered nurses, and DNP graduates (Sheer, 1994).

- Educate your family members and friends regarding your degree and the defined terms. They are often patients too, at some time in their lives.

Educating Nurses: The Literature

Nurses' perceptions of the DNP degree have not yet been studied extensively. However, the attitudes of nurses toward advanced-practice registered nurses were studied.

Gooden and Jackson (2004) noted that nurses' attitudes toward nurse practitioners in the healthcare environment could affect the patient's attitude toward the nurse practitioner and have an impact on healthcare outcomes. The same may be implied regarding nurses' attitudes toward DNP graduates. Gooden and Jackson found that, overall, nurses had positive attitudes about nurse practitioners. Specifically, these authors found that nurses agreed that "nurse practitioners made a positive impact on health care" (2004, p. 363). Further, Gooden and Jackson related that nurses considered the role of nurse practitioners to be valuable, necessary, and helpful. Participants in this study had exposure to nurse practitioners in multiple settings and possessed a clear understanding of the scope of nurse practitioner practice. The nurse participants also expressed confidence in the care provided by nurse practitioners. Importantly, nurse participants also felt that nurse practitioners were a valuable resource for advice and were receptive to suggestions regarding patient care (Gooden & Jackson, 2004). DNP graduates may also be looked to as a resource for nursing within the healthcare setting. Continuing to be a resource while exhibiting receptiveness to nursing's suggestions to improve quality of care will promote credibility and trust toward DNP graduates.

Although positive attitudes toward advanced-practice registered nurses have been noted, Richmond and Becker (2005) note that these attitudes need to be cultivated by advanced-practice registered nurses. These authors suggest specific characteristics that promote an "advanced practice nurse–friendly culture" (2005, p. 58). These characteristics may also be helpful in promoting credibility and trust toward DNP graduates. Credibility and trust will facilitate receptiveness by nurses and increase credibility of the DNP degree. Richmond and Becker's (2005) characteristics of an advanced-practice registered nurse–friendly culture are as follows:

- Clarity of visions, values, and role in an effort to align the advanced-practice registered nurse with the rest of nurses
- Commitment to practice, the nursing profession, and continued professional development
- Communication with patients and families, with the healthcare team, within the medical record, and through professional presentations and publications
- Collaboration that is clearly defined and occurs across disciplines and within nursing
- Credibility through credentialing and clinical experience, and by securing payment for services
- Contributions to patient outcomes and the organization
- Confidence in oneself and as a change agent
- Complexity to become solution oriented while conveying professional serenity

Educating Nurses: An Opportunity to Role-Model

DNP graduates can employ Richmond and Becker's (2005) characteristics to establish trust in and credibility of nursing. When credibility and trust are established, nurses will be more receptive to understanding the DNP degree. Furthermore, to successfully educate other nurses about the degree, it is essential that DNP graduates set an exceptional example. What better way to educate other nurses and promote the DNP degree than to be a role model? DNP graduates garner leadership and interprofessional collaboration skills that can be employed to facilitate role-modeling for other nurses. Additionally, many of the explanations and tips provided regarding educating patients about the DNP degree may also be employed when educating nurses about the DNP degree. Please refer to **Box 12-2** for a list of tips for educating nurses about the DNP degree.

BOX 12-2

Tips for Educating Nurses About the DNP Degree

- Educate yourself and other nurses regarding the meaning of *nursing, nursing practice*, and *advanced-practice nursing*.
- Educate yourself and other nurses regarding the meaning and origins of the terms *physician, doctor*, and *medicine*.
- Develop trust and credibility with other nurses in an effort to increase receptiveness regarding the DNP degree.
- Develop trust and credibility with other nurses in an effort to promote credibility of the DNP degree.
- Lead by example and be a role model for other nurses.
- Provide in-service training for other nurses regarding the DNP degree.
- Promote professional development by presenting at conferences and providing information regarding the DNP degree.
- Join and volunteer to present at professional nursing organizations to garner nursing support of the DNP degree.
- DNP nurse educators, including those who precept students, have an opportunity to serve as role models. Those in the nurse educator role may also provide a detailed description of the DNP degree to students in every nursing program.

Educating Other Healthcare Professionals: The Literature

The literature related to healthcare professionals' attitudes and perceptions regarding the nursing profession focuses primarily on physicians' attitudes toward nurse practitioners. Fottler, Gibson, and Pinchoff (1978) specifically examined physician receptivity of nurse practitioners. Only approximately one-third (29%) of physicians who were questioned were willing to employ a nurse practitioner in their practice. Further, approximately one-half (49%) of physicians who were questioned expressed negative attitudes regarding working with nurse practitioners. The reasons for this were evaluated, and the highest reported response was a lack of incentive for physicians to work with nurse practitioners. The second most reported response was physician satisfaction with the traditional roles and relationships of nurses and physicians. The authors speculated that this may be due to physicians' tendency to "prefer certainty over uncertainty, known over unknown and current practices over innovative practices" (Fottler et al., 1978). It was noted that physicians' attitudes are not static. Rather, the authors asserted that increased experience working with nurse practitioners resulted in more positive attitudes from physicians.

More recent research has shown that physicians' attitudes become more positive with increased experience working with nurse practitioners. Aquilino, Damiano, Williard, Momany, and Levy (1999) found that, overall, physicians had supportive attitudes about nurse practitioners. Not surprisingly, this study also found that experience with nurse practitioners led to more positive attitudes about nurse practitioners. The authors related that this finding had implications for training physicians and nurse practitioners regarding interdisciplinary care (Aquilino et al., 1999). Further, Aquilino and colleagues stated that "the results of this study support initiatives to encourage interdisciplinary training as an effective way to begin the process of mutual understanding and respect between professionals that can continue throughout their practice careers" (1999, p. 227). This is reflective of the Institute of Medicine's recommendation that all healthcare professionals be formally educated to integrate interprofessional care into healthcare delivery to adequately provide services in the 21st century (Greiner & Knebel, 2003).

Educating Other Healthcare Professionals: Education Through Demonstration

The perceptions of patients, nurses, and other healthcare professionals regarding advanced-practice nursing roles have largely been influenced by previous experience with the high-quality care that is provided by advanced-practice registered nurses (Aquilino et al., 1999; Brown, 2007; Gooden & Jackson, 2004; Levine et al., 1978; Mitchell et al., 2001; Sheer, 1994). It may therefore be safe to assume that effectively educating other healthcare professionals depends on DNP graduates consistently demonstrating the value and expertise they bring to the delivery of health care. Other healthcare professionals, such as physicians, pharmacists, and physical therapists, will be more receptive to understanding the DNP degree if patient care outcomes are shown to improve. Additionally, many of the explanations and tips provided regarding educating patients and nurses about the DNP degree may be employed when educating other healthcare professionals about the DNP degree. Please refer to **Box 12-3** for a list of tips for educating other healthcare professionals about the DNP degree.

BOX 12-3

Tips for Educating Other Healthcare Professionals About the DNP Degree

- Educate yourself and other healthcare professionals regarding the meaning of *nursing, nursing practice,* and *advanced-practice nursing.*
- Educate yourself and other healthcare professionals regarding the meaning and origins of the terms *physician, doctor,* and *medicine.*
- Develop trust and credibility with other healthcare professionals in an effort to increase receptiveness regarding the DNP degree.
- Develop trust and credibility with other healthcare professionals in an effort to promote credibility of the DNP degree.
- Provide in-service training for other healthcare professionals regarding the DNP degree.
- Develop clinical projects and practice guidelines that demonstrate the use of leadership, evidence-based practice, information technology, and inter-professional collaboration.
- Make an effort to collaborate consistently with other healthcare professionals and highlight the benefits of interdisciplinary and interprofessional patient care.
- Nurse educators, including those who precept students, have an opportunity to teach students and demonstrate the importance of interprofessional collaboration with other healthcare professionals. Through demonstration, the value of interprofessional collaboration will be reinforced for both students and healthcare professionals.

Speaking Publicly About the DNP Degree

Stephen Covey (2004) asserted that communication is the most important skill in life, with the four basic forms of communication being reading, writing, speaking, and listening. Of these, speaking and listening have a synergistic effect. When one listens and speaks, communication is improved. Moreover, Covey expressed that understanding others through empathic listening is essential to being understood (2004).

Empathic listening is defined as listening with the intent to understand (Covey, 2004). Through empathic listening, one understands another's "frame of reference" (2004, p. 240). Empathic listening is facilitated by listening and evaluating first before offering a response. When a response is offered, it should be clear, specific, and in the context of understanding the other's frame of reference (2004).

Speaking publicly about the DNP degree requires DNP graduates to first understand their audience. The literature pertaining to the perceptions of advanced-practice registered nurses was provided to give DNP graduates and others a sense of the frames of reference of patients, nurses, and other healthcare professionals. When speaking to others publicly about the DNP degree, DNP graduates can first develop an understanding of others' perceptions regarding nursing and health care and employ empathic listening to communicate effectively and be understood.

Kravitz (2007) also related that when speaking publicly, one should know the concerns, interests, and beliefs of the audience. It was noted that understanding the perceptions of the audience would influence speaking strategies (2007). Additional pointers regarding speaking publicly included knowing the essence of the presentation, showing enthusiasm toward those you are speaking to, expressing passion about the topic, practicing your material, daring to be different yet professional, and making a memorable impression (2007).

With regard to speaking publicly, it would be remiss not to mention the work of Dale Carnegie, who was a pioneer in teaching others the art of public speaking. In a revised version of his work titled *Public Speaking for Success*, he shares an essential point: "When speakers have a real message in their head and heart—an inner urge to speak—they are almost sure to do themselves credit" (Carnegie & Pell, 2005, p. 41). The definitions in the beginning of the chapter were provided to ensure that DNP graduates develop a clear understanding regarding who they are and what they contribute to nursing, the delivery of health care, and society—in essence, their message. This author has often found that when speaking about the DNP degree, passion and enthusiasm are contagious. Even people who are not in health care can sense the excitement and are therefore receptive to learning about the DNP degree. Carnegie and Carnegie Hill agreed: "When you become intensely interested in your talk, you will forget your fears, you will gain self-confidence, and your enthusiasm will carry the crowd with you" (2007, p. 41). Additionally, this author has found that the sincerity expressed when speaking publicly leaves an impression on the audience: "If you speak with a deep sincerity and whole-heartedness, your hearers will be imbued by your spirit" (Carnegie & Carnegie Hill, 2007, p. 41). Whether they speak formally to a large audience or informally in a small group, DNP graduates are expected to lead, have an inner urge to speak, and share the message about their innovative and unique degree. Please refer to **Box 12-4** for a list of tips for speaking publicly about the DNP degree.

BOX 12-4

Tips for Speaking Publicly About the DNP Degree

- Know your audience's perceptions, interests, and beliefs regarding nursing and health care.
- Express an understanding of your audience's frame of reference and utilize empathic listening when presenting (Covey, 2004).
- Express a clear understanding of your topic (the DNP degree) and know your material.
- Be unique and make an impression.
- Use the leadership skills you have garnered, and be fearless.
- Share personal anecdotal stories that are relevant to your audience or topic.
- Express sincerity and interest when speaking to an audience.
- Review the AACN's "DNP Talking Points" (AACN, 2014).
- Express passion and enthusiasm about the DNP degree with every audience—it will be contagious!

Interview with a Cofounder of DNP LLC: Then and Now

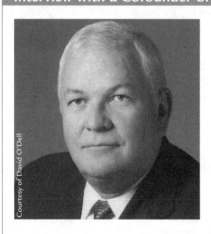

Courtesy of David O'Dell

David G. O'Dell, DNP, ARNP, FNP-BC, is the founder of D. G. O'Dell Inc. and is a cofounder and the president of Doctors of Nursing Practice Inc.

THEN . . . 2008

Dr. O'Dell, could you please describe your current position, including your nursing background?

I've been an RN since the age of 19, first with an associate's degree in nursing, later earning my BSN [bachelor of science in nursing], and evolving into an MSN [master's of science in nursing] and NP [nurse practitioner] licensure. I soon realized that to have a strong voice for change a terminal degree was needed and made an easy transition into the DNP educational route.

I currently work part-time jobs as an independent contractor with several medical groups, including internal medicine physicians, neurologists (my clinical interest is neurocognitive disorders), and also physical medicine and rehab. I have been teaching nursing students part time since 2002 and will soon accept a full-time faculty position in a local university school of nursing for undergraduate, graduate, and DNP students.

Dr. O'Dell, could you please describe what motivated you to return to school for a DNP degree?

This is a great question. After working as an NP for a few years, I realized that my role had evolved into being an extension of the physician and physician group. I was generating several hundred thousand dollars in revenue for the practice, and when I shared this information requesting an increase in salary, I was turned down. I knew my contribution was not adequately recognized, so I had to make plans for change. Returning to school was my next best step.

I realized that the bigger world of health care had greater needs and greater opportunities beyond the tasks I had grown into. I also knew I had to earn a terminal degree in order to be effective in promoting change. I looked at several PhD programs, but none felt right. When I heard about the DNP program, there were only five universities with this option. After reading what the AACN had proposed, and reviewing as many articles as I could find on this degree option, I knew that this was right for me for several reasons. First, earning a practice degree fit well with my concept of being a clinician first. The DNP degree spoke to this goal better than any other degree. Additionally, as this degree was evolving, I saw an opportunity to catch the first wave in order to be a part of a growth shift in our profession. I'm amazed daily at how the DNP degree is promoting change (sometimes through controversy). I will invest the rest of my professional career as a DNP trying to positively influence the healthcare delivery system and promote the growth of advanced nursing practice. My evolution into being a DNP was right on time for me.

Dr. O'Dell, could you please describe how earning your DNP degree has influenced your nursing practice?

My nursing practice in terms of patient care has become much easier now that I better understand the larger picture of the healthcare system and more clearly see my role as a clinician. I'm more confident in all patient interactions and know that I can incorporate sound judgment based on evidence in my decisions. The clinical hours required for my residency were more than most DNP programs require now, but I don't regret the extra experience and hands-on learning. I'm much better for the experience.

My nursing practice has taken on a much different tone since my MSN days. I'm more intrigued and capable to make change and provide leadership to whatever group that I choose to belong. I've seen more opportunity to contribute.

Dr. O'Dell, could you please describe the history of DNP LLC, including how you became involved with this venture?

Like many good things in life, sometimes events evolve through serendipity. In the first semester of the DNP program at the University of Tennessee Health Science Center College of Nursing, one of the core classes was philosophy of science. We had several projects to develop, and the online chats between and among classmates were amazing. Even though we didn't see each other face to face often, the daily (and sometimes several times per day) conversations online built a bond that will always be with us. One of the conversations spun off into comments that there was no publication of DNP literature (because the degree was so new) and that there was no mechanism to communicate among other DNPs and DNP students. Someone mentioned the need for creating such an organization, and others chimed in agreeing to the idea, but we put it aside as we were not in a position to act on these notions.

About a year later in an advanced leadership course, our assignments were to develop either a grant application or a business plan. A few of us picked up on the idea of forming an organization from the online conversation about a year earlier, and we moved it forward. By the end of that semester we had a business plan. Before that semester was complete we had incorporated and began our website that opened within 4 months of incorporation. We're very fortunate to have put into place many of our business plan ideas and have modified others as the environment and culture of DNP education and communication needs have changed.

Dr. O'Dell, what are the mission and purpose of DNP LLC?

That's easy to share as this has been discussed in detail while developing our business plan, and we have revisited it several times since our inception.

The mission of Doctors of Nursing Practice LLC is to create a forum for the communication of information, ideas, and innovations to promote the growth and development of the practice doctorate degree.

The purpose (or vision) is grounded in the following principles:

- *Dedication to providing accurate and timely information*
- *Support, develop, and disseminate professional practice innovations*
- *Professional collaboration that demonstrates universal respect for others, honesty, and integrity in communications*
- *Responsive and open discussions and dialogues that promote the evolution of advanced nursing practice and the growth of the DNP degree*

You may be interested to know that as a result of this mission and purpose statement, we have created a subsidiary organization, Doctors of Nursing Practice Professional Development Inc. This is a nonprofit organization dedicated to the educational needs of advanced-practice registered nurses. One of our first group efforts is the First National Doctors of Nursing Practice Conference: Transforming Care Through Scholarly Education and Practice. This conference was in October of 2008 in Memphis, Tennessee (the birthplace of our organization). Future conferences are already being planned. We invite all who are interested to visit our websites at www.apn-dnp.com and www.DoctorsofNursingPractice .org.

Another big step for DNP LLC as an organization is the development of a professional membership-driven organization for and by DNPs. As you know, there are many issues and controversies surrounding our degree and practice. I've spoken with DNPs throughout the United States and other countries and see that the need for communication and collaboration is more important now than ever and no doubt will continue to be important in the future.

The inception, growth, and evolution of DNP LLC and its subsidiaries and efforts are directly related to the needs of this unique and growing community. I'm very proud and honored to be a part of this process and look forward to continuing to support our collective evolution.

Dr. O'Dell, what do you feel is your role to educate patients, nurses, and others about the DNP degree?

That's a tough question to answer. I see my role as being the best clinician possible in my chosen discipline and continue to support the health of individuals and communities. This is accomplished through the growth of organizations and systems designed to meet these needs. At this point in the evolution of the DNP degree, I must explain again and again what a practice degree in nursing is all about to patients and colleagues. In the future I hope that the DNP will be better understood and won't require repetitive explanations. Time will tell on that front. The message I try to convey consistently is that the DNP is exactly what it says it is: a doctor (meaning the highest level of achievement in a discipline—a teacher or guide) of nursing practice, which is a demonstration that this degree is all about the discipline of nursing. I'm amazed and sometimes concerned that others in health care (particularly physicians) do not see the forest for the trees. We are not trying to practice as physicians; rather we are well-educated and capable nursing clinicians who can meet the needs of most every patient who is likely to walk into a practice. I'm raising the bar on my game and expect other disciplines to do the same rather than trying to downgrade, discount, or obstruct professional growth. The most confident and secure physicians I've worked with had no issue with my doctorate degree.

Dr. O'Dell, what role do you envision DNP LLC having with regard to the education of others about the DNP degree?

Doctors of Nursing Practice LLC is an organization that promotes and enhances. If I had to put our product or service into one word, it would be information. *With that in mind, we have the opportunity to consistently share the past, present, and future of the DNP for anyone that may be curious. Education is about exchange, not just dissemination of data. In order for individuals or groups to grow and evolve in any venture, an exchange of thoughts is essential. We have established a venue for this purpose and have made definitive plans to continue this effort in the future.*

The first national conference will be our first collaborative effort to demonstrate what DNPs are doing in practice and education. I look forward to seeing what will happen in the future compared to these simple times of 2009.

Dr. O'Dell, what is your advice to other DNP graduates regarding educating patients, other nurses, and other healthcare professionals about the DNP degree?

I've seen many discussions about the title of doctor and the consternation that it is causing. Even though I'm smart enough to understand human nature and motivations for actions, I'm still surprised that some have challenged the title of doctor, especially when our degree and title are so clear. We are doctors of nursing practice. This is easy to convey to patients, other nurses, and any other healthcare professional. I don't have to explain what I am not. Rather, I try to consistently point out the title and what it means.

I had an interaction with a patient a few days ago that illustrates the insignificance of title. I introduced myself as a nurse practitioner with a doctor in nursing practice degree and then went on to relay some of my background before exploring his needs and goals for that particular visit. He asked me, "Are you a doctor?" I replied that I'm a nurse practitioner with a doctorate degree. He then asked me a pointed question and made this ironic statement, "Why don't other doctors tell me what they can do like you just did? I don't have any idea why they are there or what they know. A doctor doesn't mean much to me other than someone that can help me." He didn't care that I was not a physician; he just wanted to know that I could help with his problem. That reinforced my approach to anyone I talk with regarding the DNP. I'm there to help with the skills and education at the highest level of my discipline. That's all that matters to my patients.

We are prepared through our education to evaluate and manage organizations and systems. I'm proud to be associated with DNPs that are influencing huge systems, even entire countries, through their practice. We are truly an international breed of professionals that can (and do) make a difference as a result of our education and skills. Our title reflects who we are and what we do. Staying true to that title is the best way to be consistent regarding the education of our patients and colleagues.

Dr. O'Dell, do you believe there is increased awareness among patients, nurses, and other healthcare professionals regarding the DNP degree?

I think there is most definitely more awareness among all the groups you mentioned regarding the DNP degree compared to a few years ago, but I'm not naïve [enough] to think that awareness means acceptance. The dialogue about the DNP and its implications for all parties is just beginning. I don't think that even DNPs realize the potential of our future practices (clinical, leadership, educators, and researchers). As we move closer to 2015, and as more DNP graduates enter the field, we'll have greater awareness and hopefully acceptance. We are in an early phase of a paradigm shift for our nursing discipline. Our entire healthcare delivery system—our industry—is changing too. We will no doubt be a large part of this shift as nursing is such an essential player in this process. The discussion about whether or not the DNP should exist is irrelevant. We are here. The discipline and number of graduates are growing exponentially. We will not disappear. Awareness and acceptance will be an evolutionary process. This is inevitable.

Dr. O'Dell, what impact do you expect DNP graduates will have on health care in the future?

This is a great question, and many folks are watching and waiting to see what the DNP will do to or for health care. I can speculate, but certainly cannot predict, what will happen to health care in general as a result of the DNP. I think that the degree will catalyze change rather than be the specific agent of change alone. The presence of a practice doctorate in nursing has already initiated dialogue and expectation for change. Those wheels are now in motion. The mere presence of the DNP has changed the way we educate nurses and how advanced-practice nursing (in all of its forms) will be integrated into our current system of patient care. As more DNPs confer and compare how practice is changing, and as we grow in our experiences collectively, we will impact the future of health care. These are indeed exciting times. I'm proud to help direct the trajectory of our discipline just a little by working to create systems for communication and growth specific to advanced-practice nursing and the DNP degree.

NOW . . . 2014

Dr. O'Dell, we discussed your nursing background and education last time we spoke. Could you please describe your current position?

My current career position is professor and full-time faculty at Chamberlain College of Nursing in the DNP program. My professional position is president of Doctors of Nursing Practice Inc., which is a nonprofit organization that began in 2006. It is evolving and maturing to meet the needs of the growing DNP community of graduates, students, and faculty. The seventh national DNP conference took place in the fall of 2014, and we were proud to place a spotlight on expert presenters and colleagues as these conferences continues to grow. National and regional conferences are being planned along with webinars, continuing education, and a foundation to help support scholarly DNP implementation projects. An online journal is also being discussed and is in the planning stage.

Dr. O'Dell, how has your position continued to evolve since earning your DNP degree?

Without a doubt my career continues to evolve since earning the DNP degree. Academic rewards and expectations continue to grow in my current role as a college professor. Collaborating with DNP colleagues to improve outcomes through enhancing the growth and development of the DNP degree is also evolving and growing. This is an exciting time to see the advancement of our discipline and the contributions of those with a practice doctorate degree. I am honored to be a part of improving practice and the caliber of nursing colleagues both through an academic role and through Doctors of Nursing Practice Inc. Being a part of the bigger process of healthcare evolution and growth within our discipline and this degree in particular has been a great experience that continues to challenge and offer great reward.

Dr. O'Dell, are you currently practicing as a clinician, and if so how has your clinical practice evolved since earning your DNP degree?

My clinical practice is part time, yet I very much enjoy patient contact. The current practice setting affords me great flexibility in working with other clinicians. The DNP degree has afforded me much more confidence and insight into the processes and systems of healthcare delivery, and it has also provided me great opportunities to be a part of a change in services to improve processes and outcomes. It is a very rewarding environment, and my DNP degree, along with my FNP [family nurse practitioner] designation, have been essential in this practice.

Dr. O'Dell, could you describe the current progress and growth of DNP LLC?

The Doctors of Nursing Practice Inc. organization has evolved in many ways. The first is the transition from DNP LLC to DNP Inc. We are now a nonprofit organization with the mission of improving healthcare outcomes by promoting and enhancing the practice doctorate degree. The national conferences have remained our main focus, yet a strategic plan developed over these past 2 years is being implemented. The five areas of interest and expansion for DNP Inc. include national and regional conferences and webinars, continuing education, a foundation to help support and promote DNP colleagues to complete and implement their scholarly projects, an online journal, and assisting colleagues in developing practices in their respective areas of interest. The DNP Inc. website continues to grow and evolve and will move into another generation of content and interactive capabilities by the end of the third quarter of 2014. Plans for refining and expanding services are in place. These plans are not possible without the great volunteer efforts of colleagues all over the country, with some in other countries. The organization is growing in direct relationship to the growing number of DNP programs, graduates, and interactions with professional organizations and delivery systems. These are truly exciting times.

Dr. O'Dell, when we last spoke we talked about the role of DNP LLC in educating others about the DNP degree. To date, DNP LLC has had an impressive impact on informing others about the DNP degree. Why do you think that is, and what are your plans to continue the influence of the organization?

Doctors of Nursing Practice Inc. is proud to take part in promoting education and the dissemination of information for and about the DNP degree. This is an evolutionary process. For example, in the past few years the need to identify and define the DNP degree has evolved into a demonstration of exemplars of practice. Most DNP students and graduates are learning to be comfortable with their new degree and evolving roles as a result of the degree. These graduates, students, and their faculty are producing great work. As a discipline and a degree, we are transitioning into an era of exemplars and investment in complex systems on many levels to include policy, informatics, academia, and of course clinical practice.

Disseminating the activities and thoughts of the DNP-prepared professional through forums, blogs, groups, and events is one way of helping all who are interested in the DNP degree to grow and develop. Assisting each other in sharing expertise, accomplishments, and scholarly insights is another way that the DNP Inc. organization is helping to support colleagues. The strategic plans for the near- and long-term future will assist in the building of the DNP community across all professional organizations while building a scholarly social foundation for future contributions.

The social capital that has developed over these past few years is beginning to show its abilities to speak clearly and share insights and directives for changes to improve healthcare outcomes. DNPs are impacting practice on many levels while influencing policy and functionality of systems. Seeing this evolution is a great pleasure for all in the DNP community, and I am very proud to see that the DNP Inc. organization has helped in this process.

Dr. O'Dell, what advice do you have for DNP graduates regarding their involvement in educating other nurses, healthcare professionals, employers, and patients about the DNP degree?

This is a great question. As all nurses know, educating patients to improve their health and collaborating with colleagues about best practices are expectations of the discipline. This is taking place with nurses of all levels of educational preparation. All DNP graduates are nurses in advanced practice that includes all of the well-identified clinical roles along with administrative roles, expertise in policy and informatics, and systems change. It is a natural next step for all DNP graduates to provide either direct or indirect support in the education of our nursing colleagues—again, at all levels of educational preparation. Not all DNP graduates are destined to work in an academic setting, and to move in that direction requires extra efforts and skills to meet the need of being an effective faculty member. As we all know, the term doctor *means teacher. To have earned that title reflects not only the accomplishment of specific courses, but designates the holder of that degree to be the pinnacle of expertise in his or her field of study. To teach is the next progressive and logical step. This teaching is not only within our discipline but must include our patients and their families, groups, and specific populations. Also we are ethically and morally charged to influence regional, state, national, and international political processes. Collaborating with all disciplines both within and outside of health care is our obligation as DNP-prepared nurses.*

I'll end my response by asking a hypothetical question of all that read this response: can you identify a time in the history of the profession that had a greater potential for the nursing discipline to influence health care and society? We are standing on the shoulders of giants, and the addition of the DNP degree is one more push and opportunity to be a part of a process that is much bigger than all of us.

Interviews with DNP-Prepared Educators, Clinicians, and DNP Textbook Authors

PERSPECTIVE OF AN FNP AND ASSISTANT PROFESSOR

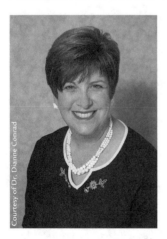

Courtesy of Dr. Dianne Conrad

Dianne Conrad, DNP, RN, FNP-BC, teaches full time in a DNP program that prepares adult and older adult nurse practitioners. In addition, she maintains her practice as an FNP.

Dr. Conrad, could you please describe your educational and professional background, including your current position?

I have had a long journey of nursing education through my career. I obtained a diploma, a BSN, and an MS in nursing and was prepared as a medical–surgical clinical nurse specialist. I became a family nurse practitioner after obtaining a postmaster's certificate, and I have been practicing since 1997 with a specialty in diabetes, becoming a certified diabetes educator and obtaining board certification in advanced diabetes management. I earned a doctor of nursing practice degree in 2011 at Madonna University in Livonia, Michigan, as one of their first postmaster's cohort.

Since 2011 I have continued to practice as an FNP as well as a full-time assistant professor at Grand Valley State University in Grand Rapids, Michigan, teaching in the DNP program preparing adult and older adult nurse practitioners.

Dr. Conrad, what led you to your decision to return to school for a DNP degree?

I have always been a lifelong learner and was waiting until nursing developed a practice doctorate that prepared the advanced-practice nurse at the doctoral level. After reviewing the AACN essentials and the program at Madonna University, I felt that the DNP degree would add value and depth to my professional nursing journey. Obtaining the DNP degree reawakened my nursing professional identity after over 15 years of focus on the medical aspects of my practice as a nurse practitioner.

The DNP degree has prepared me to address the challenges in the healthcare field and confidently sit at the table with my colleagues who have other healthcare doctorates to address individual patient, system, population, and policy issues.

Dr. Conrad, how has your career evolved since earning a DNP degree?

The DNP degree has opened so many doors to my personal and professional development as a nurse. Though teaching was not my goal prior to obtaining the DNP degree, the academic appointment has allowed me to influence and shape the trajectory of the evolving practice doctorate in my own university, the state, and nationally. My scholarly activity after graduation has focused on development of a model of nursing and use of the electronic health record in the primary care Patient Centered Medical Home. However, my scholarly work has also included defining and clarifying the role of the practice doctorate locally, nationally, and internationally through publications, presentations, and serving on state-level boards and task forces. Networking at the national DNP conferences has led to new collegial relationships and invitations to present and plan educational opportunities at the national level. The doctoral preparation in policy and advocacy has been invaluable in preparing for and serving on local and statewide boards in healthcare organizations. However, the greatest satisfaction professionally has been to see students realize their potential as doctorally prepared advanced-practice nurses.

PERSPECTIVE OF A PRIMARY CARE DNP
AND ASSISTANT PROFESSOR

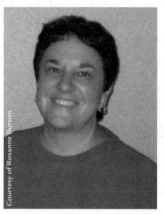

Rosanne Burson, DNP, ACNS-BC, CDE, provides support services to patients with chronic disease and consults and provides support to those who are creating innovative approaches to chronic disease management. She is also an assistant professor who teaches in a DNP program and at the graduate and undergraduate levels.

Dr. Burson, could you please describe your educational and professional background, including your current position?

I have been a lifelong learner, starting with a diploma in nursing, followed by a BSN, an MSA [master of science in administration and an MSN (adult health CNS [clinical nurse specialist]). In 2011 I completed a DNP as well as a postmasters certificate in teaching. I have had varied professional background experiences that started in acute care from the operating room, as a perfusionist, within the surgical and cardiovascular intensive care units, as well as a nurse educator and a manager. I have been in the community since 1996 as an APRN [advanced-practice registered nurse] and a CDE [certified diabetes educator] with a focus in chronic disease. I worked in primary care, diabetes education programs, the pharmaceutical industry, and as an entrepreneur, first with Diabetes Partner. Since 2010 I have been working in partnership with Dr. Moran and our company, My Self-Management Team Inc. We work in primary care to provide support services to patients with chronic disease, as well as consult and provide support to those that are creating innovative approaches to chronic disease management.

I am also an assistant professor at University of Detroit Mercy, educating in the DNP program, as well as the graduate and undergraduate levels.

Dr. Burson, what led you to your decision to return to school for a DNP degree?

All of my decisions to return to school have involved the potential to open new doors. I had been considering returning to school in order to open up the opportunity to teach at the university level. I received a flyer in the mail that highlighted the courses that would be involved in the DNP. The course topics were of great interest to me. When I spoke to the director of the program (Dr. Nancy O'Connor) she talked about the doctor of nursing practice moving nursing forward, which resonated with me.

Dr. Burson, how has your career evolved since earning a DNP degree?

There has been a wonderful evolution of my career since earning the degree. Of course, our business was built on our scholarly project and has offered the opportunity to influence the direction of self-management support for patients and providers. The degree has made a reality of a faculty position, influencing multiple areas of nursing, particularly the DNP student. And finally, our scholarship work has really grown to influence understanding of the DNP's potential to move healthcare forward.

PERSPECTIVE OF AN ASSISTANT PROFESSOR IN DNP, GRADUATE, AND BSN PROGRAMS

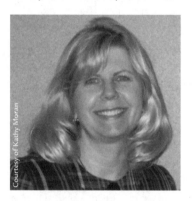

Courtesy of Kathy Moran

Kathy Moran, DNP, RN, CDE, is committed to moving the nursing profession forward as an advocate, role model, and mentor.

Dr. Moran, could you please describe your educational and professional background, including your current position?

As a young woman I started my nursing journey as a licensed practical nurse, and then went on to receive an associate degree in nursing. I explored a variety of areas in nursing during this time including cardiology, neurology, oncology, obstetrics, and home care before I found my niche in diabetes education and management. Working with this population has truly been a labor of love for me; like many professionals with a diabetes specialty I had personal life experiences that drew me to this area of practice. During this period of time, I worked as a certified diabetes educator and diabetes program coordinator at a small community hospital where I cared for patients with diabetes across the life span. A few years later I accepted a position with the State of Michigan where I was responsible for providing diabetes-specific continuing education for healthcare professionals across the state, as well as pioneering collaborative partnerships to strengthen diabetes prevention in Michigan. As my nursing career advanced, I recognized there was a need to finish my bachelor's and then master's degree in nursing. Shortly after, I was offered a position at a large healthcare system in Detroit managing their outpatient diabetes education and wound care programs. In this role, I also served as the diabetes education program coordinator for the four hospital-based diabetes programs within the healthcare system. This experience prepared me for my next role managing a national clinical team for a medical device company. It was at this point in my career that I decided it was time to pursue a terminal degree in nursing. After graduating with my DNP degree I was offered a position as assistant professor in the McAuley School of Nursing at the University of Detroit Mercy where I currently teach. My responsibilities in this role include teaching nursing courses across the curriculum—in the BSN program, the graduate nursing program, as well as in the DNP program.

Dr. Moran, what led you to your decision to return to school for a DNP degree?

My long-term goal had always been to teach nursing. I wanted to mentor, inspire, and positively influence nurses of the future. So, a few years ago, while I was reflecting on how blessed I have been throughout my nursing career, with excellent role models and many opportunities, I really started to feel that I had arrived at the point in my personal life and professional career where I could work toward that next goal . . . and begin to pay it forward. So, I started on my journey . . .

During that time, I looked at many terminal degree programs, but none of them really spoke to my personal career goals until the doctor of nursing practice degree was introduced . . . for me, that program was a perfect fit. And in May of 2011, I graduated with my DNP degree from Madonna University.

Dr. Moran, how has your career evolved since earning a DNP degree?

As a DNP-prepared nurse and educator, I approach my practice through a much broader lens. I am committed to moving the nursing profession forward as an advocate, role model, and mentor. I also believe that I have expanded my ability to influence change within health care as an individual and through collaborative efforts with my colleagues and scholarship partners. It is critical, especially during this period of flux in the U.S. healthcare system, that DNP-prepared nurses take a seat at the table where decisions affecting the health of our nation are being made. Finally, as a result of my expanded skill set in inter- and intraprofessional collaboration, leadership, and entrepreneurism, I have successfully started and now operate a small business with my colleague, Dr. Burson, providing chronic disease management and education in the primary care setting.

INTERVIEW WITH A DNP SCHOLARSHIP TEAM

DRS. KATHY MORAN, DIANNE CONRAD, AND ROSANNE BURSON are a scholarship team who authored a textbook titled *The DNP Scholarly Project: A Framework for Success.*

Dr. Moran, you and your colleagues Dr. Burson and Dr. Conrad collaborated on a textbook titled *The DNP Scholarly Project: A Framework for Success.* How was the idea for this wonderful resource developed, and what made you decide to publish this textbook?

When I was going through my DNP program, I recognized that there were limited resources available to guide students through the development of a scholarly project at the doctoral level. This was a concern to me on several levels (1) because of how difficult it is for the student, but also (2) because of the extra burden on both the faculty and practice partners who work with DNP students on these scholarly projects when a frame of reference is not available. Shortly after graduation, my colleagues, Dr. Rosanne Burson and Dr. Dianne Conrad, and I had a discussion regarding our shared experiences around this topic. We quickly realized that it was time that we utilize the skills developed during the course of our doctoral work to write a proposal for a textbook to Jones & Bartlett Learning outlining what we thought would address the identified gaps in the literature. This was the beginning of what would soon become The DNP Scholarly Project: A Framework for Success.

Drs. Moran, Burson, and Conrad, do you feel that this textbook influences the education of others regarding the DNP degree? If so, how?

Absolutely. While our ultimate goal was to provide a resource for students, faculty, and practice partners to use when embarking on the scholarly project journey, we also realized that it would be a venue to articulate the value of the DNP-prepared nurse. Since the release of the textbook, we have had multiple opportunities on local, state, and national levels to demonstrate *to others the value of the DNP degree through scholarship activities that we believe move the profession of nursing forward and have a positive impact on the health of the nation. We continue to model our work as a* scholarship team *nationally.*

Drs. Moran, Burson, and Conrad, what are your future plans to educate others about the DNP degree?

As a scholarship team, we continue to define and clarify the attributes and contributions of the DNP-prepared advanced-practice nurse in all advanced-practice roles to fellow faculty, nursing colleagues, students, policy makers, patients, and the public through modeling, mentoring, presentations, and publications. We have engaged in the scholarly work of developing a concept analysis of the practice doctorate to clearly define the antecedents and attributes that lead to producing the DNP outcomes affecting individuals, patients, populations, and policy in health care. We continue to influence the development of the Michigan DNP Network and contribute to the National DNP organization with conference planning and presentations of our scholarly work. We have organized an ongoing statewide initiative in Michigan to bring together all nine universities with DNP programs to dialogue with their practice partners on optimal preparation of DNP students and how the DNP-prepared nurse can influence positive outcomes through innovations in the organizational setting.

The advanced-practice knowledge of evidence-based practice, population health, informatics, interprofessional collaboration, and advocacy have allowed us to effectively continue practice-focused DNP projects after graduation with successful outcomes.

Drs. Moran, Burson, and Conrad, what advice do you have for DNP students and graduates regarding educating others about the DNP degree?

In all of the venues that we have had the opportunity to converse, there is a definite need to understand the DNP degree. This includes our nursing colleagues from PhD to undergraduate students, our interprofessional team members such as physicians, other practice partners, administrators, and the public. There are so many ways to participate in this education. Be courageous, creative, and available. It starts from being able to articulate within a few minutes the value and purpose of the DNP degree, to scholarly writing and presentations, and through demonstration. We encourage our DNP colleagues to consider a scholarship team. This is a wonderful way to accomplish the important work of scholarship and dissemination. Most important, though, is the demonstration that the DNP is affecting outcomes in the health of our population, the care of patients, and the cost of health care. The more we demonstrate, the more headway we will make in understanding the impact of the DNP. There are opportunities to be at the table right now, but everyone wants to be there. We need to show that we have the leadership skills and the implementation ability that will make a difference. The last point of advice is that we need to continue to present the DNP as an umbrella for all areas of advanced nursing practice—clinicians, executives, and policy experts. There is so much work to do, and we need to pull together all of our incredible and varied strengths to move health care forward.

A Personal Note: My Experience Educating Others About the DNP Degree

In 2007 I graduated from Oakland University with a DNP degree. Two months after graduating, I realized I did not understand the impact of this degree on my role as a clinician, a nurse leader, or in health care. I figured if I did not fully understand how to integrate my new skills and perspectives, my colleagues who had just earned a DNP degree may not either. That was the beginning of an amazing journey that has led me here—providing a third edition of a textbook dedicated to educating others about the DNP degree.

My responsibility to educate others did not stop with the development of this textbook. Since graduating I have been committed to educating others formally in university settings, at conferences, and in publications about the DNP degree. However, my most important tool in educating others has been leading by example and role-modeling the impact of DNP-prepared nurses. Every day I have opportunities to share with patients, other healthcare professionals, and leadership in my organization the contributions and perspectives of DNP-prepared nurses. I charge all of you who are reading this text to start your journey educating others about the DNP degree by understanding your degree and role-modeling through your contributions to nursing and health care.

SUMMARY

- Educating patients, nurses, and other healthcare professionals about the DNP degree is the responsibility of all DNP graduates.
- It is necessary that DNP graduates have a clear understanding of the terms *nursing, nursing practice, advanced-practice nursing, medicine, physician, doctor, practice doctorate*, and *doctor of nursing practice*.
- Overall the literature has shown patients to have favorable attitudes and perceptions of advanced-practice registered nurses (Brown, 2007; Levine et al., 1978; Mitchell et al., 2001; Sheer, 1994). This information provides insights for DNP graduates to develop strategies when educating patients about the DNP graduate's role and educational preparation.
- The literature has shown that nurses look to advanced-practice registered nurses as a resource and value their contribution to health care (Gooden & Jackson, 2004). DNP graduates can also be a resource for nursing and act as role models for nurses. This will increase DNP graduates' credibility and nurses' receptiveness toward the DNP degree.
- Physicians' attitudes toward nurse practitioners have evolved. Research has shown that physicians' attitudes improve when physicians work with nurse practitioners (Aquilino et al., 1999). Therefore, in an effort to effectively educate healthcare professionals about the DNP degree, DNP graduates should continue to collaborate with other healthcare professionals and provide interdisciplinary care. This will also demonstrate improvement in patient care outcomes.
- Empathic listening, or listening with the intent to understand (Covey, 2004), can enable the DNP graduate to understand the audience's frame of reference, which will allow the audience to understand the DNP graduate's message.
- When preparing to speak publicly about their educational preparation, DNP graduates should be very clear about their message.
- DNP graduates should always convey sincerity and enthusiasm to their audience when presenting information about their educational preparation.

REFLECTION QUESTIONS

1. Do you have a clear understanding of nursing as a discipline, science, and profession?

2. Do you have a clear understanding of the differences between nursing and medicine?

3. How do you think patients perceive nursing, advanced-practice nursing, and the DNP degree?

4. What can be done to increase patients' understanding of nursing and the DNP degree?

5. Do you think other nurses have a clear understanding of the DNP degree, including the rationale for a practice doctorate in nursing?

6. If not, what do you think can be done to increase nursing's understanding of the DNP degree?

7. How do you think other healthcare professionals perceive nursing and the DNP degree?

8. What can be done to increase other healthcare professionals' understanding of nursing and the DNP degree?

9. Do you agree that it is every DNP graduate's responsibility to educate others about the DNP degree?

10. What strategies do you think DNP graduates can use to increase overall awareness and understanding of the DNP degree?

REFERENCES

American Association of Colleges of Nursing. (2006a). *DNP roadmap task force report*. Retrieved from http://www.aacn.nche.edu/dnp/roadmapreport.pdf

American Association of Colleges of Nursing. (2006b). *Essentials of doctoral education for advanced nursing practice*. Retrieved from www.aacn.nche.edu/publications/position/DNPEssentials.pdf

American Association of Colleges of Nursing. (2014). DNP talking points. Retrieved from http://www.aacn.nche.edu/dnp/about/talking-points

American Nurses Association. (1995). *Nursing's social policy statement*. Washington, DC: Author.

Aquilino, M., Damiano, P., Williard, J., Momany, E., & Levy, B. (1999). Primary care physician perceptions of the nurse practitioner in the 1990s. *Archives of Family Medicine, 8*(3), 224–227.

Bailey, J. (2003). The story of "doctor, " "physician," and "surgeon." *Journal of the National Medical Association, 85*(6), 489–490.

Brown, D. (2007). Consumer perspectives on nurse practitioners and independent practice. *Journal of the American Academy of Nurse Practitioners, 19*(10), 523–529.

Brown, S. (1998). A framework for advanced practice nursing. *Journal of Professional Nursing, 14*(3), 157–164.

Bryant-Lukosius, D., DiCenso, A., Browne, G., & Pinelli, J. (2004). Advanced practice nursing roles: Development, implementation, and evaluation. *Nursing and Health Care Management and Policy, 48*(5), 519–529.

Carnegie, D., & Carnegie Hill, M. (2007). *Tips for public speaking.* Sausalito, CA: E & E.

Carnegie, D., & Pell, A. (2005). *Public speaking for success: Revised and updated version.* New York, NY: Penguin.

Covey, S. R. (2004). *The 7 habits of highly effective people.* New York, NY: Free Press.

Edmunds, M. (1988). Promoting visibility for the nurse practitioner role. *Nurse Practitioner, 13*(3), 53–55.

Fottler, M., Gibson, G., & Pinchoff, D. (1978). Physician attitudes toward the nurse practitioner. *Journal of Health and Social Behavior, 19*(3), 303–311.

Gooden, J., & Jackson, E. (2004). Attitudes of registered nurses toward nurse practitioners. *Journal of American Academy of Nurse Practitioners, 16*(8), 360–364.

Greiner, A. C., & Knebel, E. (Eds.). (2003). *Health professions education: A bridge to quality.* Washington, DC: National Academies Press.

Griffiths, Y., & Padilla, R. (2006). National status of the entry-level doctorate in occupational therapy. *American Journal of Occupational Therapy, 60*(5), 540–549.

International Council of Nurses. (1998). *Position statement: Scope of nursing practice.* Retrieved from http://www.icn.ch/images/stories/documents/publications/position_statements/B07_Scope_Nsg_Practice.pdf

International Council of Nurses. (2014). *Definition of nursing.* Retrieved from http://www.icn.ch/about-icn/icn-definition-of-nursing

Knowles, E. (2006). *The Oxford dictionary of phrase and fable.* Retrieved from http://www.encyclopedia.com/topic/doctor.aspx

Kravitz, L. (2007, January). Public speaking 101. *IDEA Fitness Journal,* 108–109.

Levine, J., Orr, S., Sheatsley, D., Lohr, J., & Brodie, B. (1978). The nurse practitioner: Role, physician utilization, patient acceptance. *Nursing Research, 27*(4), 245–254.

Marriner-Tomey, A. (1990). Historical development of doctoral programs from the middle-ages to nursing education today. *Nursing and Health Care, 3*(11), 132–137.

Medicine. (2007). In *New Oxford American Dictionary* (2nd ed.). [Computer software]. Cupertino, CA: Apple.

Medicine. (2014). In *Merriam-Webster's online dictionary.* Retrieved from http://www.merriam-webster.com/dictionary/medicine

Mitchell, J., Dixon, H., Freeman, T., & Grindrod, A. (2001). Public perceptions of and comfort level with nurse practitioners in family practice. *Canadian Nurse, 97*(8), 20–26.

Montoya, I., & Kimball, O. (2006). Marketing clinical doctorate programs. *Journal of Allied Health, 36*(2), 107–112.

Newman, M. (1975). The professional doctorate in nursing: A position paper. *Nursing Outlook,* *23*(11), 704–706.

Nichols, C., O'Connor, N., & Dunn, D. (2014). Exploring early and future use of DNP prepared nurses within healthcare organizations. *The Journal of Nursing Administration, 44*(2), 74–78.

Physician. (2014). In *Merriam-Webster's online dictionary.* Retrieved from http://www.merriam-webster.com/dictionary/physician

Richmond, T., & Becker, D. (2005). Creating an advanced practice nurse–friendly culture: A marathon not a sprint. *AACN Clinical Issues, 16*(1), 58–66.

Royeen, C., & Lavin, M. (2007). A contextual logical analysis of the clinical doctorate for health practitioners: Dilemma, delusion, or de facto? *Journal of Allied Health, 36*(2), 101–106.

Sheer, B. (1994). Reshaping the nurse practitioner image through socialization. *Nurse Practitioner Forum, 5*(4), 215–219.

Skinner, H. (1970). *Medical terms* (2nd ed.). New York, NY: Hafner.

Upvall, M., & Ptachcinski, R. (2007). The journey to the DNP program and beyond: What can we learn from pharmacy? *Journal of Professional Nursing, 23*(5), 316–321.

Whitemore, S., & Jaffe, L. (1996). Public perceptions of nurse practitioners. *Nurse Practitioner, 21*(2), 19–20.

CHAPTER 13

Shaping Your Brand: Marketing Yourself as a DNP Graduate

Lisa Astalos Chism

The number of students enrolled in doctor of nursing practice (DNP) programs continues to increase. From 2012 to 2013 the enrollment numbers increased from 11,575 to 14,699. During that same time period, the number of DNP graduates increased from 1,858 to 2,443 (American Association of Colleges of Nursing [AACN], 2014a). Despite these increasing numbers, the DNP degree is still new to many outside of and within the nursing profession. It is therefore likely that the DNP degree will be new to potential employers of DNP graduates. DNP graduates have a responsibility not only to educate others about the DNP degree, but also to develop unique strategies to market themselves as DNP graduates.

Many DNP graduates may not have a background in marketing; therefore, some basic marketing concepts are reviewed in this chapter. These concepts include the definition of marketing and branding, becoming what is sometimes referred to as a "marketpreneur" (Mackey & Estala, 2008), and creating a mission and vision statement that is unique to DNP graduates. General marketing strategies are discussed in relation to the DNP graduate, as well as unique marketing strategies with specific suggestions that this author has used to market herself as a DNP graduate.

Marketing Versus Branding

Marketing has been defined by the American Marketing Association (AMA) as "an organizational function and a set of processes for creating, communicating, and delivering value to customers and for managing customer relationships in ways that benefit the organization and its stakeholders" (AMA, 2011). Marketing also describes various concepts, such as business development, through advertising, brand and logo design, making sales calls, and designing websites, brochures, packaging, and business cards (Haim, 2005). Beals describes a more in-depth definition of marketing as a "*process,* from planning to execution, which identifies consumers for a specific product or service, communicates how the product satisfies consumer wants and needs and spurs the consumer to make a purchase" (2008, p. 7).

Conversely, Putnam (1990) describes three functions that are not inclusive of marketing, but rather are various functions of marketing. Advertising is noted to be one function of marketing, but it is not equivalent to marketing. Promotion, or making potential clients aware of your business, is also noted to be a function of marketing, but it is not inclusive of marketing. Finally, sales may or may not be a part of marketing (Putnam, 1990). Sales generally involves interactions with potential clients to explain the benefits of products or goods (Dayhoff & Moore, 2004).

Branding, a component of marketing, is an essential marketing strategy. A brand consists of a "trademark, a distinctive name, and a combination of images that creates associations and expectations in the minds of consumers" (Beals, 2008, p. 8). Beals related that "in your lifelong self-marketing campaign, *you* are the 'brand' . . . the work you do and the value you add are your *product*" (2008, p. 8).

Why develop a brand for yourself? Despite the fact that DNP graduates practice within the healthcare or academic arena, the world continues to become a more competitive place. According to Beals (2008), one may develop a brand for the following reasons:

- To benefit your career
- To increase personal recognition
- To improve your reputation
- To promote your employer's business
- To obtain new clients or patients
- To advance your own social beliefs or cause

DNP graduates may develop a brand to share the unique talents, skills, and knowledge they bring to their career environment. DNP graduates' brands may be unique to the role or setting in which they practice. DNP graduates in academic settings may develop a brand based on a curriculum they develop or on their areas of expertise. DNP graduates in clinical settings may develop brands based on their specialties, such as additional certifications.

For example, one of this author's colleagues, Ms. Christine Rymal, MSN, ANP, BC, CLT, practices in a breast health setting and holds additional certification as a lymphedema specialist (CLT). Ms. Rymal has created a brand and has a unique niche within her setting as a lymphedema specialist. Because of her brand, Ms. Rymal is regularly consulted by multiple providers within her setting and has developed a successful practice (personal communication, March 10, 2011). Developing a brand is one method DNP graduates can employ to market their unique product.

DNP Graduates as Marketpreneurs

Mackey and Estala (2008) describe *marketpreneurship* as employing leadership and innovation when marketing. Specifically, these authors refer to nurse practitioners as "marketpreneurs" who "use their imagination to build relationships and focus on target markets" (Mackey & Estala, 2008, p. 14). As innovators and leaders, marketpreneurs have a "vision they can articulate and sell this vision to others" (2008, p. 14). Additionally, a marketpreneur has "desire, determination, dedication/commitment, and a focus on success" (2008, p. 14).

DNP graduates are charged to become marketpreneurs. The DNP degree is an innovative degree that emphasizes leadership in practice. DNP graduates may develop a mission and a vision and apply these when developing their brand. The innovative contributions to improving practice and leadership skills that DNP graduates embody will foster their success as marketpreneurs.

Mission Statement

A mission statement has been defined as "a sentence describing a company's function, markets and competitive advantages; a short written statement of your business goals and philosophies" (Entrepreneur, 2014). Further, "a mission statement defines what an organization is, why it exists, its reason for being" (Entrepreneur, 2014). DNP graduates may develop their own mission statement based on their setting or specialty. For example, this author has a clinical practice and specializes in breast and menopausal health. The following is her mission statement: "To provide expertise, empathy, and compassion while evaluating and caring for patients' breast and menopause health issues."

Developing a mission statement enables DNP graduates to define exactly what they bring to their setting and decide how their unique talents and skills may be marketed. A mission statement will also help DNP graduates define their focus and channel their efforts to achieve their mission.

Vision Statement

A vision statement has been defined as an "aspirational description of what an organization would like to achieve or accomplish in the mid-term or long-term future" (Business Dictionary, 2014). DNP graduates may also develop their own vision statement when they graduate to guide them toward their long-term goals. This author's vision statement is as follows: "Develop expertise regarding the DNP degree and serve as a consultant providing pedagogical materials nationally and internationally while maintaining a clinical practice specializing in caring for patients' breast and menopause health issues."

By developing a vision statement, DNP graduates will begin to actualize their goals and develop their new roles within their setting.

Marketing Strategies

The marketing literature offers several marketing strategies. Specifics of each strategy will depend on your setting or practice site (Mackey & Estala, 2008). The following sections offer insights for DNP graduates to begin developing their own marketing strategies that are most appropriate for their settings.

Rogers's Diffusion of Innovations Theory

Dr. Everett Rogers is widely known as the creator of the Diffusion of Innovations Theory. His work stems from his personal interest in understanding why farmers in Iowa (including his father) resisted using new inventions in their fields. Instead, these farmers adopted innovations over a period of time. Dr. Rogers earned a degree in agriculture, followed by a PhD in sociology and statistics, from Iowa State University and wrote the book *Diffusion of Innovations* in 1962.

Diffusion is defined as "the process in which an innovation is communicated through certain channels over time among the members of a social system" (Rogers, 2003, p. 5). An innovation is defined by Rogers as "an idea, practice, or project that is perceived as new by an individual or other unit of adoption" (2003, p. 12). According to Rogers (2003), diffusion of innovations occurs when consequences are shared with all parties; in other words, the advantages and disadvantages must be shared to reduce uncertainty regarding an innovation. Second, communication must take place between parties regarding the innovation. Rogers defines communication as "a process in which participants create and share information with one another in order to reach a mutual understanding" (2003, p. 5).

In summary, Rogers describes the diffusion of innovations process as "an information-seeking and information-processing activity, where an individual is motivated to reduce uncertainty about the advantages and disadvantages of an innovation" (2003, p. 172). This process involves five steps: (1) knowledge, (2) persuasion, (3) decision, (4) implementation, and (5) confirmation (Rogers, 2003). This process has been used to explain the *tipping point*, or the time when an idea or innovation catches fire and spreads throughout a population (Orr, 2003). The development of the DNP degree is an example of the Diffusion of Innovations Theory in action. At one point the degree was an idea, or innovation, and it has now been adopted as the educational preparation for advanced-practice registered nurses (APRNs) with more than 153 programs now offered nationwide, and 160 more are in development (AACN, 2014b). DNP graduates may have followed this theory while deciding whether to adopt this degree as their own academic preparation, weighing the advantages and disadvantages and communicating with others to make their decision. DNP graduates may have employed knowledge, persuasion (with their families and colleagues), decision making, implementation, and finally confirmation when making the decision to return to graduate school. DNP graduates may employ this process when marketing themselves to new employers or others.

The Four Ps

The literature also discusses the Four Ps as a marketing strategy. Landrum (1998) relates the Four Ps to Rogers's (2003) work and describes the Four Ps as product, price, place, and promotion. Landrum (1998) describes the product as the APRN, the price as the cash flow involved, the place as the setting of the practice, and the promotion as advertising to promote the services provided by the APRN. Haim also describes these Four Ps in the literature. Product is described as the service offered by the APRN, price is described as how much is charged for the service, place is described as the location of the practice, and promotion is described as the process of presenting your practice to target markets (Haim, 2005).

DNP graduates may adapt this strategy to their own practice setting or career environment. They may consider themselves or their services as the product, their contribution or cash flow as the price, their practice setting as the place, and their promotion as the process of communicating the benefits and advantages of adding a DNP-prepared APRN nurse to a particular organization.

Beals's Rules

Beals relates self-marketing to playing a game. As with any game, there are basic rules to self-marketing, including positive thinking, developing expertise, being prepared, having the right attitude, counting everyone, realizing you are being watched, embracing professionalism, and communicating clearly (Beals, 2008).

Beals describes positive thinking as believing "you are a strong, talented person who has something worth marketing" (2008, p. 17). DNP graduates should adopt a positive attitude when marketing themselves. They should also realize that a positive outlook will have an impact on their success and become contagious.

Developing an expertise is a given for many DNP graduates because APRNs are already experts in their field. DNP graduates are challenged to not be shy about their expertise and beat their own drum regarding their expertise. This includes becoming active as a speaker or writing articles, columns, or blog posts professionally. By drawing attention to their area of expertise, DNP graduates become known as experts in their field.

Being prepared involves always being ready to embrace an opportunity for self-marketing (Beals, 2008). DNP graduates may embrace this rule whenever they are in networking situations. This includes conferences or meet-and-greet events when there are opportunities to market themselves.

The rule that everyone counts refers to trying to impress everyone, not only those who appear to be influential (Beals, 2008). Everyone in professional settings counts when DNP graduates are marketing themselves. It is important for DNP graduates to make a positive impression on everyone they encounter, especially when in professional settings.

Beals (2008) compares the rule that you are being watched to the dramatic arts when actors stay in character: "As a professional trying to market yourself, you must always stay in your professional 'character'" (Beals, 2008, p. 26). Beals (2008) further points out that what one does or says when no one is watching may hurt your career. DNP graduates should heed this rule and always maintain professionalism, even when they think no one is paying attention. It is very difficult to undo unprofessional behavior and repair one's reputation and legitimacy after the damage is done.

Embracing professionalism emphasizes that "behavior and image are critical parts of self-marketing" (Beals, 2008, p. 27). In addition, how one treats others will reflect professionalism. Although assertive behavior may be necessary to succeed, aggressive behavior may have a long-term negative effect on your career. "A truly professional person is nice, sincerely nice, and consistently nice" (Beals, 2008, p. 28). This rule is excellent advice for DNP graduates. After graduation others may be waiting to see how DNP graduates assimilate into their roles. It would be easy for others to develop a negative perception of DNP graduates if they are aggressive in their behavior.

Communicating clearly refers to thinking about what one is going to say before anything is said (Beals, 2008). DNP graduates should employ this rule whenever speaking publicly, especially about their degree. Further, many DNP graduates will be in leadership roles, and what they say will be listened to. DNP graduates have a responsibility to make sure what they say is accurate, concise, and clear.

Unique Strategies for DNP Graduates

The preceding section reviewed marketing strategies that may apply to any professional. These strategies are adaptable to any setting in many career choices. The following sections review unique strategies this author has found to be effective in marketing one's self as a DNP graduate after graduation and beyond.

The Introduction

It is imperative that DNP graduates know who they are and can describe their degree so they can develop a concise introduction. The introduction is essential to communicating to others the value that a DNP-prepared APRN adds to the practice, academic, or organizational setting.

The introduction has sometimes been referred to as the elevator pitch (Beals, 2008; Mackey & Estala, 2008). The elevator pitch is a brief statement that takes

60 seconds or less to introduce yourself to someone, including why you are unique and what your expertise is. The elevator pitch "gets to the point and places an image in the listener's mind . . . it should be brief, descriptive, and paint an interesting picture" (Beals, 2008, p. 29). DNP graduates should base their elevator pitch on the DNP degree and their setting or expertise. This author has used the following elevator pitch:

> I am a nurse practitioner specializing in breast health, menopause, and related health issues. My background includes caring for geriatric and women's health populations in various settings. I currently practice in an academic, multidisciplinary, comprehensive breast center. My educational preparation includes a doctor of nursing practice degree, which has prepared me as a nurse leader and given me additional skills in information technology, evidence-based practice, and healthcare policy, which in turn enables me to address the challenges of a complex healthcare environment.

In addition, this author has an elevator pitch to explain *why* a DNP was pursued. When asked, "Why a DNP? What are you going to do with that?" this author responds as follows:

> The Institute of Medicine has called for higher education in all health professions, including nursing. Also, the National Academy of Sciences has endorsed nurses earning practice doctorates. Personally, earning a DNP was about personal and professional growth. I am a nurse leader charged to improve nursing practice through the additional skills I have acquired. I am committed to the advancement of the nursing profession and the promotion of the nurse practitioner role.

The Interview

Most DNP graduates have already had experience interviewing for positions either in the practice or academic setting. However, interviewing as a DNP graduate will be a unique experience for DNP graduates. A few key pointers are worth mentioning.

Kathleen D. Pagana, PhD, RN, wrote a very informative book titled *The Nurse's Etiquette Advantage* (2008). Dr. Pagana offers many pearls of wisdom regarding etiquette that DNP graduates can use as a guide when marketing themselves. Throughout an interview, Pagana (2008) recommends the following discussion points:

- What experiences do you have that qualify you for the position?
- What distinguishes you from other candidates?
- What are your strengths?
- What are your weaknesses?
- What are your long-term goals?
- What experiences have you had working with others in teams?

These discussion points were included because of their pertinence to what DNP graduates may offer in any setting. DNP graduates may tailor their responses based on their experiences and how these experiences may enhance the position they are applying for. Also, additional skills acquired in a DNP program may be added as other strengths a graduate may highlight throughout the interview.

Appearances

Appearances matter when marketing one's self as a DNP graduate, especially while the DNP degree is still relatively new to others. "No matter what people say, you are judged by the way you dress" (Pagana, 2008, p. 43). Further, Pagana states that "whether you are interviewing for a job, giving a presentation, or asking for a promotion, the way you dress is important to your overall presentation" (2008, p. 42).

Generally, underdressing may cause embarrassment, and overdressing may cause intimidation. Sloppy or inappropriate attire may imply that one does not value personal appearance or care that appearance may affect the overall organization. DNP graduates may pay attention to what others are wearing in the organization they wish to be a part of. If one is seeking an academic position, notice what type of attire seems appropriate in that setting (Pagana, 2008). If one is seeking an organizational leadership position, note what others are wearing in that setting.

Most APRNs in a practice setting wear a lab coat over their professional clothes. One way to make sure DNP graduates are marketing themselves is to include "DNP" after their name. This author has taken this a step further by spelling out "Doctor of Nursing Practice" under her name on her lab coat. This is done in an effort to further explain and point out the DNP degree and what the initials stand for. Even this subtle effort explains to others in the elevator, in the hallway, or in line to get coffee what the *DNP* after her name means.

Networking

Some additional guidance is offered here that may assist DNP graduates when networking. The following recommendations refer to conversing with others at networking events.

When engaging in initial small talk at a networking event, Pagana suggests using the acronym *OAR* to aid conversation. *O* stands for observation—make a comment about the event in general; *A* stands for ask a question, such as "Have you been here before?"; and *R* stands for revealing something personal, such as "This is my first time at this event" (Pagana, 2008). This acronym may help when one is a bit nervous and in an unfamiliar group.

Also, when talking with many different professionals at a networking event, a good rule of thumb is to be courteous, respectful, and considerate of others' feelings. "Good manners are for good business and bad manners may mean no business" (Pagana, 2008, p. 22). DNP graduates should avoid going from person to person, handing out business cards and shaking hands with as many people as possible. This may convey insincerity and lack of interest in folks as individuals (Pagana, 2008). In addition, DNP graduates should avoid monopolizing conversations with others. This is when the elevator pitch comes in handy, especially if others ask about the DNP degree. DNP graduates may quickly and concisely explain their degree and not monopolize the conversation unless asked further specific questions about the degree. Finally, DNP graduates should employ good listening skills when networking. "A good listener can make a person feel as if they are the only person in the room" (Pagana, 2008, p. 27).

Becoming a Voice in the Community and Professionally

Marketing one's self as a DNP graduate involves exposing one's self to the public. The following recommendations refer to self-marketing by becoming active in the community and professionally.

DNP graduates should become active speakers in various settings. This may include joining a speaker's bureau related to one's specialty. DNP graduates may demonstrate their expertise and educate others about their degree. This will also promote one as an expert and facilitate creating a brand.

DNP graduates may volunteer to speak at community events to the lay public. This will share their expertise and educate others about their degree. Additionally, volunteering to speak at community events may lead to other volunteer activities in the community that may create opportunities to promote DNP graduates' expertise. One of this author's colleagues, Ms. Catherine Nichols, MSN, ANP, BC, is a DNP student and speaks regularly in her community. Ms. Nichols has spoken about breast health at Girl Scout events and has given educational talks at her church (personal communication, March 14, 2011).

Another way for DNP graduates to market themselves is writing for a local newspaper, journal, or professional organization. DNP graduates may write about topics related to their specific expertise or about the DNP degree. This will also promote DNP graduates' expertise and facilitate developing a brand. This author joined a professional journal's blog as an expert on the DNP degree. After blogging successfully on topics related to the DNP degree, this author offered to write a regular column related to the DNP degree. As a blog expert, columnist, and author of DNP-related topics, this author is developing a brand as a DNP expert.

Finally, DNP graduates should maintain memberships and become active in professional organizations. This affiliation promotes the DNP graduate's professionalism and provides numerous networking opportunities. By becoming active in various professional organizations, the DNP graduate is also able to promote the DNP degree.

The Media as a Marketing Avenue

DNP graduates have an opportunity to use the media to market themselves and highlight their expertise. Media opportunities may vary from radio and television appearances to participation in mainstream media publications and interviews. Importantly, because of the potential for high visibility in media opportunities, DNP graduates should be well prepared for these opportunities because they will likely be accessible to a wide audience for extended periods of time through the Internet.

DNP graduates will want to make a connection with their audience. Jacobs (2003) offered the Four Cs of communication when addressing the media:

1. Connect: Recognize the importance of connecting with everyone, including crew members, producers, and audience. Offer a handshake and make sure to smile.

2. Conform to the medium: Everything you say is on the record, so make sure you are concise.

3. Control the interview: Preplan for the interview and practice. Prepare for your least favorite question and plan how you will redirect it back to your key messages.

4. Correct: Correct misinformation in the moment and turn a negative spin into a positive one.

In addition, use anecdotes to tell your story and get your key messages across (Kenig, 2004). Avoid attacking the media with general statements. Also, avoid jargon or phrases that the general public may not understand, such as advanced-practice nurses (Kenig, 2004). Finally, much like the elevator pitch, develop a 30-second message about your practice that you wish to convey and that describes the focus of your practice (Kenig, 2004).

Appearances in general were discussed earlier in the chapter. Jacobs (2003) also referenced specific recommendations regarding your appearance during an interview with the media. These recommendations include the following:

- Keep your hands out of your pockets and use your hands when you wish to make a point.
- Wear your hair neatly and avoid touching your hair during the interview.
- Stand in a well-balanced stance and avoid rocking or pacing.
- Focus your attention on one person, make eye contact, complete the thought, then move on to the next person. (Jacobs, 2003)

DNP graduates may use the media to market themselves and provide an avenue to educate the public about the DNP degree. These opportunities should be embraced; however, DNP graduates should also take time to prepare and make the best impression possible. Media exposure can be accessed easily by others and for many years to come.

Involvement in Policy

Healthcare policy is included in the AACN *Essentials of Doctoral Education for Advanced Nursing Practice* (AACN, 2006) and is a part of DNP curricula. Healthcare policy defines many aspects of advanced-practice nursing, and DNP graduates are charged to become involved in healthcare policy. This involvement also fosters promotion of the DNP degree. Hall related that "educating legislators, corporate executives, and the public about NPs [nurse practitioners] is the key to success in both advancing and marketing the profession" (2000, p. 323). DNP graduates should heed these words and remember that educating legislators is also essential to promoting and marketing the DNP degree. The nursing profession, including DNP graduates, will benefit from our policy makers knowing about and understanding the DNP degree.

Specific Marketing Tools

DNP graduates may have already developed various marketing tools to promote their practice, academic appointment, or position within an organization. However, when a DNP graduate returns to the workplace or applies for a new position, these tools should be modified. The following section discusses a few relevant marketing suggestions for DNP graduates.

Most DNP graduates already have business cards with their prior degree and title displayed. Upon graduation, the DNP graduates should develop new business cards with a few pertinent changes. First, their new degree should be included as part of their credentials. This is sometimes referred to as the alphabet soup that appears after an APRN's name. Regardless, it is necessary that "DNP" be added. Generally, the highest degree is listed as the first credential (likely DNP), followed by advanced-practice designations or certifications, additional certifications, and membership as a fellow of a professional organization, if applicable. For example, this author has a DNP degree, is a board-certified gerontological nurse practitioner, is certified as a menopause practitioner, and was inducted as a fellow of the American Academy of Nurse Practitioners in 2011. Therefore the name and credentials are as follows: Lisa Astalos Chism, DNP, GNP, BC, NCMP, FAANP. Although one's credentials may be extensive, it is important to display them proudly. One adjustment this author added is explanations on her business cards under her name and credentials:

Lisa Astalos Chism, DNP, GNP, BC, NCMP, FAANP
Doctor of Nursing Practice
Gerontological Nurse Practitioner
Certified Menopause Practitioner

This gives patients, colleagues, and others an explanation of the listed credentials. Finally, when adding DNP after one's name, it is not necessary or appropriate to add "Dr." in front of one's name because Dr. is a title, not a credential.

Sometime after graduating with a DNP degree, this author applied for a new position. As part of her marketing tools, this author developed a pamphlet describing the DNP-prepared nurse practitioner. It describes what makes the DNP-prepared nurse practitioner unique and includes brief details about the DNP degree. The pamphlet has been a valuable marketing tool, especially during the time when the DNP degree was very new (2007). DNP graduates may develop their own pamphlet as part of their marketing tools to describe their specialties and the DNP degree.

Pagana (2008) recommended the use of thank-you notes after an interview or pertinent meeting. This author also found it useful to design and order stationery with her new credentials listed with her name. It is recommended that the stationery be generic so it can be used for any occasion, both professional and personal. Stationery is a professional yet warm way to communicate with others, especially when a more personal form of communication is warranted.

Finally, as technology advances, many APRNs with their own businesses, practices, or pedagogical materials have a website. This marketing tool may be helpful for DNP graduates to create, especially if developing a consulting business or their own practice. DNP graduates may devote a section of the website to explain the DNP degree and use the opportunity to market themselves as DNP-prepared consultants, providers, or educators.

A summary of tips for marketing yourself as a DNP graduate can be found in **Box 13-1**.

A Personal Note: My Involvement in Marketing

Since joining my institution, I have had the pleasure of being very involved in marketing at many levels. This involvement has helped me realize how important marketing is to nursing, advanced-practice nursing, and the DNP degree. Hence, I dedicated this chapter to marketing in the current edition of this text and included new information about marketing.

My educational background did not prepare me for involvement in marketing, but I have learned some key pointers along the way. I have shared what I have learned about marketing tools, such as spelling out your credentials on business cards and developing a pamphlet. The most exciting (and scary) marketing opportunities have been my involvement in the media. I have been fortunate enough to be invited to do radio interviews, television news interviews, and sporting events to promote breast health and menopause awareness. Looking back at my first interviews, it is clear that I needed practice. Each time I am presented with these opportunities, I am better at

BOX 13-1

Tips for Marketing Yourself as a DNP Graduate

- Develop your brand based on your specialty and setting. Engage in activities that will help develop your brand, such as writing and speaking on topics related to your expertise.

- Develop an elevator pitch (Mackey & Estala, 2008) to briefly introduce yourself and explain the DNP degree.

- Dress for success and model your attire after those in positions you aspire to.

- Add "DNP" to your credentials on your lab coat if you work in a clinical setting.

- While conversing at networking events, be courteous, respectful, and considerate of others' feelings. Also, do not monopolize conversations, and remember to be a good listener.

- Get involved speaking about your expertise or the DNP degree in your community and professionally.

- Start writing in your community or for professional journals. Examples include local newspaper articles, blogging, columns, and professional manuscripts.

- Get involved in healthcare policy by staying current about the issues or contacting or volunteering for your local legislator and educating him or her about the DNP degree.

- Customize your business cards to include "DNP" and possibly "Doctor of Nursing Practice" under your name to explain what DNP means.

- Develop a pamphlet to explain your expertise and specialty, including what the DNP degree is.

- After graduation, order personalized stationery with your name and credentials. Stationery may be used to send a thank-you note or communicate with others in a professional yet warm way.

- Create a website to explain your business, practice, or pedagogical materials, including an explanation of the DNP degree.

- Embrace involvement in media opportunities. Take the time to prepare for interviews and other opportunities.

calming my nerves and presenting a clear message. Importantly, I find the advice of others, such as Pagana (2008), Kenig (2004), and Jacobs (2003), to be very valuable.

My advice to DNP students and graduates is to seize every opportunity and practice, practice, practice. Always be prepared and consult with others regarding your appearance. Dress for the event and remember that you are representing others.

I have done interviews where I wished I could have crawled under the table, and in others I could have talked forever—I don't recommend either of these behaviors! But I never said no when asked. When others know they can count on you, they tend to ask you back. Media is a very powerful marketing tool—embrace the opportunity and grow from it. You will not regret it!

Interviews with Nurse Marketers

PERSPECTIVE OF A MEDIA EXPERT

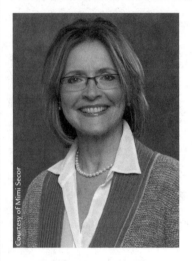

Mimi Secor, MS, M.Ed, FNP-C, NCMP, FAANP, is a media expert, nurse practitioner, and DNP student.

Ms. Secor, can you please describe your educational and professional background, including your experience in media and nursing?

As a family nurse practitioner for the past 37 years specializing in women's health, I currently hold a master's degree in nursing, I am a DNP student, and I am board certified by ANCC [American Nurses Credentialing Center]. I also hold a master's degree in education and national board certification as a certified menopause practitioner (CNMP) with the North American Menopause Society (NAMS). I have practiced in emergency, urgent care, family practice, urban, and rural settings, college health, prisons, and private practice settings. I owned and operated an independent NP practice for 12 years in Cambridge, Massachusetts, and practiced in rural Alaska for 7 years. My media experience has included being interviewed on Good Morning America, *by reporters for the* Wall Street Journal, *the* Boston Globe, *and staff of magazines including* Bridal Guide *and* Cosmopolitan, *and by reporters for many national radio and print publications. I have hosted a nationally syndicated radio show for 2.5 years and cohosted a national* ReachMD *radio show for 2 years. I have received several awards, including most recently the 2012 Lifetime Achievement Award from the Massachusetts Coalition of Nurse Practitioners.*

Ms. Secor, can you describe why you decided to return to school to earn a DNP degree?

Courtesy of Mimi Secor

As a nurse practitioner clinician, educator, and national leader, I felt the need to expand my education in order to attain the new educational standard of a practice doctorate. I feel strongly that the complexity of the rapidly changing healthcare system requires nurse practitioners to not only possess expert clinical skills, but also advanced competencies in evidence-based practice, healthcare policy, informatics, leadership, organizational development, communications, and healthcare finance. This is a tall order that I believe will be facilitated by more NPs possessing doctoral degrees.

Ms. Secor, since returning to graduate school, how has your perspective of nursing changed?

I increasingly appreciate the advanced competencies required to engage in evidence-based practice and how my master's degree did not sufficiently prepare me for this level of rigorous clinical practice. I also appreciate the emerging role of the NP as a leader in the healthcare system; an expert in informatics, management, finance, communications, strategic planning, research, and much more. Finally, as the United States moves toward universal healthcare coverage, nurse practitioners will need to help manage the burgeoning healthcare costs, while at the same time ensuring improved patient care outcomes. We will need to focus more on prevention and helping our patients practice effective self-care. Of course, this is our specialty and passion, so it comes naturally to us.

Ms. Secor, could you describe how DNP graduates may use the media to enhance the nursing profession?

We must increasingly use the media to convey important patient education information to the masses and also to enhance the image of the NP and NPs' roles in the nursing profession. This dual mission is long overdue, and it should be a priority for all NPs. Media outreach will help improve the health of our patients, while also combating the still-pervasive problem of our invisibility in the media. If we each become involved with the media, we will no longer be perceived as the best-kept secret in health care. This initiative is long overdue.

Ms. Secor, what advice do you have for DNP graduates regarding the unique opportunities they may have to become involved in media?

DNP graduates have a unique opportunity to utilize the media as a vehicle to communicate to patients, community leaders, stakeholders, and other healthcare professionals. As leaders in our healthcare systems and communities, our expert opinions will be sought after by members of the media, and so we will need to be media savvy in order to effectively communicate our messages.

PERSPECTIVE OF A BUSINESS OWNER

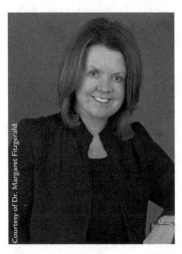

Courtesy of Dr. Margaret Fitzgerald

Margaret Fitzgerald, DNP, FNP-BC, NP-C, FAANP, CSP, FAAN, DCC, is a nurse practitioner and business owner of Fitzgerald Health Associates.

Dr. Fitzgerald, could you please describe your current practice and educational background?

My educational background is as follows:
1993–2006: Case Western Reserve University, Cleveland, Ohio, Frances Payne Bolton School of Nursing, Doctor of Nursing Practice, GPA 4.0
1984–1986: University of Lowell, Lowell, Massachusetts, Master of Science in Nursing, Family and Community Health, Family Nurse Practitioner Role Preparation, Honors GPA
1977–1983: Salem State College, Salem, Massachusetts, Division of Continuing Education, Bachelor of Science in Nursing, with Honors
1968–1970: Northern Essex Community College, Haverhill, Massachusetts, Associate Degree in Science, Nursing Major
Family nurse practitioner: Greater Lawrence Family Health Center, Lawrence, Massachusetts. Primary healthcare provider in a family-centered healthcare center serving an ethnically diverse, inner-city population.

My clinical practice experience includes obstetric, infant, child, and adult primary healthcare and same-day urgent care. I have also been a clinical preceptor for nurse practitioner and medical students. In addition, I am a former adjunct faculty with Family Practice Physician Residency Program, the first NP to hold such an appointment, sponsored by the health center (primarily responsible for teaching psychopharmacology).

I am also founder, president, principal lecturer: Fitzgerald Health Education Associates Inc. (FHEA), an NP-owned company dedicated to helping nurse practitioners and advanced-practice registered nurses achieve certification and maintain professional competence by providing live continuing education seminars, including NP Certification Exam Review, to more than 75,000 NPs throughout North America. Additional programs provided include Pharmacology Updates, Clinical Skills Workshops, Speakers School, web- and computer-based learning courses, audio and video learning modules, and books.

I have also developed and taught pharmacology and laboratory assessment programs used in six universities. Finally, I am responsible for product development, program planning, speaker development and mentorship, and liaison with NP professionals.

My editorial experience includes my work as publisher, Fitzgerald Health Education Associates' News, which is a monthly email newsletter. I am responsible for editorial oversight of a publication on healthcare issues received by more than 60,000 NPs in North America and abroad.

Dr. Fitzgerald, could you please describe your company, including what gave you the idea to start your company and the steps you took to develop it?

The earliest days of FHEA evolved from an opportunity to provide certification review for a small group of NPs who approached me to help them out. The state nursing association had for years provided such a course but was not going to do so that year due to relocating their headquarters. This helped to create the opportunity, as NPs had no local review option. This humble start, with six people around my dining room table, marked the beginnings of the company that is the industry leader and the largest company of its kind in the world.

Dr. Fitzgerald, how did you market your company in the beginning?

Early marketing was largely word of mouth, but word traveled fast! That first year I ended up giving the course a second time, since word traveled throughout the eastern Massachusetts area. Given that this was pre-Internet, before wide use of email, and the number of NPs was quite low nationwide, relatively few options existed for getting information out about our programs. However, by the early 1990s we were exhibiting at most major NP meetings and advertising in the major NP journals. Our earliest advertising was done largely on a barter basis. Indeed, we continue to barter for select services in exchange for disturbing promotional materials at our courses.

Dr. Fitzgerald, how has your marketing plan changed over time as your company has grown?

By 1998 we had a website and online store, only 4 years after Amazon. By the early 2000s we had an email newsletter, a point that distinguishes FHEA from the competition and is currently the most widely distributed NP-focused monthly newsletter, with more than 60,000 subscribers. We maintain a presence in print ads, online, focused email promotion, a print and online product and conference catalog, and exhibit at most major state, regional, and national NP meetings. We also maintain an active presence with the National Organization of Nurse Practitioner Faculties through a variety of activities. Our Facebook page has thousands of followers, and we are branching into Twitter.

The FHEA faculty are featured speakers at numerous NP meetings across the country. Personally, I speak about 100 times a year, both for FHEA and other organizations. This helps maintain a high profile in the relatively small market that comprises the NP population in North America.

Dr. Fitzgerald, what do you believe are the successful ingredients for a great marketing plan?

In this digital age, the adage "be everywhere all the time" still holds. But the consumer can be simply bombarded with information. Focusing promotion is critical.

Dr. Fitzgerald, do you believe DNP graduates should market themselves as well as the DNP degree?

All nurses need to market themselves, period. Those of us who have earned the DNP to date are pioneers in this educational preparation and need to have a strong understanding of the significance of the shift in the education of advanced-practice registered nurses. We need to be able to say what it is we do, how we do it, and what are our outcomes.

Dr. Fitzgerald, what advice do you have for DNP graduates to market themselves and the DNP degree?

Truly understand the significance of being in the earliest cohorts earning the degree. Soon, all newly graduating APRNs will follow. Setting the DNP as the entry into advanced-practice nursing helps recognize the rigor of current master's-level education in nursing while providing a venue for the APRN student to study areas not currently included, or presented in a less formal fashion, in the current programs; this includes but is not limited to education in evidence-based practice, quality improvement, and systems leadership. The DNP also offers an alternative to research-focused doctoral programs. DNP-prepared nurses can facilitate the implementation of the science developed by researchers prepared in PhD and other research-focused doctorates.

Another important factor is the need for APRNs to achieve educational parity with other professions including law, dentistry, social work, pharmacy, medicine, and physical therapy that have established the practice doctorate as entry into practice. This parity is critically important to NP advancement in the area of healthcare policy and leadership. The NP profession has survived and thrived since the transition from the certificate to master's level as entry into practice. I believe the transition to the DNP will yield similar results.

Over the years, requirements for the profession of nursing have evolved, consistent with needs of the healthcare environment. Nurses prepared at the doctoral level with a blend of clinical, organizational, economic, and leadership skills are most likely to be able to critique nursing and other clinical scientific findings and design programs of care delivery that are locally acceptable and economically feasible, and that have a significant impact on healthcare outcomes. This will help advance the NP profession beyond its current considerable reach.

SUMMARY

- DNP graduates have a responsibility not only to educate others about the DNP degree, but also to develop unique strategies to market themselves as DNP graduates.

- Marketing has been defined by the AMA as "an organizational function and a set of processes for creating, communicating, and delivering value to customers and for managing customer relationships in ways that benefit the organization and its stakeholders" (AMA, 2011).

- Marketing is also defined as a "*process,* from planning to execution, which identifies consumers for a specific product or service, communicates how the product satisfies consumer wants and needs and spurs the consumer to make a purchase" (Beals, 2008, p. 7).

- Branding, a component of marketing, is an essential marketing strategy. A brand consists of a "trademark, a distinctive name, and a combination of images that creates associations and expectations in the minds of consumers" (Beals, 2008, p. 7).

- DNP graduates may develop a brand to share what unique talents, skills, and knowledge they bring to their career environment.

- Marketpreneurship is employing leadership and innovation when marketing (Mackey & Estala, 2008).

- A mission statement has been defined as "a sentence describing a company's function, markets and competitive advantages; a short written statement of your business goals and philosophies" (Entrepreneur, 2014).

- Developing a mission statement enables DNP graduates to define exactly what they bring to their setting and decide how their unique talents and skills may be marketed.

- A vision statement has been defined as an "aspirational description of what an organization would like to achieve or accomplish in the mid-term or long-term future" (Business Dictionary, 2014).

- DNP graduates may develop their own vision statement when they graduate to guide them toward their long-term goals.

- The Diffusion of Innovations Theory is "an information-seeking and information-processing activity, where an individual is motivated to reduce uncertainty about the advantages and disadvantages of an innovation (Rogers, 2003, p. 172).

- The Four Ps, a marketing strategy, are product, price, place, and promotion (Haim, 2005; Landrum, 1998).

- Beals (2008) describes the eight rules of self-marketing as positive thinking, developing an expertise, being prepared, having the right attitude, counting everyone, realizing you are being watched, embracing professionalism, and communicating clearly.
- An elevator pitch is a brief introduction that takes 60 seconds or less to introduce yourself and explain why you are unique and what your expertise is.
- When talking with many different professionals at a networking event, a good rule of thumb is to be courteous, respectful, and considerate of others' feelings.
- DNP graduates should become active speakers in various settings as part of self-marketing.
- Healthcare policy defines many aspects of advanced-practice nursing, and DNP graduates are charged to become involved in healthcare policy as part of their marketing strategy.
- DNP graduates may have already developed various marketing tools to promote their practice, academic appointment, or position within an organization. When a DNP graduate returns to the workplace or applies for a new position, these tools (business cards, pamphlets, stationery, website) should be adapted to include the DNP degree.
- DNP graduates should embrace opportunities in the media to promote their specific practices, specialties, and expertise as well as the DNP degree.

REFLECTION QUESTIONS

1. What marketing strategies or tools have you used to market yourself?

2. Do you feel it is important for DNP graduates to market themselves differently after graduating with a DNP degree?

3. What will your mission statement be after graduation?

4. What will your vision statement be after graduation?

5. How do you think Dr. Rogers's Diffusion of Innovations Theory applies to the momentum of the DNP degree?

6. Do you agree with Beals's eight rules of self-marketing? How would you apply these rules to marketing yourself after you graduate with a DNP degree?

7. What is your elevator pitch going to be?

8. Do you agree that involvement in healthcare policy is important to marketing the DNP degree?

9. What types of marketing strategies or tools will you use after graduating with a DNP degree?

10. Are you comfortable exploring media opportunities to promote yourself and the DNP degree? If not, how may you better prepare for these opportunities?

REFERENCES

American Association of Colleges of Nursing. (2006). *Essentials of doctoral education for advanced nursing practice*. Retrieved from http://www.aacn.nche.edu/publications/position/DNPEssentials.pdf

American Association of Colleges of Nursing. (2014a). *DNP fact sheet*. Retrieved from http://www.aacn.nche.edu/media-relations/fact-sheets/dnp

American Association of Colleges of Nursing. (2014b). Program directory. Retrieved from http://www.aacn.nche.edu/dnp/program-schools

American Marketing Association. (2011). Dictionary. Retrieved from http://www.marketing-power.com/_layouts/Dictionary.aspx?dLetter=M

Beals, J. (2008). *Self marketing power: Branding yourself as a business of one*. Omaha, NE: Keynote.

Business Dictionary. (2014). Vision statement. Retrieved from http://www.businessdictionary.com/definition/vision-statement.html

Dayhoff, N. E., & Moore, P. S. (2004). CNS entrepreneurship: Marketing 101. *Clinical Nurse Specialist, 18*(3), 123–125.

Entrepreneur. (2014). Mission statement. Retrieved from http://www.entrepreneur.com/encyclopedia/mission-statement

Haim, A. (2005). *Marketing kit for dummies* (2nd ed.). Indianapolis, IN: Wiley.

Hall, R. A. (2000). Marketing nurse practitioners is the key to lobbying. *Journal of Pediatric Health Care, 14*(6), 321–323.

Jacobs, T. (2003, October). The essence of ICE: Impress, connect, engage (manage the media). Program and abstracts of the National Association of Nurse Practitioners in Women's Health, Savannah, GA.

Kenig, S. M. (2004). Impress, connect, engage: A media expert's guide for nurse practitioners. Retrieved from http://www.medscape.org/viewarticle/465855

Landrum, B. (1998). Marketing innovations to nurses, part 2: Marketing's role in the adoptions of innovations. *Journal of Wound, Ostomy and Continence Nursing, 25*(5), 227–232.

Mackey, T. A., & Estala, S. (2008). Marketing your nurse-managed practice: Become a "marketpreneur." *Clinical Scholars Review, 1*(1), 13–17.

Orr, G. (2003). *Diffusion of innovations*, by Everett Rogers (1995) [Review]. Retrieved from http://www.stanford.edu/class/symbsys205/Diffusion%20of%20Innovations.htm

Pagana, K. D. (2008). *The nurse's etiquette advantage*. Indianapolis, IN: Sigma Theta Tau International.

Putnam, A. O. (1990). *Marketing your services*. New York, NY: Wiley.

Rogers, E. M. (2003). *Diffusion of innovations* (5th ed.). New York, NY: Free Press.

CHAPTER 14

Where Do We Go from Here?
The Future of the DNP Degree

Lisa Astalos Chism

The rapid evolution toward a practice doctorate in nursing has truly been astonishing. Initially this evolution was met with much debate in the literature. Early discussions seemed to focus on the advantages and disadvantages of a practice doctorate in nursing. Later discussions reflected the accelerated growth of doctor of nursing practice (DNP) degree programs across the country and implications of the DNP degree. The impact of the DNP degree on the future of nursing education remains to be seen; however, one can speculate that as a practice doctorate becomes accepted as the terminal degree in nursing practice, the profession of nursing is likely to benefit from the increased standards of educational preparation and the recognition of nursing's expertise in healthcare delivery.

A discussion of the debate regarding the DNP degree provides interesting dialogue when considering the future of nursing education. Therefore, highlights of this debate are reviewed in this chapter. The future of the DNP degree is influenced by the growth of the DNP degree, faculty availability, program development, and student enrollment. Additional factors influencing the future of the DNP degree, such as nurse residencies and an update from the American Association of Colleges of Nursing (AACN), are also discussed. The current literature about DNP education and recommendations for the next steps regarding the DNP degree are also reviewed. Finally, it is proposed that DNP graduates will shape the future by meeting societal needs. This chapter concludes with comments regarding the role DNP graduates will fulfill in meeting the societal needs evident within this challenging healthcare environment.

Nursing's Debate Regarding the DNP Degree

Early publications regarding the DNP degree reflect the position that it was largely unknown whether a practice doctorate in nursing would be accepted. A practice doctorate in nursing was mentioned in the 1970s (Newman, 1975), but earlier attempts to implement such a degree failed. A review of early arguments related to the DNP degree may provide insights regarding why a practice degree in nursing seems to have finally taken root. The current literature related to the role of the DNP graduate in research is also reviewed to provide insight regarding more recent dialogue related to the DNP degree.

An editorial by Dracup and Bryan-Brown (2005), with a response from Burman, Hart, and McCabe (2005), pointedly illustrated key early issues and rebuttal regarding the DNP degree. Dracup and Bryan-Brown's article, titled "Doctor of Nursing Practice—MRI or Total Body Scan?," has been cited numerous times in arguments against the DNP degree. Dracup and Bryan-Brown discussed the following key issues:

- "A new nursing degree will add to the public's confusion about educational requirements in nursing" (2005, p. 279).
- Practice doctorates "will threaten the already tenuous supply of nurses who pursue a PhD" (2005, p. 279).
- The DNP degree will "enlarge the gap that already exists between academic and clinical nursing and increase discord within the profession" (2005, p. 280).

This editorial presented an opportunity for Burman and colleagues (2005) to respond with these counterpoints:

- The DNP degree will not enlarge the gap that exists between academic and clinical nursing but will instead do the opposite. In fact, this degree will "bridge the practice–research chasm that has haunted nurses professionally" (2005, p. 463). Further, this degree may "bring together the spectral ends of the continuum of professional life: The academician researcher and the clinician" (2005, p. 463).
- The DNP degree will not force nurses to choose between a research doctorate and a practice doctorate. This choice already occurs frequently, and claims that this will worsen with a practice doctorate are unsubstantiated. "Nurse educators should be able to be clinicians, at the highest degreed level, with or without a mantle of research layered over their shoulders" (2005, p. 463).
- "The DNP gives nursing the opportunity to reconceptualize what advanced practice nursing is and should be to develop the core sciences of true advanced nursing practice" (2005, p. 464).

Sperhac and Clinton (2004) thoroughly presented some of the pertinent challenges and advantages related to the DNP degree. One challenge noted was the dissemination of accurate information about the DNP degree and entry into practice.

Currently the master's degree is still required for entry into practice for advanced-practice registered nurses (APRNs). However, the DNP degree has sparked concern among APRNs regarding eligibility to practice. If and when the DNP degree is mandated for entry into practice, individual state boards will have to reflect these standards (Sperhac & Clinton, 2004).

Another challenge presented by Sperhac and Clinton (2004) is the confusion regarding titles. The nursing doctorate (ND), doctor of nursing science (DNS and DNSc), and doctor of nursing practice (DrNP and DNP) degrees have all been referred to as practice doctorates in the past. However, the AACN has recommended that one title, doctor of nursing practice, be used (AACN, 2006a). Further, the ND will be phased out. In the future, two degrees will represent the highest level of education in nursing: the DNP and the PhD (Sperhac & Clinton, 2004).

The question of higher compensation for additional education was also presented by Sperhac and Clinton. Although patient outcomes have been shown to improve with care provided by APRNs, increased compensation should not be an expectation of those seeking a DNP degree. Rather, "market forces shall prevail and incomes may be commensurate with demographic characteristics, geographic areas, and the rules of supply and demand" (Sperhac & Clinton, 2004, p. 292).

An advantage of the DNP degree was presented as increased educational preparation that will meet the needs of a complex healthcare environment, which requires a knowledge base that integrates a growing set of skills and level of expertise. Most master's degree programs that prepare APRNs are increasing in length to meet these needs. Many master's degrees in nursing are frequently found to be lengthier than practice doctorates in many other fields, such as pharmacy, audiology, and physical therapy (Sperhac & Clinton, 2004). The DNP degree accommodates the increased preparation required to meet the demands of a complex healthcare system and provides nursing with parity among other healthcare professionals (Sperhac & Clinton, 2004).

Finally, Sperhac and Clinton suggest that increasing educational preparation of APRNs to the doctorate level will convey a level of competence to legislators and facilitate increased scope of practice and privileges. "The public, legislators, and other stakeholders understand the significance of a doctorate and what this represents in other disciplines" (Sperhac & Clinton, 2004, p. 293). It is therefore speculated that a practice doctorate will increase parity with other disciplines with regard to legislative regulations. To date, however, the DNP degree has not changed the scope of practice of APRNs on a federal or state level.

Chase and Pruitt discussed the DNP movement as "innovation or disruption" and asked the question, "Does the DNP movement provide an innovation that solves a problem of complexity by providing a simpler solution to problems or does it add increasing complexity and enhance the position of key stakeholders?" (2006, p. 156). In an attempt to answer this question, the authors posited several issues related to the adoption of the DNP degree.

First, the point was made that the nursing professoriate has finally achieved senior ranks in academia at leading universities. The AACN has stated that additional education is needed for DNP graduates to pursue roles in education. Chase and Pruitt asserted that "by preparing graduates whose credentials will not prepare them for full preparation in the academic community, the DNP degree disrupts the flow of graduates to a single terminal degree" (2006, p. 157).

Chase and Pruitt (2006) also related concerns regarding titling and licensure. It was noted that although the DNP is an academic degree, it remains unclear how certifying bodies will credential DNP graduates. The point was also made that if there is no change in the scope of practice of DNP graduates, how will health care delivered by DNP graduates differ from that delivered by APRNs without a DNP degree (Chase & Pruitt, 2006)?

Issues related to curriculum development were also described by Chase and Pruitt (2006). The lack of course work devoted to the development of the nursing discipline was mentioned as a concern. The variance that exists among current DNP degree curricula and outcomes was noted by these authors. Finally, a concern regarding the addition of nurse residency programs to the DNP degree course work was raised. "The idea that a doctoral program would have a training mentality with a residency attached does not move doctoral education forward; it looks backward and borrows from other professions" (2006, p. 159).

Hathaway, Jacob, Stegbauer, Thompson, and Graff (2006) specifically addressed Chase and Pruitt's (2006) concerns. They explained that the practice doctorate in nursing is both innovation and disruption, not one or the other. It was noted that the movement of the DNP degree is "predictable" given that "DNP programs enable nurses to move competently upmarket in today's complex practice environment" (Hathaway et al., 2006, p. 488) in an effort to fulfill unmet needs of a changing market. Further, Hathaway and colleagues purport that any change causes disruption, but that should not prevent innovation from occurring. Moreover, it will undeniably take time to validate the contributions of DNP graduates to health care. Hathaway and colleagues further asserted that "society must recognize that world changing innovations cannot always be built around quantitative science" (2006, p. 488).

The number of nurses pursuing doctoral study has been an issue for nursing. With the adoption of the DNP degree, there has been an increase in the number of nurses returning to school for doctoral work. Hathaway and colleagues (2006) pointed out that this includes PhD enrollment as well. Nurses enrolled in doctoral programs have increased the number of nurses discussing doctoral study, which has increased the number of nurses pursuing PhD degrees (Hathaway et al., 2006). The increased number of nurses pursuing doctoral degrees is fulfilling a previously unmet need and is therefore an advantage of the DNP degree.

Chase and Pruitt criticized the addition of a practice doctorate in nursing by stating, "To now support a degree that allows graduates to be recognized as doctoral prepared when the same level of rigor in their preparation has not been required risks dismantling the hard work of doctoral educators over the past 50 years" (2006, p. 159). Hathaway and colleagues responded to this criticism by stating, "This claim discredits all individuals who hold professional degrees" (2006, p. 490). Hathaway and colleagues further asserted that "the discipline of nursing, like other health science disciplines needs both research scientists and practice-scientists" (2006, p. 490). Additionally, the DNP degree fosters the theory–research–practice feedback loop, which has been a goal of nursing for years (Hathaway et al., 2006). Moreover, nursing science will advance more rapidly to continue to build the discipline of nursing by having experts in both the research and practice realms (Hathaway et al., 2006).

More recent literature discussed concerns regarding DNP graduates and research. Florczak (2011) published an essay related to the DNP graduate conducting research. This essay described the concerns of a PhD-prepared nurse referred to as Katie. Katie appeared disturbed by the idea of DNP graduates and PhD-prepared nurses working together and voiced concerns about being in a consultant role to the DNP graduate. Further, Florczak related that "Katie's anxiety began to intensify as she read some of the studies conducted by nurses without research experience" (2011, p. 17).

Katie seemed threatened by the DNP graduate, yet the literature clearly states that a partnership should exist between PhD-prepared nurses and DNP graduates. Edwardson (2010) related that PhD-prepared researchers and DNP graduates should work interdependently, each drawing from the other's expertise. "Rather than obsessing about the relative proportion of PhD faculty members, the more cogent issue may be how can the practice expertise of the DNP faculty complement and supplement the research and scholarship of the PhD prepared faculty" (2010, p. 138).

Others also related that PhD researchers and DNP graduates should complement one another when engaged in research endeavors. Vincent, Johnson, Velasquez, and Rigney related that "as practitioner-researchers, DNP prepared nurses are uniquely qualified to reduce the research-to-practice gap" (2010, p. 28). These authors also stated that "DNP prepared nurses transform knowledge generated in research into feasible studies and application" (2010, p. 30).

Conclusion

A review of the arguments related to the DNP degree provides insights regarding the issues that have shaped the progression of this innovative degree. Interestingly, it seems that each time a concern related to the adoption of a practice doctorate was argued, a thoughtful and valid response was formulated. Newer concerns related to the role of the DNP graduate's role in research also seem unfounded because PhD and DNP graduates have been found to complement each other. Issues related to the DNP degree will likely continue to provide interesting debate in the future literature.

The Future of the DNP Degree

The future of the DNP degree may be influenced by various factors such as the growth of DNP programs, faculty availability, program development, and student enrollment. These factors are fluid and continue to shift as the momentum of this degree continues. The current literature regarding areas of consensus and controversy regarding the DNP degree is reviewed in this section, along with future developments such as nurse residencies and an update from the AACN.

The Growth of DNP Programs

It seems that the number of DNP programs continues to grow at an astounding rate. The AACN maintains a frequently updated list of all approved DNP programs across the country (AACN, 2014c). It reflects new programs and developing programs. At the time of this writing, 241 DNP programs are currently enrolling students at schools of nursing nationwide, and an additional 59 DNP programs are in the planning stages (AACN, 2014a). Programs will vary in their clinical content; however, the AACN *Essentials of Doctoral Education for Advanced Nursing Practice* (AACN, 2006b) should be used as a guide for program content. Prospective students are encouraged to research DNP degree programs when deciding which one most accurately fulfills their needs. Additionally, prospective students will be able to assess specific program curricula by visiting the website of each school's DNP program (AACN, 2014c).

Faculty Availability

Although DNP programs seem to be abundant, the incredible growth of this degree may present new issues related to faculty availability. This has been a pervasive problem for schools of nursing and is a valid concern. The AACN reported that schools of nursing turned away 79,659 applicants across the country in 2012 (AACN, 2014b). The reasons cited include insufficient numbers of faculty, insufficient numbers of clinical sites, limited classroom space, limited preceptors, and budget constraints (AACN, 2014b). Additionally, a survey reported by the AACN in 2013 noted that out of 680 schools of nursing, there were more than 1,358 vacancies for faculty positions (AACN, 2014b). In addition, a large number of current faculty members are considering retirement. It was projected that between 200 and 300 doctorally prepared faculty will be eligible for retirement each year from 2003 through 2012, and between 220 and 280 master's-prepared nurse faculty will be eligible for retirement from 2012 through 2018 (AACN, 2014b). Ideally, the influx of new DNP graduates will help meet the need for clinical faculty positions. Who better to teach nursing than those who are currently practicing? Nursing is a practice discipline, and although a need will always exist for nursing scientists to broaden the nursing knowledge base, expert clinicians clearly have a role in nursing education.

The development of numerous DNP programs across the country presents a similar dilemma: As these new programs are developed, who will educate DNP students? Should DNP graduates teach future DNP graduates? This notion may require paradigm shifts for both universities and nursing faculties. Acceptance of nursing faculty members with practice-focused doctorates has been varied. Until parity between the two doctorates (PhD and DNP) is established, this will continue to be a controversial concern among universities and nursing faculty. While this particular paradigm shift evolves, DNP graduates can shape the future by continuing to combine nursing scholarship and practice.

Program Development

DNP curricula are guided by the *Essentials of Doctoral Education for Advanced Nursing Practice* outlined by the AACN (2006b). In an effort to decrease ambiguity regarding nurse practitioner curriculum development, the National Organization of Nurse Practitioner Faculties (NONPF) has designed curriculum templates for DNP programs to help guide course development (2013). The National Association of Clinical Nurse Specialists has developed *Core Practice Doctorate Clinical Nurse Specialist Competencies* that may also help guide curriculum development for CNS-focused DNP programs (2009).

It is important to note that although there may be variations among programs with regard to length, clinical components, and course structure, the content and length of programs should be somewhat unified for DNP programs to establish credibility. Moreover, a concern has been noted that programs may become too research intensive, which would result in the DNP degree becoming more similar to a PhD degree, much like what happened to the DNS degree. DNP program lengths should also remain unified. Current master's degree programs in nursing have traditionally become longer with regard to credit hours. DNP programs should maintain consistency regarding credit hours and length. This will also increase the likelihood that the content of DNP programs is consistent. Program development was also addressed during the Committee on Institutional Cooperation's (CIC) Dean's Conference on the Doctor of Nursing Practice and during the AACN summer board meeting in 2013. A summary of the CIC dean's conference and the AACN board recommendations regarding the DNP will be discussed in the AACN update section of this chapter.

Student Enrollment

Student recruitment does not seem to be an issue thus far; however, this author has noted that many APRNs are still cautious about the DNP degree. Through a professional online blog that specifically addressed concerns related to the DNP degree (Advance Healthcare Network for NPs and PAs, 2014), this author noted that APRNs are concerned about the time commitment, cost, and marketability of a DNP degree. Many APRNs who inquired about the DNP degree expressed a lack of understanding about how the DNP degree will improve their practice.

Despite the concerns, current enrollment has continued to increase. From 2012 to 2013 the number of students enrolled in DNP programs increased from 11,575 to 14,699. During that same time period, the number of DNP graduates increased from 1,858 to 2,443 (AACN, 2014a). In addition, the AACN fall 2013 survey found that DNP enrollment was up 21.6% from 2012 to 2013. The DNP graduates who were interviewed for this book shared that their motivation for returning to school was to pursue a practice-focused doctorate and to develop expertise in leadership, evidence-based practice, policy, and population health. Nursing had been discussing a practice-focused doctorate for decades. Many DNP graduates and prospective students expressed to this author that they had been waiting for a practice-focused doctorate to meet their practice needs and professional goals. The practice-focused doctorate seems to have filled a niche within nursing, especially among APRNs who aspire to pursue additional educational preparation but also wish to maintain a practice-oriented career.

The success, productivity, and enthusiasm of current DNP graduates will also help to determine whether others continue to pursue this degree. It is imperative that DNP graduates publish their doctoral work after graduation to share their contributions to nursing from a practice-oriented perspective. It is also important that DNP graduates continue to stay involved in nursing scholarship by maintaining interests in clinical research projects and pursuing leadership and educational opportunities (formal or informal). The enthusiasm regarding a practice-focused doctorate seems to have grown over the past decade. This will also contribute to the momentum of future enrollment in DNP programs. DNP graduates should continue to be proactive about their degree by maintaining their enthusiasm and contributions to the nursing profession and society.

A Word About Nurse Residencies

Many DNP programs offer a residency, or clinical experience, within their programs. NONPF addressed the number of clinical hours required in DNP programs and for postmaster's and postbachelor's degrees. The organization published a document titled *Clinical Education Issues in Preparing Nurse Practitioner Students for Independent Practice: An Ongoing Series of Papers* (2010). NONPF has recommended a minimum of 500 hours post-BSN for nurse practitioner students. However, it is acknowledged that additional clinical hours will be required to achieve the DNP competencies outlined by NONPF. Therefore, many DNP programs have integrated residencies or role-immersion experiences that focus specifically on the skills outlined in the NONPF competencies and the AACN essentials. Clinton and

Sperhac related that "generally these residencies provide the student with a mentored experience that is intended to assist them in acquiring the DNP competencies" (2009, p. 349). To review each program's requirements for residencies or clinical hours, prospective students may go to the AACN DNP program list and click the school name to visit the website of each DNP program (AACN, 2014c).

An Update from the AACN

In 2010 the AACN published *The Doctor of Nursing Practice: A Report on Progress*. This report confirmed that 2015 is the target date for adoption of the DNP degree as entry into advanced nursing practice. It was also acknowledged that great progress toward the 2015 goal had been made, with significant program growth and student enrollment.

Since the publication of this report, the CIC Dean's Conference on the Doctor of Nursing Practice convened in August 2013 to review the developmental status of this degree (AACN, 2014d; Grey, 2013). Areas of consensus and controversy were identified. Consensus was noted regarding significant interest in the DNP degree. Another area of consensus included the intent of the DNP degree to expand the role of APRNs (Grey, 2013). Areas of controversy were varied but seemed to focus on what the DNP end product is. For example, controversy existed regarding the focus of DNP programs and whether they are preparing nurses as leaders or APRNs (Grey, 2013). Controversy also surrounded inconsistencies in content and clinical hours or residencies across DNP programs. Capstone projects were also found to be controversial with various experiences and projects among programs (Grey, 2013). Finally, controversy was noted regarding the outcomes of DNP programs. Specifically, many DNP graduates have moved into administrative or education roles. This poses the question of whether the original goals of the DNP degree are being attained (Grey, 2013).

As a follow-up to the CIC dean's conference, the AACN decided that more dialogue was needed, so it developed the DNP Summit, which was held in April 2014. The purpose of the summit was to explore program plans of study, clinical practicums, scholarly projects, outcomes of DNP programs, and revisions of the essentials document (AACN, 2014d). Areas of agreement were consistent with the CIC dean's conference and included the importance of the DNP degree to the advancement of the discipline. It was also agreed that the DNP is intended to enhance advanced-practice roles and prepare experts in population-based practice, leadership, and policy (AACN, 2014d). Regarding the AACN essentials, it was recommended that they be maintained and expanded. For example, it was recommended that Essential IV include self-care management (e.g., telehealth and web-based apps). Additionally, it was recommended that Essential VII include the roles of nurse executive, community health, and others (AACN, 2014d).

As a result of the DNP Summit, a task force was formed regarding the implementation of the DNP degree (AACN, 2014d). The intent of this task force is to formulate a white paper to clarify expectations of the DNP scholarly project and practice requirements of the DNP degree. Specifically, the task force is charged with the following:

1. Describing the current state of DNP scholarly products, challenges, and variability among program requirements.

2. Defining resources needed to support development of quality DNP products, including mentorship, oversight, access to data, and practice sites.

3. Designing recommendations for scholarship of DNP graduates and how this translates into program expectations.

4. Identifying the term to be used for the final DNP scholarly product.

5. Developing a set of recommendations and exemplars for DNP scholarly products, e.g., single project, group project, portfolio, or a series of products.

6. Evaluating the current landscape regarding program length; and clarifying or reaffirming the DNP Essentials statements regarding program duration for post-baccalaureate and post-master's DNP programs.

7. Examining the current challenges for meeting DNP practice hour requirements.

8. Clarifying the purpose or intent of the DNP practice requirements in preparing graduates for an area of advanced nursing practice.

9. Constructing the nature of the collaborative relationship that should be established to facilitate the development of DNP students, including DNP practice expectations for the schools, practice partners, and mentors.

10. Formulating recommendations for integrative and collaborative DNP practice experiences that meet the DNP Essentials.

11. Highlighting exemplary opportunities and innovations for intra (DNP and PhD) and inter-professional learning and practice. (AACN, 2014d)

The task force convened in January 2014 and plans to present its findings to the AACN in June 2015.

The DNP Degree and Societal Needs

Societal needs have historically affected the development of healthcare innovations. The nurse practitioner movement in the 1970s occurred as a result of societal needs for more primary care providers, especially in underserved, impoverished areas. Although this movement was initially met with opposition, nurse practitioners have consistently proven to be high-quality healthcare providers (Mundinger et al., 2000).

The DNP movement may be compared to the nurse practitioner movement in that societal needs were noted, and nursing responded by increasing "nursing's capacity to lead and improve the health of the nation" (Brown et al., 2006, p. 132). The Institute of Medicine (IOM) has recommended that healthcare professionals' educational preparation focus on specific needs in health care, such as expertise in leadership, information technology, interprofessional collaboration, and evidence-based practice (Greiner & Knebel, 2003; IOM, 2010). The AACN *Essentials of Doctoral Education for Advanced Nursing Practice* (2006b), which guides the curriculum of DNP programs, specifically addresses these topics. Additionally, a complex and chronically ill population has driven the need for increased preparation of healthcare professionals. Caring for this type of population requires expert healthcare providers who can "work across disciplines, mobilize resources, and coordinate care interventions" (Brown et al., 2006, p. 132).

Societal needs also require that healthcare professionals develop an awareness of the disparities that exist in health care today. DNP programs "will enable graduates to apply a social justice framework to guide leadership efforts in multiple arenas" (Brown et al., 2006, p. 132) and address the unique needs associated with healthcare disparities. DNP graduates' "enhanced ability to integrate multicultural awareness and knowledge into their healthcare practices and programs will encourage them to challenge social, cultural, economic and political inequities as major determinants of health" (Brown et al., 2006, p. 132). Caring for individuals and communities with health disparities continues to be a prominent and growing need in health care and society. DNP graduates have an opportunity to improve the care of these populations through expertise in leadership, the development of health policies, and the use of evidence-based practice measures to design healthcare delivery specific to these populations' needs.

Over the past several decades, societal needs have influenced the necessity for nursing to deliver safe, effective, high-quality health care. It is therefore prudent to reflect on nursing's social policy statement, which describes the goals and purpose of nursing in relation to societal needs. The practice of nursing is "based on a social contract that acknowledges professional rights and responsibilities as well as mechanisms for public accountability" (American Nurses Association [ANA], 1995, p. 3). Further, "professional nursing's scope of practice is dynamic and continually evolving, characterized by a flexible boundary responsive to the changing needs of society and the expanding knowledge base of applicable theoretical and scientific domains" (ANA, 2010, pp. 16–17). Through the knowledge and expertise garnered in a DNP program, graduates expand their knowledge base to meet the changing needs of society. DNP graduates' preparation enables them to utilize information technologies, provide evidence-based practice, develop healthcare policies, and provide leadership in an effort to meet the societal needs of a multicultural, complex healthcare environment. Whether fulfilling roles as leaders, clinicians, researchers, healthcare policy advocates, educators, or an integration of these roles, DNP graduates are on the cutting edge of shaping the future of healthcare delivery.

Interview with an Innovative DNP Program Director: Then and Now

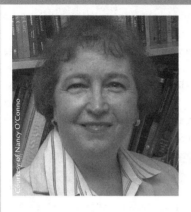

Nancy O'Connor, PhD, APRN, BC, is professor and chair of Nursing Graduate Programs and director of the Nurse Practitioner Program at Madonna University in Livonia, Michigan.

THEN . . . 2008

Dr. O'Connor, could you please describe your nursing background, including your current position?

I graduated from Henry Ford Hospital's School of Nursing diploma program in Detroit, Michigan, in 1974. My first nursing position was in the coronary care unit. I had an interest in developing long-term relationships with patients, so I pursued a position in cardiac rehab. This allowed me to see patients over time and become more involved in health prevention. I completed my bachelor's degree at Madonna University in Livonia, Michigan, which proved to be a wonderful experience. I received credit for my previous experience as an RN and was able to build on this foundation. I then began a master's in nursing program at Wayne State University in Detroit, Michigan. At that time, the program was a health nurse clinician program, which led me to become a nurse practitioner. I graduated with an MSN [master's of science in nursing] from Wayne State University in 1980. During my master's program, I approached the director of the program and suggested that due to the length and intensity of the program (52 credits), it should actually be a clinical doctorate program. Even then I felt that the current master's degrees in nursing were beyond the scope of other master's degrees because of the theoretic and clinical content required to fulfill the role of a nurse practitioner.

I then pursued a career as an adult primary care nurse practitioner and held various positions, including working on a grant-funded project as an NP [nurse practitioner] in chronic disease care, and eventually ran three outpatient NP clinics in Detroit, Michigan. This led me back to Wayne State University, where I began teaching in a nurse practitioner program. I was able to combine teaching and practice in a primary care nursing services program at Detroit Receiving Hospital in a joint practice–faculty appointment. Eventually, my interest in teaching led me to pursue graduate school once again, and I began doctoral study at Wayne State University in 1989.

During my doctoral study I became interested in exploring what made NP practice unique and why NPs made such a difference in health care. I developed a theory inductively through my practice experiences, which is linked to Orem's self-care deficit theory. My theory focused on self-care enhancement strategies for patients. While attempting to develop this theory, I independently studied qualitative research methods but found that the intensive research focus took me further away from patient care. While pursuing my doctorate in nursing at Wayne State University, I also taught in an adult health nurse practitioner program at Oakland University in Rochester, Michigan.

I graduated in 1995 with a PhD in nursing and was faced with a common dilemma: I felt I could not adequately balance teaching, research, and practice while attending to all three in an ethical way. Because of my strong desire to teach, I accepted a faculty position at Madonna University in 2000. I helped to develop additional NP programs at Madonna and became the chair of Nursing Graduate Programs and program director of Nurse Practitioner Programs. Since I joined as NP program director, we have added the acute care nurse practitioner track and the palliative care nurse practitioner track. I am also very excited that in May 2009 we will be starting our new doctor of nursing practice program. This is the first doctoral program in any field here at Madonna. We were officially approved last March by the North Central Higher Learning Commission and became an accredited program. Eventually, we will be phasing out the nurse practitioner master's degree programs, and the program will be offered as a postbaccalaureate degree.

Dr. O'Connor, could you please share how you think nursing education has evolved over the years?

We are getting better about responding to the needs nursing can fill and also getting more realistic about meeting those needs. This is evidenced by the second-degree nursing programs; we are capturing those interested in nursing with a former skill set and still able to bring them into nursing. On a graduate level, we have done well with our master's degrees in nursing. We have created a generation of highly educated, master's-prepared nurses who are doing amazing things in health care. These individuals are the folks who will return to graduate school for a DNP degree. These nurses will want the additional skill set the DNP offers: additional knowledge in applied research and leadership. These nurses will also want recognition for their level of education and expertise in healthcare delivery. We have sensibly created a degree that is doable and value added to the experience master's-prepared nurses already have. Madonna's DNP program is innovative in that each student will have the opportunity to pursue his or her degree in an individualized way. Also, students will have the opportunity to work interprofessionally with others, such as physical therapy students, occupational therapy students, and pharmacy students. With the experiences of learning together with other professionals, the DNP graduate is poised to lead and become more system savvy. We hope to promote more PhD–DNP relationships as well through our program. This way, more research in nursing will get done by the PhDs and DNPs working in teams. This seems to be the perfect model.

I also feel that the AACN made a powerful decision with the DNP target date of 2015. By taking a stand, the AACN has empowered nursing to move forward. We may not have solved all of the problems related to entry into practice, but at least we can move forward with the DNP degree. Nurses are responding to this empowerment by applying and graduating from DNP programs across the country.

Dr. O'Connor, what do you think was the impetus for the development of the DNP degree?

The need for a practice-based terminal degree in nursing compared to having only a research-based terminal degree. Both degrees are needed for nursing to be full spectrum.

Dr. O'Connor, could you please describe why Madonna University's School of Nursing has adopted a DNP program?

We wanted to remain on the cutting edge of graduate education in nursing. We have established a program of excellent nurse practitioner faculty as well as faculty for nursing administration. This represents a certain depth and skill set of healthcare expertise. It is exciting to offer a program so closely integrated in practice. We also want to be on the forefront of the theory–practice interface. The DNP program is aligned with Madonna's mission to provide a practical, yet doctoral-level degree to serve the vulnerable and underserved populations in health care.

Dr. O'Connor, could you please describe the process involved in developing a new DNP program at Madonna University?

First, a task force was formed within the school of nursing faculty. We spent about a year and a half developing the curriculum, attending conferences relate[d] to the DNP degree, and meeting with others who were developing a DNP degree program. The program had to be approved by Madonna's governance process, college university board of trustees, and finally the North Central Higher Learning Commission. This process was completed in March 2008.

Dr. O'Connor, what were some of the challenges you experienced regarding the adoption and development of a DNP program at Madonna University?

People questioned whether nurses should be encouraged to get a DNP degree when we currently need more BSN-prepared nurses at the bedside, especially with the shortage of nursing faculty. Some felt that this was a misguided use of resources. However, most have moved forward in their thinking. People realized that you can't just offer nurses a BSN without career mobility as an option. It's not about an either/or option; nurses are needed at all levels. We reviewed our resources (faculty and library) and made sure we had the infrastructure to support doctoral study.

Dr. O'Connor, what are some of the benefits of developing a DNP degree at Madonna University?

It has been exciting work and a great teamwork opportunity for all of us. We wouldn't have followed the DNP movement so closely if we weren't developing a DNP program. Also, the DNP program offers the university recognition through the addition of the first doctoral program at Madonna University. This program also enabled us to educate our professional colleagues about what nursing is doing at all levels. Others now know about the capabilities and possibilities of nursing.

Dr. O'Connor, what do you think are the future challenges related to the adoption of multiple DNP programs across the country?

Mostly faculty shortages and the right mix of faculty. We will need enough PhD and DNP faculty to really teach at all levels. At Madonna, we are attempting to solve this resource problem by collaborating with other universities to share faculty. This will also ensure that DNP students have exposure to a wide variety of faculty. We are also providing students with a role immersion experience where they participate in a practicum experience within a healthcare system. This will bring DNP students close to the healthcare system as well as provide mentorships through leadership and policy experience. A practicum experience will also teach DNP students how to work in teams.

Dr. O'Connor, how do you think the DNP degree will affect nursing education?

It will drastically increase the number of nurses holding doctorates. It will also increase the number of PhD and DNP graduates as a result of clarifying career paths.

The DNP degree will also strengthen undergraduate nursing education. We will have access to more clinical faculty who are teaching at the undergraduate and graduate levels. The quality of teaching will escalate, and the gap between education and practice will close.

NOW . . .2014

Dr. O'Connor, we discussed your nursing background and education last time we spoke. Could you describe your current position and any additional interests you have?

I am currently a professor and chair of the nursing graduate program and director of the postmaster's DNP program at Madonna University. I am also a certified adult nurse practitioner.

Dr. O'Connor, as a DNP program director, could you describe the current state of the DNP program at Madonna University?

The postmaster's DNP program at Madonna admitted our first cohort of students in 2009, and graduated our first class in 2011. We are currently admitting our sixth cohort of postmaster's DNP students. We are in the early stages of planning our post-BSN DNP curriculum. Our alumni are positioned in academic and healthcare systems and report a high degree of satisfaction with the professional development they have experienced since obtaining the DNP degree.

Dr. O'Connor, could you please describe your perception of the current progress of the DNP degree in general?

The increasing number of nurses enrolled in DNP programs nationally is encouraging as we attempt to meet the recommendations of The Future of Nursing *report (IOM, 2010) to double the number of nurses with doctoral preparation by 2020. The fact that so many nurses have embraced the practice doctorate bodes well for forging a clinically relevant and up-to-date nursing curriculum of the future. Many DNPs will contribute to educating nurses of the future, through academic appointments, practice leadership, or joint appointments.*

Dr. O'Connor, why do you think the momentum of enrollment to DNP programs has increased over time?

Many nurses are attracted to the professional discipline of nursing because of a desire to practice clinical nursing throughout their lives. The DNP, as a terminal practice degree, creates a pathway for career mobility, diversification, and expertise development for those whose hearts, hands, and minds are primarily oriented to the betterment of clinical nursing practice through direct or indirect means.

Dr. O'Connor, what are some of the current and new challenges you face as a DNP program director?

In offering our current postmaster's curriculum, it is has been a challenge to design a program of study that is compelling and meaningful for expert nurses who are returning to the classroom after a hiatus in their formal education. Teaching methods and program delivery models must match the learner; we have found that a hybrid executive model (online with three to four on-ground meetings per semester year round) works best with students who are working adults and who are also juggling other demands of adulthood.

Dr. O'Connor, do you have any comment regarding the AACN's development of a task force regarding the implementation of the DNP degree?

I had the opportunity to participate in the DNP National Summit in April 2013 that culminated in AACN's launch of the new task force on implementation of the DNP. The task force will reflect and take action on a number of pressing issues in DNP education that have emerged across our nearly 10-year history of offering this level of education in our profession. While there is a need to monitor trends and examine extreme inconsistencies in DNP program implementation, it is my hope that the task force will not recommend too many highly prescriptive measures for DNP programs. The possibility and promise of this degree has not been fully plumbed, particularly in relation to the place of practice theory and analytical methods in the curriculum; we would be well served to avoid premature closure on these issues. Too much structure in doctoral education, whether it be research or practice focused, can curtail creativity and growth.

Dr. O'Connor, the AACN recently identified inconsistencies regarding DNP program hours and residencies. Do you agree that there are inconsistencies? If so, how do you suggest this be addressed?

The AACN's requirement for 1,000 post-BSN practicum hours within DNP programs underscores the applied and integrative nature of DNP education. With a minimum of 500 hours in direct clinical practice being the typical requirement for national APRN certification bodies, this leaves other practicum hours that can be devoted to other DNP competencies for those pursuing APRN preparation at the DNP level. The AACN's 2013 task force on DNP program implementation may expand on this recommendation and generate some model ways of implementation within programs, including the potential for residency requirements. The residency concept has particular merit for post-BSN models of DNP education.

Dr. O'Connor, the AACN also recently identified inconsistencies regarding the DNP scholarly project. Do you agree that there are inconsistencies? If so, how do you suggest this be addressed?

I agree that there are inconsistencies in the final DNP scholarly projects across programs. Some programs rely heavily on these projects for integration of a number of DNP competencies, whereas others use them to meet fewer competencies. The DNP essentials document (AACN, 2006b) notes that the final scholarly project should reflect a synthesis of student learning within the program. Conceptualization of DNP scholarship within Boyer's (1990) model of scholarship is very helpful to continue to identify expected types of scholarship that will guide DNP scholarly projects.

Dr. O'Connor, what is your advice to nurses and potential students regarding the DNP degree?

The DNP degree is a practical, innovative, and timely nursing doctoral degree of the future that will help many nurses meet their career goals, advance the practice of nursing, and provide leadership for our ailing U.S. healthcare system. Enroll now!

SUMMARY

- Although the evolution of doctoral education in nursing to a practice-focused doctorate has been discussed since the 1970s, the adoption of the DNP degree has evolved over the past decade.
- Early discussions regarding a DNP degree seemed to focus on the advantages and disadvantages of a practice doctorate in nursing.
- Early arguments against the DNP degree included the following:
  - "A new nursing degree will add to the public's confusion about educational requirements in nursing" (Dracup & Bryan-Brown, 2005, p. 279).
  - Practice doctorates "will threaten the already tenuous supply of nurses who pursue a PhD" (Dracup & Bryan-Brown, 2005, p. 279).
  - The DNP degree will "enlarge the gap that already exists between academic and clinical nursing and increase discord within the profession" (Dracup & Bryan-Brown, 2005, p. 280).
- Accurate information about the DNP degree and entry into practice needs to be disseminated. Currently the master's degree is still required for entry into practice for APRNs. However, the DNP degree has sparked concern among APRNs regarding eligibility to practice (Sperhac & Clinton, 2004).
- There is confusion regarding titles. The ND, DNS, DrNP, DNP, and DNSc degrees have all been referred to as practice doctorates in the past (Sperhac & Clinton, 2004).
- Increasing educational preparation of APRNs to the doctorate level will convey competence to legislators and facilitate an increased scope of practice and privileges (Sperhac & Clinton, 2004).
- The nursing professoriate has finally achieved senior ranks in academia in leading universities. The AACN has stated that additional education is needed for DNP graduates to pursue roles in education (Chase & Pruitt, 2006).
- Chase and Pruitt (2006) related concerns regarding titling and licensure. It was noted that although the DNP is an academic degree, it remains unclear how certifying bodies will credential DNP graduates.
- The lack of course work devoted to the development of the discipline of nursing was noted to be a concern. The variance that exists among current DNP degree curricula and outcomes was also noted (Chase & Pruitt, 2006).
- Concerns regarding the addition of nurse residency programs to the DNP degree course work have been raised (Chase & Pruitt, 2006).
- Counterarguments for the DNP program were also noted in the literature:
  - The DNP degree will not enlarge the gap that exists between academic and clinical nursing but will instead do the opposite. In fact, this degree will "bridge the practice–research chasm that has haunted

nurses professionally" (Burman et al., 2005, p. 463). Further, this degree may "bring together the spectral ends of the continuum of professional life: The academician researcher and the clinician" (Burman et al., 2005, p. 463).

- The DNP degree will not force nurses to choose between a research doctorate and a practice doctorate. This choice already occurs frequently, and claims that this will worsen with a practice doctorate are unsubstantiated. "Nurse educators should be able to be clinicians, at the highest degreed level, with or without a mantle of research layered over their shoulders" (Burman et al., 2005, p. 463).

- "The DNP gives nursing the opportunity to reconceptualize what advanced practice nursing is and should be to develop the core sciences of true advanced nursing practice" (Burman et al., 2005, p. 464).

- Increased educational preparation will meet the needs of a complex healthcare environment. This complex healthcare environment requires a knowledge base that integrates a growing set of skills and level of expertise (Sperhac & Clinton, 2004).

- With the adoption of the DNP degree, there has been an increase in the number of nurses returning to school for doctoral work (Hathaway et al., 2006).

- The DNP degree fosters the theory–research–practice feedback loop, which has been a goal of nursing for years (Hathaway et al., 2006).

- The AACN maintains an updated program list of all approved DNP programs across the country (AACN, 2014c). This list continues to grow as new programs are developed. At the time of this writing, 153 programs existed, with 160 programs in development.

- Although variations may exist among programs with regard to length, clinical components, and course structure, the content and length of programs should be somewhat unified for DNP programs to establish credibility.

- In an effort to decrease ambiguity regarding curriculum development, NONPF has designed curriculum templates for DNP programs to help guide course development (2013).

- New DNP graduates will help meet the need for clinical faculty positions. However, this will require a paradigm shift among universities and nursing faculties.

- The success, productivity, and enthusiasm of current DNP graduates will also help to determine whether others continue to pursue this degree. It is imperative that DNP graduates publish their doctoral work after graduation to share their contributions to nursing from a practice-oriented perspective.

- It is acknowledged that additional clinical hours will be required to achieve the DNP competencies outlined by NONPF. Therefore, many DNP programs have integrated residencies or role-immersion experiences that focus specifically on the skills outlined by the NONPF competencies and the AACN essentials.

■ In 2010 the AACN published *The Doctor of Nursing Practice: A Report on Progress*. This report confirmed that 2015 is the target date for adoption of the DNP degree as entry into advanced nursing practice.

■ The CIC Dean's Conference on the Doctor of Nursing Practice convened in August 2013 to review the developmental status of this degree (AACN, 2014d; Grey, 2013). Areas of consensus and controversy were identified.

■ As a follow-up to the CIC dean's meeting, the AACN decided that more dialogue was needed, so it developed the DNP Summit, which was held in April 2014. The purpose of the summit was to explore program plans of study, clinical practicums, scholarly projects, outcomes of DNP programs, and revisions of the essentials document (AACN, 2014d).

■ As a result of the DNP Summit, a task force was formed regarding the implementation of the DNP degree (AACN, 2014d). The intent of this task force is to formulate a white paper to clarify expectations of the DNP scholarly project and practice requirements of the DNP degree.

■ The DNP degree enables nursing to continue to serve societal needs, such as caring for chronically ill, complex populations and persons with health disparities.

■ The practice of nursing is "based on a social contract that acknowledges professional rights and responsibilities as well as mechanisms for public accountability" (ANA, 1995, p. 3).

■ The knowledge and expertise acquired in a DNP program assist graduates in meeting the changing needs of society. DNP graduates' preparation enables them to utilize information technologies, provide evidence-based practice, develop healthcare policies, and provide leadership in an effort to meet the societal needs of a multicultural, complex healthcare environment.

■ Whether fulfilling roles as leaders, clinicians, researchers, educators, or an integration of these roles, DNP graduates are on the cutting edge of shaping the future of nursing education and healthcare delivery.

REFLECTION QUESTIONS

1. How do you think the early arguments for and against the DNP degree have shaped the growth of the degree?

2. Which set of arguments is most compelling to you?

3. What do you think will increase credibility of the DNP degree?

4. Do you think DNP graduates should fulfill the current need for additional nursing faculty? If so, how should this occur?

5. Do you believe the current momentum of enrollment in DNP programs will continue? If so, what will ensure this momentum?

6. Do you think nurse residencies are necessary in DNP programs? What would you hope to gain from a nurse residency?

7. Do you think DNP graduates are and will continue to fulfill current societal needs? If so, in what ways?

REFERENCES

Advance Healthcare Network for NPs and PAs. (2014). Advance for NPs and PAs blog. Retrieved from http://community.advanceweb.com/blogs/nppa_1/default.aspx

American Association of Colleges of Nursing. (2006a). *DNP roadmap task force report*. Retrieved from http://www.aacn.nche.edu/dnp/roadmapreport.pdf

American Association of Colleges of Nursing. (2006b). *The essentials of doctoral education for advanced nursing practice*. Retrieved from http://www.aacn.nche.edu/publications/position/DNPEssentials.pdf

American Association of Colleges of Nursing. (2010). *The doctor of nursing practice: A report on progress*. Retrieved from http://www.aacn.nche.edu/leading-initiatives/dnp/DNPForum3-10.pdf

American Association of Colleges of Nursing. (2014a). DNP fact sheet. Retrieved from http://www.aacn.nche.edu/media-relations/fact-sheets/dnp

American Association of Colleges of Nursing. (2014b). Nursing faculty shortage. Retrieved from http://www.aacn.nche.edu/media-relations/fact-sheets/nursing-faculty-shortage

American Association of Colleges of Nursing. (2014c). Program directory. Retrieved from http://www.aacn.nche.edu/dnp/program-directory

American Association of Colleges of Nursing. (2014d). Reflections on the future of doctoral programs in nursing. Retrieved from http://www.aacn.nche.edu/dnp/JK-2014-DNP.pdf

American Nurses Association. (1995). *Nursing's social policy statement*. Washington, DC: Author.

American Nurses Association. (2010). *Nursing's social policy statement* (2nd ed.). Washington, DC: Author.

Boyer, E. L. (1990). *Scholarship reconsidered: Priorities of the professoriate*. San Francisco, CA: Jossey-Bass.

Brown, M., Draye, M., Zimmer, P., Magyary, D., Woods, S., Whitney, J., . . . Katz, J. R. (2006). Developing a practice doctorate in nursing: University of Washington perspectives and experience. *Nursing Outlook, 54*(3), 130–138.

Burman, M., Hart, A., & McCabe, S. (2005). Doctor of nursing practice: Opportunity amidst chaos. *American Journal of Critical Care, 14*(6), 463–464.

Chase, S., & Pruitt, R. (2006). The practice doctorate: Innovation or disruption? *Journal of Nursing Education, 45*(5), 155–161.

Clinton, P., & Sperhac, A. M. (2009). The DNP and unintended consequences: An opportunity for dialogue. *Journal of Pediatric Health Care, 23*(5), 348–351.

Dracup, K., & Bryan-Brown, C. (2005). Doctor of nursing practice—MRI or total body scan? *American Journal of Critical Care, 14*(4), 278–281.

Edwardson, S. R. (2010). Doctor of philosophy and doctor of nursing practice as complementary degrees. *Journal of Professional Nursing, 26*(3), 137–140.

Florczak, K. L. (2011). Research and the doctor of nursing practice: A cause for consternation. *Nursing Science Quarterly, 23*(1), 13–17.

Greiner, A. C., & Knebel, E. (Eds.). (2003). *Health professions education: A bridge to quality.* Washington, DC: National Academies Press.

Grey, M. (2013). The doctor of nursing practice: Defining the next steps. *Journal of Nursing Education, 52*(8), 462–465.

Hathaway, D., Jacob, S., Stegbauer, C., Thompson, C., & Graff, C. (2006). The practice doctorate: Perspectives of early adopters. *Journal of Nursing Education, 45*(12), 487–496.

Institute of Medicine. (2010). *The future of nursing: Leading change, advancing health.* Washington, DC: National Academies Press. Retrieved from http://www.iom.edu/Reports/2010/The-Future-of-Nursing-Leading-Change-Advancing-Health.aspx

Mundinger, M., Kane, R., Lentz, E., Trotten, A., Tsai, W., Cleary, P., . . . Shelanski, M. L. (2000). Primary care outcomes in patients treated by nurse practitioners or physicians: A randomized trial. *Journal of the American Medical Association, 283*(1), 59–68.

National Association of Clinical Nurse Specialists. (2009). *Core practice doctorate clinical nurse specialist competencies.* Retrieved from http://www.nacns.org/docs/CorePracticeDoctorate.pdf

National Organization of Nurse Practitioner Faculties. (2010). *Clinical education issues in preparing nurse practitioner students for independent practice: An ongoing series of papers.* Washington, DC: Author.

National Organization of Nurse Practitioner Faculties. (2013). Sample curriculum templates for doctorate of nursing practice (DNP) NP Education. Retrieved from http://c.ymcdn.com/sites/www.nonpf.org/resource/resmgr/imported/CurriculumTemplates2013Final.pdf

Newman, M. (1975). The professional doctorate in nursing: A position paper. *Nursing Outlook, 23*(11), 704–706.

Sperhac, A., & Clinton, P. (2004). Facts and fallacies: The practice doctorate. *Journal of Pediatric Health, 18*(6), 292–296.

Vincent, D., Johnson, C., Velasquez, D., & Rigney, T. (2010). DNP-prepared nurses as researchers: Closing the gap between research and practice. *The American Journal for Nurse Practitioners, 14*(11/12), 28–33.

A Personal Account of Integrating the *Essentials of Doctoral Education for Advanced Nursing Practice* into Practice

I. Scientific Underpinnings for Practice

- Completion and publication of my DNP scholarly project*
  - Developed and tested a middle-range nursing theory (Chism's Middle-Range Theory of Spiritual Empathy, see **Figure A-1**) in collaboration with my chair and mentor, Dr. Morris Magnan
  - Published "The Relationship of Nursing Students' Spiritual Care Perspectives to Their Expressions of Spiritual Empathy" (Chism & Magnan, 2009)

II. Organizational and Systems Leadership for Quality Improvement and Systems Thinking

- Publication of *The Doctor of Nursing Practice: A Guidebook for Role Development and Professional Issues*, the first DNP-related textbook written and edited by a DNP graduate
- Informal leadership roles as mentor, preceptor, guest lecturer
- Development of a formal leadership role as clinical director of the Women's Wellness Clinic
- Chair of the membership committee for the North American Menopause Society

III. Clinical Scholarship and Analytical Methods for Evidence-Based Practice

Scholarship through evaluation, translation, and implementation of evidence-based practice:

- Evaluation, translation, and implementation of evidence-based practice in the development of a specialty clinic within my setting (dedicated menopause clinic for breast cancer patients and survivors)
- Participation and completion of University of Michigan's Sexual Health Certificate Program with the goal of garnering evidence-based knowledge related to sexual health

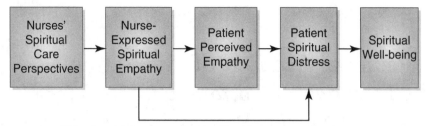

Figure A-1 Chism's middle-range theory of spiritual empathy

Scholarship through educating others:

- Assistant adjunct professor, Madonna University
    - DNP Role Development, DNP and Nursing Theory
- Guest lecture at universities around the country
    - DNP Role Development, Spiritual Care and Nursing, Menopause, Menopause and Breast Cancer
- Multiple professional peer-reviewed presentations
- Multiple professional peer-reviewed publications

IV. Information Systems and Technology and Patient Care Technology for the Improvement and Transformation of Health Care

- Assist colleagues and patients with information searches
- Promote the use of information technologies within my clinical setting

V. Healthcare Policy for Advocacy in Health Care

- Participation in professional organizations, such as American Association of Nurse Practitioners (AANP), North American Menopause Society (NAMS)
- Participated in my state's Advocacy Day to promote the passage of legislature that would directly impact the practice of nurse practitioners in my state (MINCP)
- Met with state legislatures to garner support regarding legislature that would directly impact the practice of nurse practitioners in my state (MINCP)
- Membership on specific committees within NAMS, such as scientific programming committee and membership committee, current chair of membership committee

VI. Interprofessional Collaboration for Improving Patient and Population Health Outcomes

- Collaborative practice in my clinical setting involving ongoing and frequent communication with radiologists
- Collaboration with radiologists within my clinical setting to develop new programs, such as the Women's Wellness Clinic and a quality initiative regarding the direct communication of biopsy results to patients
- Publication of a manuscript (coauthored with a physician and PhD-prepared clinical nurse specialist) describing a collaborative practice model used within my clinical setting: "The Environment of Care Model: A Paradigm Shift in Comprehensive Breast Care," *Journal of Interprofessional Care* (2014)

VII. Clinical Prevention and Population Health for Improving the Nation's Health

- Development of a specialty clinic to meet the needs of a specific population within my clinical setting (dedicated menopause clinic for breast cancer patients and survivors)
- Future development of a specialty clinic to meet the needs of a specific population within my clinical setting (sexual health clinic dedicated to the needs of breast cancer patients and survivors)

VIII. Advanced Nursing Practice

- Practice as an advanced-practice nurse in a specialty setting

NOTE

*The DNP scholarly project this author completed is not necessarily customary for the requirement of the DNP degree. This project was rooted in real-life patient interactions and an interest in Olson's and Hanchett's Middle-Range Theory of Empathic Process (1997). Through extensive mentoring from this author's PhD-prepared chair, Morris Magnan, this theory was developed and tested. Importantly, this project grew from bedside interactions and may be translated directly to improve practice—an important objective of proposed DNP scholarly projects.

REFERENCES

Chism, L. A., & Magnan, M. A. (2009). The relationship of student nurses, spiritual care perspectives to their expressions of spiritual empathy. *Journal of Nursing Education, 48*(11), 597–605.

Chism, L. A., Magnan, M. A., & Helmer, S. (2014). The environment of care model: A paradigm shift in comprehensive breast care. *Journal of Interprofessional Care.* Retrieved from http://informahealthcare.com/doi/abs/10.3109/13561820.2014.922530

Olson, J., & Hanchett, E. (1997). Nurse-expressed empathy, patient outcomes, and development of a middle-range theory. *Image: Journal of Nursing Scholarship, 29*(1), 71–76.

INDEX

Note: Page numbers followed by *b, f,* or *t* indicate materials in boxes, figures, or tables respectively.

A

AANP Political Action Committee (AANP-PAC), 160
accelerated career pathways, 183
accountability, 222
ACNP. *See* Acute Care Nurse Practitioner
activism. *See* healthcare policy and advocacy
Acute Care Nurse Practitioner (ACNP), 194
advanced nursing practice, 19–20, 39, 40, 280. *See also* clinical nursing practice
  advanced practice nursing *vs.*, 73–74
  domain of, 74
  essentials for (AACN). *See* Essentials of Doctoral Education for Advanced Nursing Practice
advanced practice nurse (APNs), 280
  DNP degree for, 284
  grandfathering of, 29, 262–263
"advanced practice nurse-friendly culture," 339
advanced practice nursing
  advanced nursing practice *vs.*, 73–74
  defined as, 333
advanced-practice registered nurses (APRNs), 72, 74, 84, 280, 301
  certification, 194
  consensus model, 288–289
  educational preparation for, 366
  friendly culture characteristics of, 339
  patients' awareness and perceptions of, 337
  positive attitudes toward, 339
  specialization as, 20
Advancing the Nation's Health Needs: NIH Research Training Programs, 185

advertising, in marketing, 364
advocacy. *See* healthcare policy and advocacy
advocate, NI specialist, 250–251
affiliative leadership style, 47, 48*t*
  case scenario, 57, 58
age of nursing faculty members, 180
AJN. See American Journal of Nursing
AMA. *See* American Marketing Association
ambiguity, appreciation of (competency), 42–43
American Academy of Nurse Practitioners (AANP), 283, 326
American Association of Colleges of Nursing (AACN), 39, 40, 71, 149–151, 157*b*, 158*b*, 279, 390
  board of directors, 282
  for DNP degree, 280
  DNP Essentials Task Force, 283
  DNP Roadmap Task Force, 262, 283
  on duration of DNP program, 182
  Essentials of Doctoral Education for Advanced Nursing Practice, 14–20, 373
  key differences between DNP and PhD/DNS/DNSc programs, 6*t*–7*t*
  on nurse faculty vacancy, 179
  Position Statement on the Practice Doctorate in Nursing, 9, 175
  on practice doctorates, 3–5, 9–11, 175–176
  on scholarship, 125
  task force, 9
  update from, 393–394
American Association of Critical-Care Nurses, 89

Boyer. *See Scholarship Reconsidered: Priorities of the Professoriate*
branding, marketing *vs.,* 363–365
breast imaging specialists, 93
Brewster, Mary, 154
broad-based APRN education, 75
BSN. *See* bachelor of science in nursing
BSN-to-DNP students. *See* bachelor of science in nursing to DNP students
Burson, Rosanne (interview), 354–358

C
C-SPAN radio, 159*b*
cable television, as health policy resource, 159*b*
capstone project. *See* final DNP project
caring
    competencies, 42–43
    defined, 209
Carnegie, Dale, 343
Carolin, Kathleen (interviews), 60–62
casuistry, 208
CCNE. *See* Commission on Collegiate Nursing Education
Center for Nursing Leadership, caring competencies, 42
certification as a lymphedema specialist (CLT), 364
certified registered nurse anesthetists (CRNAs), 23
chairperson for final project committee, 132
Chambers, Oswald, 271
change
    effective, 53–54
    experienced by DNP students, 129, 136
    inspiring and leading, 95
    resistance to evidence-based practice, 76
    technology, adoption of, 82
    unexpected leadership, 54–55
chat, ethical perils of social networks, 222–223
chief nursing officers (CNOs), 60
clinical competence, 51
    as leadership attribute, 45*t*, 58
clinical doctorate, 334
clinical nurse leader (CNL) degree, 4

clinical nurse specialist (CNS), 57
clinical nursing practice, 54, 56–64, 71–110
    curriculum standards, 40, 72–73
    information technology in, 81–87
        case scenario, 85–87
        role of, 86*b*
    interprofessional collaboration in, 87–93
    interviews
        Kelm, Lauren, 101–102
        Nichols, Catherine, 103
        Palleschi, Maria, 106–108
        Payson, Kathleen A., 109
        Schmitt, Tonya, 98–100
    leadership scenarios, 56–60
    mentoring and precepting in, 72, 94–97
    nursing theories for, 118–120, 120*b*
    research with, 190, 194–196
    scholarship, 138–139, 141
clinical prevention, 19
clinical scholarship for evidence-based practice, 16–17
CLT. *See* certification as a lymphedema specialist
CNL degree. *See* clinical nurse leader degree
CNOs. *See* chief nursing officers
CNS. *See* clinical nurse specialist
coaching leadership style, 46, 48
coalition meeting on *doctor* title, 308, 310
code of ethics, 206, 220
collaboration, 39–40, 50. *See also* communication
    case scenarios, 56–60
    conflict management, 44
        case scenario, 56–57
        humor and, 52
        as leadership attribute, 58
    consulting others about decisions, 268–269
    curriculum standards, 40
    effective change, 53–54
    interprofessional, 18–19
        in clinical setting, 87–93
        collaboration, 40
    networking. *See* networking in research and scholarship
    publication and, 135–136
    qualities for success, 51–52
    relationship management, 44